ESSENTIALS OF FREE RADICAL BIOLOGY AND MEDICINE

ESSENTIALS OF FREE RADICAL BIOLOGY AND MEDICINE

ROBERT Z. HOPKINS

Senor Principal Scientist
Editor-in-Chief of Reactive Oxygen Species
AIMSCI Research Institute
P.O. Box 37504, Raleigh, North Carolina 27626, USA

Y. ROBERT LI

Professor of Pharmacology
Chair of Department of Pharmacology, Campbell University SOM
Buies Creek, North Carolina 27506, USA

Adjunct Professor of Biomedical Engineering and Sciences
Virginia Tech–Wake Forest University School of Biomedical Engineering and Sciences
Blacksburg, Virginia 24061, USA

Adjunct Professor of Biomedical Sciences and Pathobiology
Department of Biomedical Sciences and Pathobiology, Virginia Polytechnic Institute and State University
Blacksburg, Virginia 24061, USA

Adjunct Professor of Biology
Department of Biology, University of North Carolina
Greensboro, North Carolina 27412, USA

CELL MED PRESS, AIMSCI Inc.

ESSENTIALS OF FREE RADICAL BIOLOGY AND MEDICINE   ISBN: 978-1-68056-000-8

Cell Med Press also publishes this book in digital formats. For more information on the products of Cell Med Press, please visit the website at http://www.cellmedpress.com.

This book is printed on acid-free paper.

Printed in the United States of America

Cover illustration: Phagocytic NADPH oxidase-derived superoxide acts as a precursor of secondary reactive species for killing invading pathogens. As depicted, upon insults from invading pathogens, phagocytic cells undergo respiratory burst, resulting in the formation of superoxide ($O_2^{\cdot-}$) via activation of the membrane-associated NADPH oxidase (not shown). Superoxide undergoes dismutation to form hydrogen peroxide (H_2O_2), which, in the presence of phagocytic myeloperoxidase (MPO), reacts with chloride ion to form hypochlorous acid (HOCl), a potent oxidant and pathogen-killing compound that is also the active ingredient of household bleach. Superoxide also reacts with nitric oxide ($NO^{\cdot}$) derived from phagocytic inducible nitric oxide synthase (not shown) to form peroxynitrite ($ONOO^-$), another potent oxidant capable of killing pathogens. Lastly, iron-catalyzed Haber–Weiss reaction produces hydroxyl radicals ($OH^{\cdot}$), the most potent oxidizing species formed in biological systems. The above potent oxidants, along with other reactive species, collectively contribute to phagocytic cell-mediated innate immunity against invading microorganisms. This is a typical scenario where free radicals and related reactive species play an important physiological role.

Contents

CONTENTS IN BRIEF

CONTENTS

PREFACE

Aerobic metabolism results in the inevitable formation of a variety of free radicals and related reactive species (FRRS), with reactive oxygen species (ROS) being the most notable and extensively studied examples. Studies on the biological activities of these reactive species and their involvement in health and disease have led to the creation and development of a new scientific discipline, which is known as "Free Radical Biology and Medicine".

The past several decades have witnessed the rapid progression of the field of free radical biology and medicine. As new terminologies and concepts keep emerging as a result of ongoing active research, free radical biology and medicine has become an increasingly important subject that impacts both basic bioscience and clinical medicine. The rapidly evolving nature of this field makes it imperative to clearly define the scope of free radical biology and medicine and emphasize the essence of this scientific discipline. In this context, a concise book focusing on the fundamental principles and concepts of free radical biology and medicine would greatly facilitate both the learning of basic knowledge and the understanding of the advancement of cutting-edge research in the field. This notion has prompted the writing of "Essentials of Free Radical Biology and Medicine".

"Essentials of Free Radical Biology and Medicine" takes a unique approach to integrating the fundamental principles with high quality cutting-edge research discoveries, and the basic bioscience with clinical medicine so as to provide the reader a comprehensive picture of the field in a concise manner. Accordingly, as outlined below, the book is divided into three units with a total of 15 chapters: Unit I (Chapters 1–4): The Birth of Concepts; Unit II (Chapters 5–7): Chemical and Biological Principles; and Unit III (Chapters 8–15): Common Free Radicals and Related Reactive Species.

Unit I covers the basic concepts of free radical biology and medicine. It contains four chapters. Chapter 1 describes the discovery of molecular oxygen and the evolvement of the concept of oxygen

toxicity. The chapter also introduces the emerging concept of redox signaling and free radical physiology. To facilitate the discussion of the fundamental principles and concepts of free radical biology and medicine, Chapter 2 considers some essential terminologies in the field, defining such terms as free radicals, ROS, reactive nitrogen species (RNS), electrophiles, and antioxidants and related entities. Chapter 3 is devoted to the detailed discussion of two fundamental concepts in free radical biology and medicine, namely, oxidative stress and redox signaling. It also discusses some related concepts, including nitrative stress, nitrosative stress, redox proteome, and redox metabolome. The last chapter of Unit I introduces a newly developed concept in free radical biology and medicine, known as free radical paradigm. The chapter defines the scope of free radical paradigm and discusses the importance of this paradigm in offering a framework for understanding the basic biology of FRRS and antioxidants as well as their roles in human health and disease.

Unit II consisting of three chapters (Chapters 5–7) examines the chemical and biological principles related to FRRS. Chapter 5 describes three basic common chemical properties of FRRS, namely, free radical reactions, reaction rate constant, and reduction potential. Chapter 6 surveys the major biological sources of FRRS, including NADPH oxidases, mitochondria, and cytochrome P450 system and related proteins, among others. The chapter also considers the environmental sources of FRRS that may impact the biological systems. Chapter 7 provides an overview of the biological effects of FRRS at both molecular and cellular levels. The chapter also examines the potential physiological functions of FRRS, including immunity, redox signaling, suppression of cancer development, as well as prolongation of lifespan. This sets a stage for the subsequent discussion in Unit III of the major FRRS with regard to their roles in biology and medicine.

Unit III contains eight chapters (Chapters 8–15) devoted to the discussion of the roles of common

FRRS in biology and medicine. These include super-oxide (Chapter 8), hydrogen peroxide (Chapter 9), hydroxyl radicals (Chapter 10), peroxynitrite (Chapter 11), nitric oxide (Chapter 12), hypochlorous acid (Chapter 13), singlet oxygen (Chapter 14), and others (Chapter 15).

To help the reader study the various topics and retain new knowledge, each of the above 15 chapters is supplemented at the end with a summary of the chapter key points and a list of self-assessment questions with answers and explanations. In addition, the book also includes two appendices and a list of glossary. Appendix A lists some of the commonly used formulas or abbreviations for chemical entities in free radical biology and medicine. These include the widely accepted formulas or abbreviations for: FRRS as well as other relevant chemical species; antioxidants and related entities; and enzymes involved in the production of FRRS. Appendix B provides an overview of common cellular antioxidants and related entities that are involved in the metabolism of FRRS, focusing primarily on their basic biochemistry and major biological functions. Here it is noteworthy that peer-reviewed scholar journals of high quality are instrumental in disseminating the cutting-edge scientific findings so as to advance our scientific knowledge. In this context, the contents of this book are written primarily based on the original scientific findings published in influential peer-reviewed journals. Due to space limitations, the citation is primarily based on original and representative references.

It is hoped that this book, by integrating fundamental concepts with cutting-edge discoveries and translating essential bioscience to clinical medicine, will provide the reader a unique approach to understanding the rapidly evolving field of free radical biology and medicine. Because of the rapidly evolving nature of the field, and biomedicine as a whole, the information contained in this book is subject to change based on new scientific knowledge and clinical investigations. Although the authors of the book have checked with sources believed to be reliable and accurate at the time of publication, information included in the book may not be accurate in every respect due to the possibility of human errors and rapid changes in biomedical sciences. As such, the authors of the book do not warrant that the information contained in the work is in every respect accurate and complete. The authors disclaim all responsibility for any errors or omissions or for the results obtained from the use of the information contained in this book. The reader is advised to seek independent verification for any data, advice, or recommendations contained in the work.

"Essentials of Free Radical Biology and Medicine" would not have been possible without the original essential scientific findings published by numerous scientists in influential scholarly journals of high scientific quality. We are grateful to those (over 100 scientists worldwide) who provided us reprints of their publications and/or comments on part of the book manuscript. We are thankful for the time and effort made by the editorial personnel at Cell Med Press, AIMSCI Inc., which made the work possible and of high quality.

Robert Z. Hopkins
and
Y. Robert Li
North Carolina, USA
April 2017

UNIT I

THE BIRTH OF THE CONCEPTS

Chapter 1

Oxygen and Oxygen Toxicity: The Birth of the Concepts

ABSTRACT | Oxygen, if not specified, may refer to element oxygen (O), ground state (triplet) molecular dioxygen (O_2, commonly called molecular oxygen or simply, oxygen), or ozone (O_3). O_2 is the second most common component of the Earth's atmosphere, taking up ~21% of its volume and ~23% of its mass. O_2 was discovered by Carl Wilhelm Scheele, Joseph Priestley, and Antoine-Laurent Lavoisier about two and a half centuries ago. Despite its essentialness in aerobic life, O_2 may also cause harm. Although oxygen toxicity in animals was recognized in the 1870s, only the past few decades have witnessed the explosion in knowledge on oxygen toxicity and the underlying molecular mechanisms, especially the role of oxygen-derived free radicals and related reactive species (FRRS) in disease process. Research over the past two to three decades has also uncovered an emerging role for oxygen-derived FRRS in cell signaling and normal physiology.

KEYWORDS | Free radicals and related reactive species; Oxygen; Oxygen toxicity; Reactive oxygen species; Redox signaling

CITATION | *Hopkins RZ and Li YR. Essentials of Free Radical Biology and Medicine. Cell Med Press, Raleigh, NC, USA. 2017. http://dx.doi.org/10.20455/efrbm.2017.01*

ABBREVIATIONS | CNS, central nervous system; EPR, electron paramagnetic resonance; FRRS, free radicals and related reactive species; GOE, Great Oxidation Event; ROS, reactive oxygen species; SOD, superoxide dismutase

CHAPTER AT A GLANCE

1. OVERVIEW

Molecular dioxygen (O_2) is an essential element of aerobic life, yet incomplete reduction or excitation of O_2 during aerobic metabolisms generates diverse oxygen-containing free radicals and related reactive species (FRRS), commonly known as reactive oxygen species (ROS) (see Chapters 2 and 3 for details on FRRS and ROS). On the one hand, ROS pose a serious threat to aerobic organisms via inducing oxidative damage to cellular constituents. On the other hand, these reactive species, when their generation is under homeostatic control, also play important physiological roles (e.g., constituting an important component of immunity and participating in redox signaling). This chapter defines oxygen and the key facts about oxygen, and discusses the relationship between oxygen and emergence of early animals on Earth. The chapter then describes the discovery of oxygen by three historical figures and examines the birth of the concept of oxygen toxicity and the underlying free radical mechanisms. The chapter ends with a brief introduction to the emerging field of ROS-mediated redox signaling and physiological responses. A more detailed introduction to key concepts of free radical biology and medicine is provided in Chapter 2.

2. OXYGEN: DEFINITIONS AND KEY FACTS

2.1. Definitions

Oxygen, if not specified, may refer to: (1) element oxygen (O), which is also known as oxygen atom with an atomic number of 8 and is a member of the chalcogen group on the periodic table; (2) ground state (triplet) molecular dioxygen (O_2), which is commonly called molecular oxygen or simply, oxygen or oxygen gas; or (3) ozone (O_3), which is a pale blue gas with a distinctively pungent smell and is formed from O_2 by the action of ultraviolet light as well as atmospheric electrical discharges. Ozone is also known as trioxygen and is an allotrope of oxygen (see Section 2.3) that is present in low concentrations throughout the Earth's atmosphere. It has been suggested that ozone may be generated by antibodies via a water oxidation pathway and play a role

in phagocyte-mediated immunity [1–3]. Ozone is also present in atherosclerotic lesions and possibly formed by the antibodies and immune cells located there. The locally generated ozone might contribute to plaque formation by oxidizing cholesterol [4].

2.2. Abundance

Oxygen is a highly reactive nonmetallic element that readily forms compounds with most other elements. By mass, oxygen is the third most abundant element in the cosmos after hydrogen and helium. It is the most abundant chemical element by mass in the Earth's biosphere, air, sea, and land, constituting ~46–47% of the Earth's crust and ~86–87% of the world's oceans.

Molecular dioxygen is the second most common component of the Earth's atmosphere, taking up ~21% of its volume and ~23% of its mass. Oxygen is also the most abundant element in the human body, accounting for ~65% of total body mass.

2.3. Isotopes and Allotropes

Naturally occurring oxygen exists as three stable isotopes: ^{16}O, ^{17}O, and ^{18}O, with ^{16}O being the most abundant form (~99.8% natural abundance). Radioactive, short-lived, isotopes of oxygen with mass numbers from ^{12}O to ^{26}O have also been recently identified [5].

Allotropes are different forms of the same chemical element that exhibit different physical and chemical properties. There are several known allotropes of oxygen, with O_2 being the most familiar one. The second most familiar allotrope is the highly reactive ozone (also see Section 2.1). Other allotropes of oxygen include tetraoxygen (O_4) and the dark-red solid oxygen O_8, which are formed under very high pressures [6, 7].

2.4. Chemical and Physical Properties of O_2

2.4.1. General Properties

The molecular weight of O_2 is 31.9988 g/mol. O_2 gas is colorless, odorless, and tasteless with a density of 1.429 g/L at $0°C$. O_2 changes from a gas to a liquid at a temperature of $-182.96°C$ when it takes on a slight-

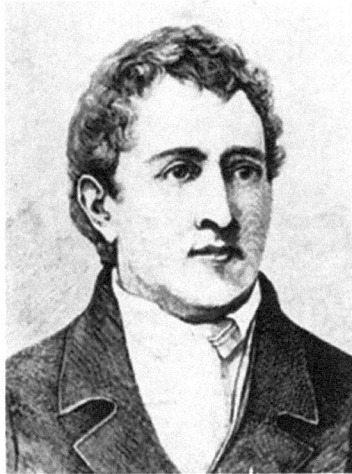

Carl Wilhelm Scheele
(1742-1786)

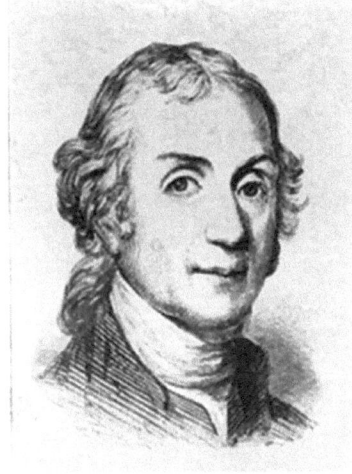

Joseph Priestley
(1733–1804)

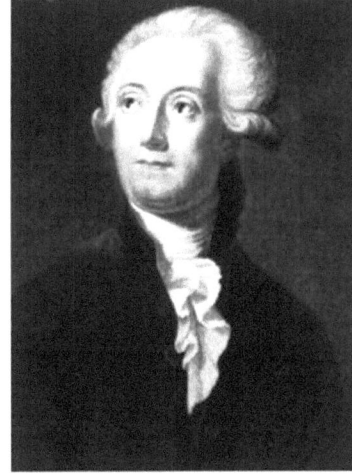

Antoine-Laurent Lavoisier
(1743-1794)

FIGURE 1.1. Historical figures who discovered oxygen. Carl Wilhelm Scheele, Joseph Priestley, and Antoine-Laurent Lavoisier are generally credited with the discovery of oxygen (source: Library of Congress; www.loc.gov).

ly bluish color. Liquid oxygen can then be solidified or frozen at a temperature of –218.4°C.

2.4.2. Triplet State

An electron configuration with two unpaired electrons, as found in O_2, occupying orbitals of equal energy is termed a spin triplet state or ground state. Hence, the oxygen in the air that we breathe is ground (triplet) state molecular dioxygen.

2.4.3. Paramagnetism

Molecular dioxygen contains two unpaired electrons and is thus paramagnetic. Paramagnetism refers to the magnetic state of a chemical species with one or more unpaired electrons. The unpaired electrons are attracted by a magnetic field due to the electrons' magnetic dipole moments. The paramagnetic feature makes it possible to detect and measure O_2 using electron paramagnetic resonance (EPR) spectrometry (also frequently called spectroscopy).

EPR spectrometry, also known as electron spin resonance (ESR) spectrometry, is a sophisticated and most specific technique for detecting substances with unpaired electrons, including free radicals and transition metal ions (see Chapter 2 for definition of free radicals).

3. OXYGEN AND ANIMALS' EMERGENCE ON EARTH

Most of us take our richly oxygenated world for granted and expect to find oxygen everywhere – after all it makes up ~21% of the modern atmosphere (also see Section 2.2). But free oxygen, at levels mostly less than 0.001% of those present in the atmosphere today, was anything but plentiful during the first half of Earth's 4.5-billion-year history [8].

The atmosphere of Earth was anaerobic until the advent of oxygenic photosynthesis. The rise of oxygen in Earth's early atmosphere and ocean led to the emergence and diversification of animals [9, 10]. Accumulating evidence suggests a permanent rise to appreciable concentrations of oxygen in the atmosphere sometime between 2.4 and 2.1 billion years ago. This increase, now popularly known as the Great Oxidation Event (GOE), left clear fingerprints in the rock record [8], and is believed to lead to the emergence of multicellular organisms and earliest animals on Earth [11].

4. DISCOVERY OF OXYGEN

Three historical figures are generally credited with the discovery of oxygen. They are Carl Wilhelm

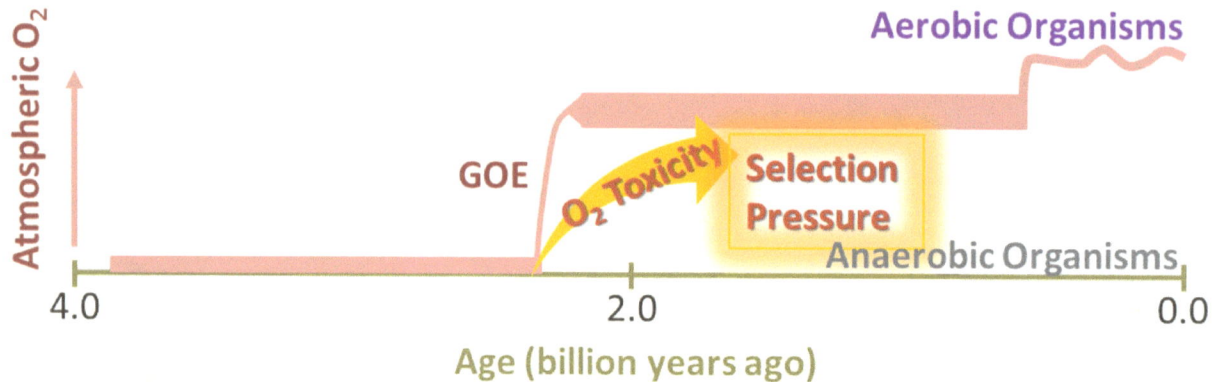

FIGURE 1.2. Oxygen and emergency of animals on Earth. The increase of oxygen in the atmosphere 2.4–2.1 billion years ago, commonly known as the Great Oxidation Event (GOE), is believed to lead to the emergence of earliest animals on Earth. On the other hand, oxygen toxicity is thought to exert evolutional pressure contributing to the diversification of animals. Organisms that could not accommodate to the challenge of oxygen toxicity evolved into anaerobes. This scheme is based primarily on ref. 8.

Scheele, Joseph Priestley, and Antoine-Laurent Lavoisier (**Figure 1.1**).

4.1. Carl Wilhelm Scheele

Between 1771 and 1772, Scheele (1742–1786), a Swedish chemist, did a series of experiments with mercuric oxide and potassium nitrate. On heating the two he obtained a gas that caused candles to burn more brightly. He did not, however, rush to publish his observation until 1777.

4.2. Joseph Priestley

Working independently in 1774, Priestley (1733–1804), an English radical Unitarian minister and chemist, observed that a gas was liberated when he heated the mineral mercuric oxide. In the atmosphere of this gas, a candle burned more brightly and a mouse could live longer than when sealed in a comparable volume of ordinary air. He reported this remarkable experiment in 1775, which was two years earlier than did Scheele (also see Section 4.1). Priestley did not have much training in chemistry, and was unable to abandon the phlogiston theory of his time (the theory stated that all combustible material contains something known as a phlogiston, that on heating, is transformed into fire). By heating a burnt substance, such as mercury oxide, Priestley believed that he was removing phlogiston from the atmosphere into the mercury, thereby purifying the air. As such, he referred to the gas as "dephlogisticated air".

4.3. Antoine-Laurent Lavoisier

Inspired by Priestley's experiment conducted in 1775, Lavoisier (1743–1794), a French chemist, began his own experiment with the gas during the same year, and came to agree that air contained an element that supported life and combustion. Lavoisier noted its tendency to form acids by combining with many different substances and incorrectly believed it to be a component of all acids, and hence named the gas oxygen ("*oxygène*" in French), meaning acid former. In fact, the word oxygen comes from Greek words: oxus (acid) and gennan (generate).

5. DISCOVERY OF OXYGEN TOXICITY

5.1. An Evolutionary View

The accumulation of O_2 in Earth's atmosphere as well as ocean changed the environment for, and therefore changed the selection pressures on, all living organisms. It also increased the mutation rate and therefore hastened subsequent evolution. Advantages could be gained by using O_2 to increase the useful energy derivable from foodstuffs, to carry out novel metabolic transformations, to solubilize and detoxify numerous compounds, and even to generate heat and light [12]. But there was a price to pay for these benefits and that was to provide defenses against the considerable toxicity of oxygen, a paramagnetic gas (also see section 2.4.3). Those organisms that suc-

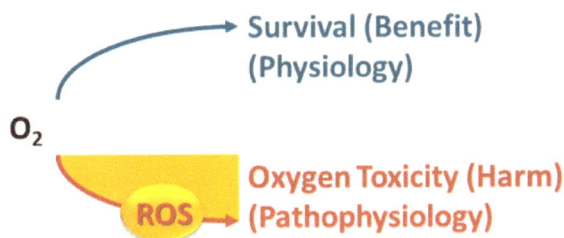

FIGURE 1.3. Free radical mechanisms of oxygen toxicity. On the one hand, oxygen is essential for aerobic life. On the other hand, utilization of oxygen also inevitably results in the formation of reactive oxygen species (ROS). The ROS, when their formation is abnormally increased, may cause oxidative damage to cellular constituents, which constitutes the molecular basis of oxygen toxicity.

FIGURE 1.4. Reactive oxygen species (ROS) in physiology. The involvement of ROS in physiology is two-fold: On the one hand, ROS derived from O_2 contribute to killing of pathogenic microorganisms by phagocytic cells, thereby promoting the survival of the host. On the other hand, ROS act as second messengers to activate cell signal transduction, leading to desired physiological responses.

ceeded in developing the requisite defenses could reap the benefits, and they gave rise to the enormous variety of aerobic life forms that are now so evident on Earth. Those that could not accommodate to the challenge of oxygen toxicity evolved into anaerobic organisms [12] (**Figure 1.2**).

Interestingly, a recent study reports that multicellular animals live in deep hypersaline anoxic basins of the Mediterranean Sea, suggesting that certain forms of multicellular animals may live entirely without oxygen [13].

5.2. Joseph Priestley's Conjecture on Oxygen's Harm

Priestley, who discovered oxygen, an element essential to life, was himself among the first to suggest that there might be adverse effects of the gas. In 1775, he conjectured that "though pure dephlogisticated air [oxygen] might be very useful as a medicine [for sick persons], it might not be so proper for us in the usual healthy state of the body; for, as a candle burns out much faster in dephlogisticated than in common air, so we might, as may be said, live out too fast, and the animal powers be too soon exhausted in this pure kind of air".

Priestley's speculation on oxygen toxicity was subsequently proved correct, and it is now well-established that oxygen therapy is like a two-edged sword – at one edge, oxygen is essential to human survival, whereas at the other edge, the same gas may cause injury and even death at an elevated partial pressure [14].

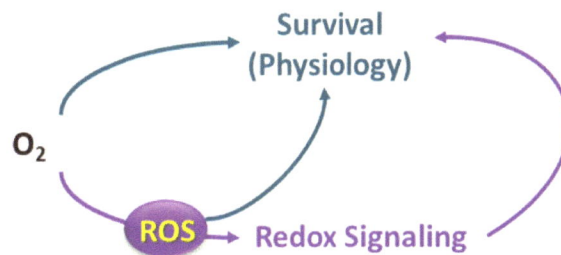

5.3. Historic Overview of Oxygen Toxicity in Experimental Animals

The first important contribution to oxygen toxicity was made in 1878 by Paul Bert (1833–1886), a French physiologist. His pioneer work has withstood the test of time in a most impressive manner. He showed that oxygen at increased pressures was highly poisonous and that no living matter was exempt. Larks exposed to 15–20 atmospheres of air convulsed and finally died. In a large series of experiments, Bert showed that the oxygen tension was the decisive factor in the immediate effect of air or of any mixture of nitrogen and oxygen. This is why the central nervous system (CNS) effect of hyperbaric oxygen is sometimes called the "Paul Bert effect".

Subsequently in 1899, James Lorrain Smith (1862–1931), a Scottish pathologist demonstrated that animals breathing oxygen at moderately high tensions over prolonged periods suffered severe and finally fatal pulmonary damage, and as such, the pulmonary oxygen toxicity is also known as the "Lorrain Smith effect" [15]. In fact, the CNS and pulmonary effects remain as the major features of oxygen toxicity in both experimental animals and human subjects.

5.4. Historic Overview of Oxygen Toxicity in Humans

Although oxygen therapy has been used in medical practice for over two centuries, the recognition of oxygen toxicity as an important clinical problem is relatively recent. Reports in the early 1950s linked oxygen therapy to retrolental fibroplasia (also known as retinopathy of prematurity) in premature infants [16]. It was shown in the early 1970s that breathing 50–100% oxygen at one atmosphere was potentially toxic to the lungs [17]. Since then, the toxic effects of oxygen on other organs and systems of the body have also been recognized. These include the eyes, liver, heart, kidneys, blood, and endocrine system [18]. Meanwhile, progress has been made to understand the molecular basis of oxygen toxicity.

5.5. Free Radical Mechanisms of Oxygen Toxicity

Although the harmful effects of oxygen were noticed in 1878, insights into the molecular mechanisms of oxygen toxicity were provided in several articles published during 1950s and 1960s. In 1954, Rebeca Gerschman and associates published an article in the Science magazine, hypothesizing that oxygen poisoning and radiation injury have at least one common basis of action, possibly through the formation of oxidizing free radicals [19].

Another important event in the investigation of oxygen toxicity was the finding by Joe M. McCord and Irwin Fridovich in 1969 of an enzymatic function of a protein containing both copper and zinc, which then was known alternatively as erythrocuprein, hepatocuprein, or cerebrocuprein [20]. The function of this enzyme is the catalysis of dismutation of superoxide anion radical ($O_2{}^{\cdot-}$) (superoxide for simplicity) to produce hydrogen peroxide and molecular oxygen, and it is known as superoxide dismutase (SOD) (see Appendix B for detailed description of SOD). This discovery has triggered extensive investigations into the free radical mechanisms of oxygen toxicity (**Figure 1.3**). Substantial evidence accumulated over the past several decades supports a critical involvement of free radicals and related reactive species, especially ROS, in the pathophysiology of a variety of human diseases.

5.6. Discovery of ROS Physiology

Four years after the discovery of SOD by McCord and Fridovich, Bernard Babior and colleagues reported in 1973 that one of the principal bactericidal actions of leukocytes was the enzymatic generation of superoxide [21]. Now we know that superoxide formed from the NADPH oxidase of phagocytic cells during respiratory burst and the resulting hydrogen peroxide and hypochlorous acid constitute an important mechanism of innate immunity against path-

ogenic microorganisms [22, 23]. More recently, mitochondria-derived ROS are shown to also be required for antigen-specific T cell activation [24, 25]. In addition to the antimicrobial activity, ROS have been demonstrated to play an important role in redox regulation of cell growth, differentiation, apoptosis, autophagy, and senescence [26–28], as well as longevity [29–31]. Notably, self-renewal of certain stem cells may actually require ROS [32, 33]. Elucidation of the physiological roles of ROS along with their harmful effects over the past decades has greatly broadened the concepts of oxidative stress and redox signaling (**Figure 1.4**) (also see Chapter 2).

6. SUMMARY OF CHAPTER KEY POINTS

- Oxygen, if not specified, may refer to element oxygen (O), ground state (triplet) molecular dioxygen (O_2), or ozone (O_3). O_2 was discovered by Carl Wilhelm Scheele, Joseph Priestley, and Antoine-Laurent Lavoisier over 240 years ago.
- By mass, oxygen is the third most abundant element in the cosmos after hydrogen and helium. It is the most abundant chemical element by mass in the Earth's biosphere, air, sea, and land, as well as the human body.
- Naturally occurring oxygen exists as 3 stable isotopes: ^{16}O, ^{17}O, and ^{18}O, with ^{16}O being the most abundant form. Radioactive, short-lived, isotopes of oxygen with mass numbers from ^{12}O to ^{26}O have also been identified. Allotropes of oxygen include O_2 and O_3, as well as the recently identified dark-red solid oxygen O_8.
- O_2 has two unpaired electrons and is paramagnetic. As such, O_2 can be measured by electron paramagnetic resonance (EPR) spectrometry.
- A permanent rise of oxygen in the atmosphere sometime between 2.4 and 2.1 billion years ago, known as the Great Oxidation Event (GOE), is believed to lead to the emergence of multicellular organisms and earliest animals on Earth.
- The accumulation of O_2 in Earth's atmosphere as well as ocean changed the environment for, and therefore changed the selection pressures on, all living organisms. Metabolic advantages, such as efficient production of energy from foodstuffs could be gained by using O_2, but the organisms would need to pay a price—that was the evolvement of defenses against oxygen toxicity.
- Organisms that succeeded in developing the requisite defenses could reap the benefits, and they gave rise to the enormous variety of aerobic life forms

that are now so evident on Earth. Those that could not accommodate to the challenge of oxygen toxicity evolved into anaerobic organisms.

■ Joseph Priestley, who discovered oxygen, an element essential to life, was himself among the first to conjecture in 1775 that there might be adverse effects of the gas.

■ The first important contribution to oxygen toxicity was made in 1878 by Paul Bert, who demonstrated the CNS toxicity of high oxygen tensions in animals, and as such, the CNS effect of hyperbaric oxygen is also referred to as the "Paul Bert effect".

■ In 1899, James Lorrain Smith demonstrated the pulmonary injury caused by high oxygen tensions in animals, and, hence, pulmonary oxygen toxicity is also known as the "Lorrain Smith effect".

■ Recognition of oxygen toxicity as a clinical problem began in the early 1950s, and now oxygen toxicity is a well-recognized clinical problem of oxygen therapy. Also in the 1950s, scientists began looking into the molecular mechanisms of oxygen toxicity. The subsequent discovery of SOD in 1969 triggered an explosion of investigations on free radical mechanisms of oxygen toxicity.

■ Over the past 4–5 decades since the discovery of SOD, substantial evidence supports ROS as important contributors to the pathogenesis of a wide variety of human diseases. On the other hand, the past 2–3 decades have also witnessed the emergence and evolvement of the concept that ROS also play important physiological roles (e.g., constituting innate immunity and participating in redox signaling).

7. SELF-ASSESSMENT QUESTIONS

7.1. Ozone (trioxygen), an allotrope of oxygen, is present in low concentrations throughout the Earth's atmosphere. Recent work suggests that ozone may be produced by which of the following pathways in biological systems?

A. Antibody-mediated water oxidation
B. Dismutation of superoxide by SOD
C. One-electron oxidation of dioxygen
D. One-electron reduction of hydrogen peroxide
E. Reaction between superoxide and oxygen atom

7.2. Which of the following is the most abundant element in the human body?

A. Carbon

B. Hydrogen
C. Iron
D. Nitrogen
E. Oxygen

7.3. Naturally occurring oxygen exists as three stable isotopes. Which of the following is the most abundant form?

A. ^{12}O
B. ^{16}O
C. ^{18}O
D. ^{20}O
E. ^{26}O

7.4. Paramagnetism refers to the magnetic state of a chemical species with one or more unpaired electrons. Which of the following gases can be detected by electron paramagnetic resonance (EPR) spectrometry?

A. Argon
B. Helium
C. Hydrogen
D. Nitrogen
E. Oxygen

7.5. Superoxide dismutase catalyzes the dismutation of superoxide, leading to the formation of hydrogen peroxide and molecular oxygen. This antioxidant enzyme was discovered in 1969 by which of the following scientists?

A. Bernard Babior
B. Carl Scheele
C. Joe McCord
D. Paul Bert
E. Rebeca Gerschman

7.6. Chronic granulomatous disease (CGD) is a genetic disorder that results from an inability of phagocytic cells to produce bactericidal superoxide through an enzyme known as NADPH oxidase, leading to recurrent life-threatening bacterial and fungal infections. Which of the following scientists first discovered the bactericidal action of phagocyte-derived superoxide?

A. Bernard Babior
B. Carl Scheele
C. Irwin Fridovich
D. James Lorrain Smith
E. Paul Bert

ANSWERS AND EXPLANATIONS

7.1. The answer is A. Ozone may be generated by antibodies via a water oxidation pathway and play a role in phagocyte-mediated innate immunity. Ozone may also be formed in atherosclerotic plaques.

7.2. The answer is E. Oxygen is the most abundant element in the human body, accounting for ~65% of the total body mass. This oxygen mass is largely derived from the body water.

7.3. The answer is B. ^{16}O is the most abundant form of naturally occurring oxygen isotopes, accounting for ~99.8% natural abundance.

7.4. The answer is E. Molecular dioxygen contains two unpaired electrons and is thus paramagnetic. Because of this, molecular dioxygen is actually a di-radical species.

7.5. The answer is C. The superoxide dismutation function of a protein containing both copper and zinc (i.e., SOD), which then was known alternatively as erythrocuprein, hepatocuprein, or cerebrocuprein, was discovered by Joe M. McCord and Irwin Fridovich and this discovery was reported in the Journal of Biological Chemistry in 1969.

7.6. The answer is A. Bernard Babior and colleagues reported for the first time that one of the principal bactericidal actions of leukocytes was the enzymatic generation of superoxide. This finding was published in the Journal of Clinical Investigation in 1973.

REFERENCES

1. Marx J. Immunology. Antibodies kill by producing ozone. *Science* 2002; 298(5597):1319.
2. Lerner RA, Eschenmoser A. Ozone in biology. *Proc Natl Acad Sci USA* 2003; 100(6):3013–5.
3. Yamashita K, Miyoshi T, Arai T, Endo N, Itoh H, Makino K, Mizugishi K, Uchiyama T, Sasada M. Ozone production by amino acids contributes to killing of bacteria. *Proc Natl Acad Sci USA* 2008; 105(44):16912–7.
4. Wentworth P, Jr., Nieva J, Takeuchi C, Galve R, Wentworth AD, Dilley RB, DeLaria GA, Saven A, Babior BM, Janda KD, Eschenmoser A, Lerner RA. Evidence for ozone formation in human atherosclerotic arteries. *Science* 2003; 302(5647):1053–6.
5. Lunderberg E, DeYoung PA, Kohley Z, Attanayake H, Baumann T, Bazin D, Christian G, Divaratne D, Grimes SM, Haagsma A, Finck JE, Frank N, et al. Evidence for the ground-state resonance of ^{26}O. *Phys Rev Lett* 2012; 108(14):142503.
6. Militzer B, Hemley RJ. Crystallography: solid oxygen takes shape. *Nature* 2006; 443(7108):150–1.
7. Klotz S, Strassle T, Cornelius AL, Philippe J, Hansen T. Magnetic ordering in solid oxygen up to room temperature. *Phys Rev Lett* 2010; 104(11):115501.
8. Lyons TW, Reinhard CT, Planavsky NJ. The rise of oxygen in Earth's early ocean and atmosphere. *Nature* 2014; 506(7488):307–15.
9. Mills DB, Ward LM, Jones C, Sweeten B, Forth M, Treusch AH, Canfield DE. Oxygen requirements of the earliest animals. *Proc Natl Acad Sci USA* 2014; 111(11):4168–72.
10. Knoll AH, Sperling EA. Oxygen and animals in Earth history. *Proc Natl Acad Sci USA* 2014; 111(11):3907–8.
11. Gramling C. Geochemistry. Low oxygen stifled animals' emergence, study says. *Science* 2014; 346(6209):537.
12. Fridovich I. Oxygen toxicity: a radical explanation. *J Exp Biol* 1998; 201(Pt 8):1203–9.
13. Danovaro R, Dell'Anno A, Pusceddu A, Gambi C, Heiner I, Kristensen RM. The first metazoa living in permanently anoxic conditions. *BMC Biol* 2010; 8:30.
14. Grainge C. Breath of life: the evolution of oxygen therapy. *J R Soc Med* 2004; 97(10):489–93.
15. Donald KW. Oxygen poisoning in man. *Br Med J* 1947; 1(4506):667–672.
16. Ingalls TH, Purshottam N. Oxygenation and retrolental fibroplasia. *N Engl J Med* 1954; 250(15):621–9.
17. Wolfe WG, DeVries WC. Oxygen toxicity. *Annu Rev Med* 1975; 26:203–17.
18. Thomson L, Paton J. Oxygen toxicity. *Paediatr Respir Rev* 2014; 15(2):120–3.
19. Gerschman R, Gilbert DL, Nye SW, Dwyer P, Fenn WO. Oxygen poisoning and x-irradiation: a mechanism in common. *Science* 1954; 119(3097):623–6.
20. McCord JM, Fridovich I. Superoxide dismutase: an enzymic function for erythrocuprein (hemocuprein). *J Biol Chem* 1969; 244(22):6049–55.
21. Babior BM, Kipnes RS, Curnutte JT. Biological

defense mechanisms: the production by leukocytes of superoxide, a potential bactericidal agent. *J Clin Invest* 1973; 52(3):741–4.

22. Nathan C, Shiloh MU. Reactive oxygen and nitrogen intermediates in the relationship between mammalian hosts and microbial pathogens. *Proc Natl Acad Sci USA* 2000; 97(16):8841–8.

23. Kuhns DB, Alvord WG, Heller T, Feld JJ, Pike KM, Marciano BE, Uzel G, DeRavin SS, Priel DA, Soule BP, Zarember KA, Malech HL, et al. Residual NADPH oxidase and survival in chronic granulomatous disease. *N Engl J Med* 2010; 363(27):2600–10.

24. Sena LA, Li S, Jairaman A, Prakriya M, Ezponda T, Hildeman DA, Wang CR, Schumacker PT, Licht JD, Perlman H, Bryce PJ, Chandel NS. Mitochondria are required for antigen-specific T cell activation through reactive oxygen species signaling. *Immunity* 2013; 38(2):225–36.

25. Okoye I, Wang L, Pallmer K, Richter K, Ichimura T, Haas R, Crouse J, Choi O, Heathcote D, Lovo E, Mauro C, Abdi R, et al. T cell metabolism. The protein LEM promotes CD8$^+$ T cell immunity through effects on mitochondrial respiration. *Science* 2015; 348(6238):995–1001.

26. D'Autreaux B, Toledano MB. ROS as signalling molecules: mechanisms that generate specificity in ROS homeostasis. *Nat Rev Mol Cell Biol* 2007; 8(10):813–24.

27. Sena LA, Chandel NS. Physiological roles of mitochondrial reactive oxygen species. *Mol Cell* 2012; 48(2):158–67.

28. Kawagishi H, Finkel T. Unraveling the truth about antioxidants: ROS and disease: finding the right balance. *Nat Med* 2014; 20(7):711–3.

29. Scialo F, Sriram A, Fernandez-Ayala D, Gubina N, Lohmus M, Nelson G, Logan A, Cooper HM, Navas P, Enriquez JA, Murphy MP, Sanz A. Mitochondrial ROS produced via reverse electron transport extend animal lifespan. *Cell Metab* 2016; 23(4):725–34.

30. Hanzen S, Vielfort K, Yang J, Roger F, Andersson V, Zamarbide-Fores S, Andersson R, Malm L, Palais G, Biteau B, Liu B, Toledano MB, et al. Lifespan control by redox-dependent recruitment of chaperones to misfolded proteins. *Cell* 2016; 166(1):140–51.

31. Wang Y, Hekimi S. Mitochondrial dysfunction and longevity in animals: untangling the knot. *Science* 2015; 350(6265):1204–7.

32. Morimoto H, Iwata K, Ogonuki N, Inoue K, Atsuo O, Kanatsu-Shinohara M, Morimoto T, Yabe-Nishimura C, Shinohara T. ROS are required for mouse spermatogonial stem cell self-renewal. *Cell Stem Cell* 2013; 12(6):774–86.

33. Liu J, Finkel T. Stem cells and oxidants: too little of a bad thing. *Cell Metab* 2013; 18(1):1–2.

Chapter 2

Essential Terminologies in Free Radical Biology and Medicine

ABSTRACT | In chemistry, a free radical is any atom or a group of atoms that has at least one unpaired electron and is generally unstable and highly reactive. Free radicals and related reactive species (FRRS) are key players in the field of free radical biology and medicine, a scientific discipline that deals with the involvement of FRRS as well as antioxidants in biology and medicine with an emphasis on their roles in health and disease. While FRRS comprise various chemical groups, the most important one in biology and medicine is the reactive oxygen species (ROS), which may be defined simply as reactive chemical species that are derived from molecular oxygen during various metabolic processes. ROS is one of the most encountered terms in free radical biology and medicine.

KEYWORDS | Antioxidants; Free radicals; Phase 2 proteins; Reactive oxygen species; Reactive nitrogen species

CITATION | Hopkins RZ and Li YR. Essentials of Free Radical Biology and Medicine. Cell Med Press, Raleigh, NC, USA. 2017. http://dx.doi.org/10.20455/efrbm.2017.02

ABBREVIATIONS | FRRS, free radicals and related reactive species; RCS, reactive chlorine species; RNS, reactive nitrogen species; ROS, reactive oxygen species

CHAPTER AT A GLANCE

1. OVERVIEW

To understand a discipline, it is imperative to know the basic terminologies in that particular field. This chapter defines the field "free radical biology and medicine", and considers the commonly encountered terms in the field, including free radicals, reactive oxygen species, reactive nitrogen species, reactive chlorine species, electrophiles, antioxidants, phase 2 enzymes or proteins, as well as antioxidative/anti-inflammatory defenses. The terms and concepts of oxidative stress and redox signaling are covered separately in Chapter 3.

2. FREE RADICAL BIOLOGY AND MEDICINE

Free radical biology and medicine is a relatively new field. To define it, we need to first consider the definitions of biology and medicine. The word biology is defined as the science of life and living things (e.g., plants and animals), studying their structure, function, growth, origin, evolution, and distribution. On the other hand, the word medicine refers to the science or practice of the diagnosis, treatment, and prevention of disease. Modern medicine develops primarily as a result of our profound understanding of human and animal biology at the molecular and cellular levels. Free radical biology and medicine may be defined as a field that studies the biological effects of free radicals and related reactive species as well as antioxidants with an emphasis on the involvement of these reactive species and antioxidants in health and disease.

3. FREE RADICALS AND RELATED SPECIES

3.1. Free Radicals

The term free radical refers to any chemical species capable of independent existence that contains one or more unpaired electrons. An unpaired electron refers to the one that occupies an atomic or molecular orbital by itself. Superoxide ($O_2^{\cdot-}$) as introduced in Section 5.5 of Chapter 1, is a free radical. It is called superoxide anion radical because of its negative charge. The superscript dot indicates the unpaired electron. In general, free radicals are reactive species in biological systems. However, as described below, reactive species are not necessarily free radicals. The term biological system is often used, but frequently ill-defined. In this book, a biological system refers to a system consisting of biological entities or processes, such as organs, tissues, cells, or biomolecules, or combinations of them. Biomolecules are molecules produced by living cells, including proteins, carbohydrates, lipids, and nucleic acids.

3.2. Reactive Oxygen Species

Reactive oxygen species (ROS) is a term frequently used in free radical biology and medicine. This term can be simply defined as oxygen-containing reactive species. It is a collective term to include superoxide, hydrogen peroxide (H_2O_2), hydroxyl radical ($OH^{\cdot}$), singlet oxygen ($^1O_2$), peroxyl radical ($LOO^{\cdot}$), alkoxyl radical ($LO^{\cdot}$), lipid hydroperoxide (LOOH), peroxynitrite ($ONOO^-$), hypochlorous acid (HOCl), and ozone (O_3) [1]. Although ROS is a widely used term in free radical biology and medicine to describe oxygen-containing reactive species, other alternative terms also exist in the literature, including reactive oxygen metabolites (ROMs), reactive oxygen intermediates (ROIs), and oxygen radicals. Among the above terms, ROS is most commonly used in the literature (**Table 2.1**).

3.3. Oxygen Radicals

Among the ROS listed above in Section 3.2, some contain unpaired electrons, and thus belong to free radicals. They are hence also called oxygen radicals or oxygen free radicals. Examples of oxygen radicals include superoxide, hydroxyl, peroxyl, and alkoxyl radicals. On the other hand, some ROS do not contain any unpaired electrons, and as such, they are not free radicals. Examples of the non-radical ROS include hydrogen peroxide, peroxynitrite, hypochlorous acid, and ozone.

As illustrated in **Figure 2.1** and further discussed in Chapter 14, singlet oxygen can exist in two states: the delta state ($^1\Delta_g$) and sigma state ($^1\Sigma_g^+$). ($^1\Sigma_g^+$)$^1O_2$ is a free radical because it contains two unpaired electrons with opposite spin directions. On the other hand, ($^1\Delta_g$)$^1O_2$ is a non-radical. Due to its highly unstable nature, ($^1\Sigma_g^+$)$^1O_2$ is generally regarded to lack biological significance. Thus, in free radical biology and medicine, the term singlet oxygen, if not specified, usually refers to the $^1\Delta_g$ state.

3.4. Reactive Nitrogen Species

Similar to ROS, the term reactive nitrogen species (RNS) has been coined to include nitric oxide ($NO^{\cdot}$),

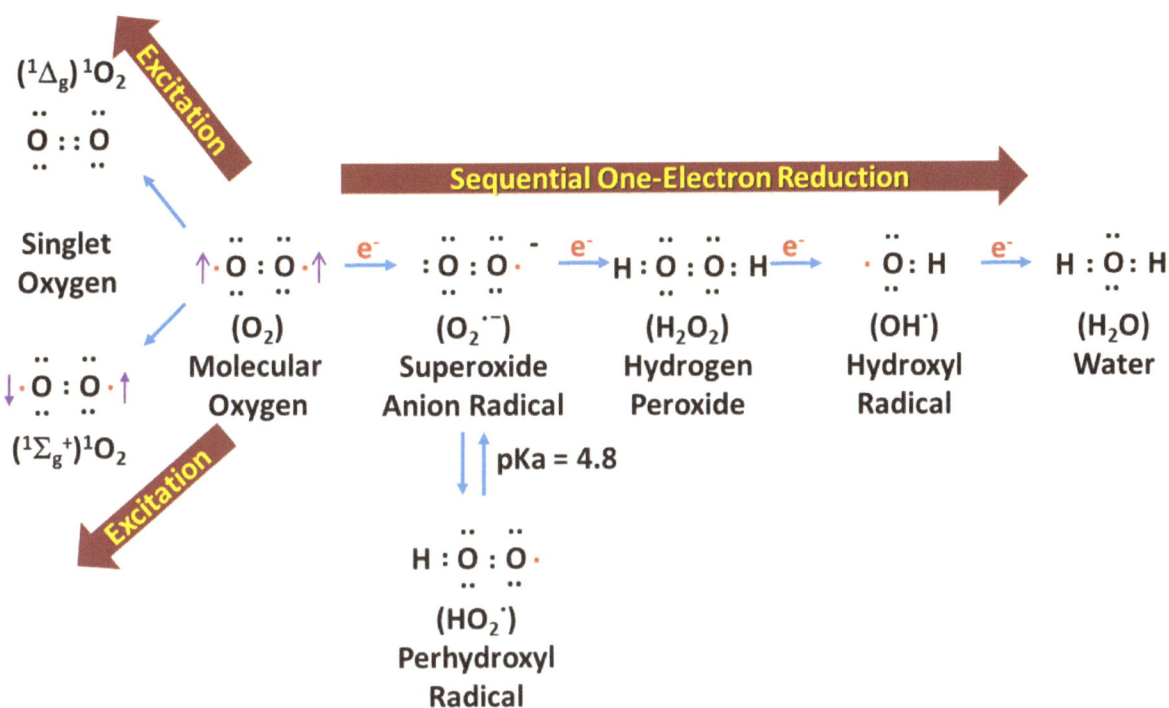

FIGURE 2.1. Excitation and univalent reduction of molecular oxygen to yield reactive oxygen species (ROS) in biological systems. As indicated, ground state molecular oxygen (O_2) is a free radical (it is actually a di-radical) because it contains two unpaired electrons. O_2 is much less reactive than ROS due to spin restriction caused by the same spin direction of its two unpaired electrons. O_2 can be excited to form singlet oxygen ($^1O_2$). There are two states of singlet oxygen: delta and sigma. The sigma state singlet oxygen is a free radical due to the existence of two unpaired electrons, whereas the delta state is a non-radical. One electron reduction of O_2 gives rise to superoxide anion radical ($O_2^{\cdot-}$), which then undergoes another one electron reduction to yield hydrogen peroxide (H_2O_2). One electron reduction of hydrogen peroxide generates hydroxyl radical ($OH^\cdot$), which can then be reduced by one electron to form water. Perhydroxyl radical ($HO_2^\cdot$) is a protonated form of superoxide anion radical.

peroxynitrite, nitrogen dioxide radical ($NO_2^\cdot$), and other oxides of nitrogen or nitrogen-containing reactive species. Because RNS are almost exclusively oxygen-containing species, by definition, they may also be classified as ROS. For example, peroxynitrite is classified as either an ROS or an RNS. The chemistry and biology of peroxynitrite are discussed in Chapter 11.

3.5. Reactive Chlorine Species

The term reactive chlorine species (RCS) refers to chlorine-containing reactive species, with hypochlorous acid (HOCl) as a prototype. As compared to ROS and RNS, the term RCS is less frequently used in free radical biology and medicine. The chemistry and biology of HOCl are discussed in Chapter 13.

3.6. Reactive Oxygen and Nitrogen Species

As noted earlier, the RCS hypochlorous acid and the RNS peroxynitrite are also classified into the ROS category. Indeed, the ROS category comprises the most commonly encountered free radicals and related species in biology and medicine. Due to the increasingly recognized biological effects of nitric oxide and related nitrogen-containing species, the term RNS has been coined and becoming more commonly used in the literature (**Table 2.1**). Frequently, the compound term "reactive oxygen and nitrogen species (ROS/RNS)" is employed to refer to a group of ROS and RNS commonly seen in biological systems. Nevertheless, because all biologically relevant RNS are exclusively also oxygen-containing species (and hence can be called ROS by definition),

TABLE 2.1. The number of entries in PubMed (https://www.ncbi.nlm.nih.gov/pubmed) involving the use of "reactive oxygen species" and other related terms in title/abstract

Term	Entries
Reactive oxygen species	81,679
Reactive oxygen intermediates	1,880
Reactive oxygen metabolites	1,155
Oxygen radicals	5,059
Reactive nitrogen species	2,201
Reactive chlorine species	30

Note: The number of entries as of November 21, 2016.

and for simplicity, the term ROS is used throughout the book to include both ROS and RNS.

3.7. Electrophiles

ROS are reactive species capable of causing damage to biomolecules, including proteins, lipids, and nucleic acids, leading to cell and tissue injury. Reactions of these reactive species with biomolecules also generate a large array of secondary electrophilic products (also known as electrophiles), including α,β-unsaturated aldehydes, ω-6 and ω-3 unsaturated fatty acids, as well as nitro-fatty acids. The term electrophile refers to an electron-deficient species that undergoes covalent reactions by accepting an electron pair from an electron-rich biomolecule (also known as a nucleophile). Electrophilic species can also be derived from biotransformation of xenobiotics. The term xenobiotic can be defined as any substance that does not occur naturally in the human body. While high levels of electrophiles, especially α,β-unsaturated aldehydes are able to cause overt cell and tissue injury, at non-cytotoxic levels, these electrophilic species can interfere with cell signaling [2, 3]. Notably, the endogenously formed electrophilic 8-nitroguanosine 3′,5′-cyclic monophosphate also acts as a second messenger for nitric oxide-mediated signal transduction [4, 5].

4. ANTIOXIDANTS AND RELATED TERMS

4.1. Antioxidants

Mammals including humans have evolved a series of antioxidant defenses to protect vital biomolecules from ROS and related species-mediated damage. In addition, a number of components derived from the dietary sources also possess antioxidant activities in biological systems. The term antioxidant can be defined as any substance that can prevent, reduce, or repair the ROS-induced damage of a target biomolecule. In free radical biology and medicine, the target molecules usually include proteins, lipids, and nucleic acids.

There are many different kinds of antioxidants in biology and medicine, and they are classified in various ways. For example, the superoxide dismutase mentioned above is an endogenous antioxidant enzyme, whereas vitamin C is a widely known antioxidant derived from the dietary sources.

4.2. Phase 2 Enzymes or Proteins

Phase 1 and phase 2 (also written as phase I and Phase II) reactions are related to biotransformation (also known as metabolism) of xenobiotics. Phase 1 biotransformation reactions include oxidation, reduction, and hydrolysis. Phase 2 biotransformation involves primarily conjugation reactions, such as conjugation with endogenous cellular ligands (e.g., glutathione and glucuronic acid). Glutathione S-transferase and UDP-glucuronosyltransferase catalyze conjugation with glutathione and glucuronic acid, respectively. These enzymes along with many others involved in phase 2 biotransformation reactions of xenobiotics are classically referred to as phase 2 proteins or enzymes. Recently, the term phase 2 proteins is expanded to include not only the above conjugation-catalyzing enzymes, but also NAD(P)H:quinone oxidoreductase, epoxide hydrolase, dihydrodiol dehydrogenase, γ-glutamylcysteine ligase, heme oxygenase-1, leukotriene B4 dehydrogenase, aflatoxin B1 dehydrogenase, and ferritin [6]. Some of the above phase 2 proteins, such as γ-glutamylcysteine ligase, heme oxygenase-1, and ferritin are typically classified as antioxidants (see Appendix B). Thus, the compound term "antioxidative/phase 2 proteins" is frequently encountered in free radical biology and medicine. Indeed, many phase 2 proteins possess antioxidant activities. Appendix B describes the various types of antioxidants in biology and medicine.

4.3. Antioxidative/Anti-Inflammatory Defenses

Free radicals and related species, including ROS are mediators of inflammatory responses. In addition, ROS also activate cell signaling, augmenting production and release of proinflammatory cytokines, thereby perpetuating the inflammatory responses. As we know well-controlled inflammatory responses are part of our body's innate immunity, protecting against invading pathogens. However, overstimulated or prolonged inflammatory responses cause tissue injury, and as such, constitute a major pathophysiological mechanism of a wide variety of human diseases [7]. Due to the fact that ROS and inflammation are intimately intertwined [8, 9], many antioxidant enzymes or proteins, as well as non-protein antioxidants also possess anti-inflammatory activities [10]. Hence, the compound term "antioxidative/anti-inflammatory defenses" is sometimes used to describe these antioxidative molecules.

5. SUMMARY OF CHAPTER KEY POINTS

- Free radical biology and medicine may be defined as a field that studies the biological effects of free radicals and related reactive species (especially ROS) as well as antioxidants with an emphasis on the involvement of ROS and antioxidants in health and disease.
- Free radical refers to any chemical species capable of independent existence that contains one or more unpaired electrons. ROS is a collective term to include superoxide, hydrogen peroxide, hydroxyl radical, singlet oxygen, peroxyl radical, alkoxyl radical, lipid hydroperoxide, peroxynitrite, hypochlorous acid, and ozone. Some ROS, such as superoxide and hydroxyl radicals are free radicals; others such as hydrogen peroxide and peroxynitrite are non-radical ROS, but can give rise to free radicals upon their further metabolisms in biological systems.
- The term RNS has been coined to include nitric oxide, peroxynitrite, nitrogen dioxide radical, and other oxides of nitrogen or nitrogen-containing reactive species. Because RNS are almost exclusively oxygen-containing species, by definition, they may also be considered as ROS.
- Due to the potential harmful effects of ROS, aerobic organisms have evolved a series of antioxidant defenses to protect vital biomolecules from ROS-mediated damage. The term antioxidant refers to any substance that can prevent, reduce, or repair the ROS-induced damage of a target biomolecule at physiologically relevant concentrations.
- As ROS and inflammation are intimately intertwined, many antioxidants also possess anti-inflammatory activities. Hence, the compound

term "antioxidative/anti-inflammatory defenses" is sometimes used to describe these antioxidants.

6. SELF-ASSESSMENT QUESTIONS

6.1. A free radical is a chemical species capable of independent existence that contains one or more unpaired electrons. Which of the following chemical species is a free radical?

A. Hydrogen peroxide
B. Hypochlorous acid
C. Ozone
D. Peroxynitrite
E. Superoxide

6.2. Metabolism of molecular dioxygen gives rise to a number of oxygen-containing reactive species, known as reactive oxygen species (ROS). Which of the following best describes the property of ROS?

A. All ROS are also reactive nitrogen species
B. All ROS are non-radicals
C. ROS only exist in biological systems
D. Some ROS are free radicals
E. HOCl is also a reactive nitrogen species

6.3. Which of the following species is a non-radical reactive oxygen species?

A. Molecular dioxygen
B. Nitric oxide
C. Ozone
D. Sigma state singlet oxygen
E. Superoxide

6.4. Which of the following species can be considered as either a reactive oxygen or a reactive nitrogen species of non-free radical nature?

A. Hydrogen peroxide
B. Hypochlorous acid
C. Nitric oxide
D. Nitrogen dioxide
E. Peroxynitrite

6.5. Which of the following is a reactive nitrogen species of free radical nature?

A. Hydrogen peroxide
B. Hypochlorous acid
C. Nitrogen dioxide

D. Peroxyl radical
E. Peroxynitrite

ANSWERS AND EXPLANATIONS

6.1. The answer is E. Among the listed species, only superoxide is a free radical. Superoxide is also known as superoxide anion radical and contains an unpaired electron. None of the other species listed contains an unpaired electron, and as such, does not meet the criterion for being a free radical.

6.2. The answer is D. Reactive oxygen species (ROS) include both radicals and non-radicals. Superoxide is a typical oxygen free radical, whereas hydrogen peroxide is a typical non-radical ROS.

6.3. The answer is C. Among the species listed, only ozone does not contain an unpaired electron. Molecular dioxygen is a di-radical because it contains two unpaired electrons. Sigma state singlet oxygen is a free radical, but the delta state single oxygen is a non-radical.

6.4. The answer is E. Peroxynitrite is a non-radical species that arises from the reaction of superoxide and nitric oxide and can be considered as either a reactive oxygen species (ROS) or a reactive nitrogen species (RNS). Nitrogen dioxide is a free radical, and by definition, it can also be considered as either an ROS or an RNS.

6.5. The answer is C. Both nitric oxide and peroxynitrite are common reactive nitrogen specicies (RNS). Nitric oxide is a free radical because it contains an unpaired electron. On the other hand, peroxynitrite does not contain any unpaired electron and is thus a non-radical RNS.

REFERENCES

1. Halliwell B. Antioxidants in human health and disease. *Annu Rev Nutr* 1996; 16:33–50.

2. Trevisani M, Siemens J, Materazzi S, Bautista DM, Nassini R, Campi B, Imamachi N, Andre E, Patacchini R, Cottrell GS, Gatti R, Basbaum AI, et al. 4-Hydroxynonenal, an endogenous aldehyde, causes pain and neurogenic inflammation through activation of the irritant receptor TRPA1. *Proc Natl Acad Sci USA* 2007; 104(33):13519–24.

3. Ruef J, Rao GN, Li F, Bode C, Patterson C, Bhatnagar A, Runge MS. Induction of rat aortic smooth muscle cell growth by the lipid peroxidation product 4-hydroxy-2-nonenal. *Circulation* 1998; 97(11):1071–8.

4. Sawa T, Zaki MH, Okamoto T, Akuta T, Tokutomi Y, Kim-Mitsuyama S, Ihara H, Kobayashi A, Yamamoto M, Fujii S, Arimoto H, Akaike T. Protein S-guanylation by the biological signal 8-nitroguanosine 3',5'-cyclic monophosphate. *Nat Chem Biol* 2007; 3(11):727–35.

5. Ito C, Saito Y, Nozawa T, Fujii S, Sawa T, Inoue H, Matsunaga T, Khan S, Akashi S, Hashimoto R, Aikawa C, Takahashi E, et al. Endogenous nitrated nucleotide is a key mediator of autophagy and innate defense against bacteria. *Mol Cell* 2013; 52(6):794–804.

6. Talalay P. Chemoprotection against cancer by induction of phase 2 enzymes. *Biofactors* 2000; 12(1–4):5–11.

7. Noubade R, Wong K, Ota N, Rutz S, Eidenschenk C, Valdez PA, Ding J, Peng I, Sebrell A, Caplazi P, DeVoss J, Soriano RH, et al. NRROS negatively regulates reactive oxygen species during host defence and autoimmunity. *Nature* 2014; 509(7499):235–9.

8. Zhang K, Kaufman RJ. From endoplasmic-reticulum stress to the inflammatory response. *Nature* 2008; 454(7203):455–62.

9. Zhou R, Yazdi AS, Menu P, Tschopp J. A role for mitochondria in NLRP3 inflammasome activation. *Nature* 2011; 469(7329):221–5.

10. Roth TL, Nayak D, Atanasijevic T, Koretsky AP, Latour LL, McGavern DB. Transcranial amelioration of inflammation and cell death after brain injury. *Nature* 2014; 505(7482):223–8.

Chapter 3

Oxidative Stress and Redox Signaling

ABSTRACT | Free radicals and related reactive species (FRRS), particularly reactive oxygen species (ROS), are double-edged swords. On the one hand, when their production overwhelms the normal antioxidant defenses in a biological system, excessive amounts of ROS cause potential oxidative damage to cellular constituents, creating a condition known as oxidative stress. Likewise, excessive production of reactive nitrogen species may cause nitrative and nitrosative stress. In contrast to their overproduction causing oxidative stress, ROS, when their production is tightly regulated under certain conditions, may act as important carriers of cell signal transduction, leading to desired physiological responses. This concept is commonly known as redox signaling. Oxidative stress and redox signaling are thus the two opposite edges of the double-edged swords represented by ROS and related species.

KEYWORDS | Nitrative stress; Nitrosative stress; Oxidative stress; Reactive oxygen species; Redox metabolome; Redox modulation; Redox proteome; Redox signaling

CITATION | Hopkins RZ and Li YR. Essentials of Free Radical Biology and Medicine. Cell Med Press, Raleigh, NC, USA. 2017. http://dx.doi.org/10.20455/efrbm.2017.03

ABBREVIATIONS | cAMP, cyclic adenosine monophosphate; FRRS, free radicals and related reactive species; GSH, reduced form of glutathione; GSSG, oxidized form of glutathione (also called glutathione disulfide); RNS, reactive nitrogen species; ROS, reactive oxygen species

CHAPTER AT A GLANCE

1. OVERVIEW

Free radicals and related reactive species, especially reactive oxygen species (ROS), are capable of causing oxidative damage in biological systems upon their over production. On the other hand, these same species, under certain conditions, may act as signaling molecules to participate in cell signal transduction. This chapter defines oxidative stress and related concepts. It also introduces the concept of redox signaling, an emerging area of active research in free radical biology and medicine.

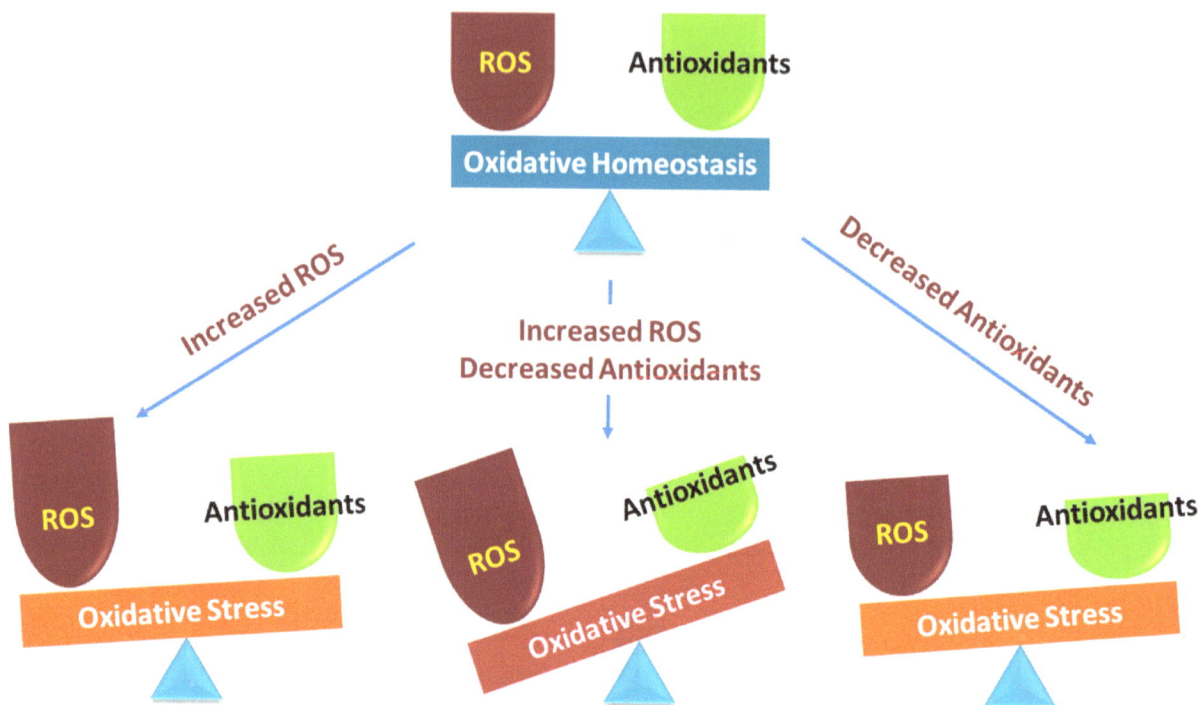

FIGURE 3.1. Schematic illustration of oxidative stress. As depicted, oxidative stress is caused by either increased formation of reactive oxygen species (ROS) or decreased antioxidant defenses, or both. It is important to distinguish oxidative stress from redox signaling. Oxidative stress emphasizes the potential detrimental effects of increased ROS, whereas redox signaling underlines the involvement of ROS in cell signaling transduction leading to physiological responses.

2. OXIDATIVE STRESS AND RELATED CONCEPTS

2.1. Oxidative Stress

Oxidative stress is an important concept in biology and medicine. The term was initially coined in 1985 by Helmut Sies (a highly respected German scientist) and defined in his book, titled: "Oxidative Stress" (Academic Press, London, UK, 1985). It refers to a condition where the levels of ROS significantly overwhelm the capacity of antioxidant defenses, leading to potential damage in a biological system. Oxidative stress condition can be caused by either increased ROS formation or decreased activity of antioxidants or both in a biological system. Oxidative stress condition is associated with oxidative damage to biomolecules, including proteins, lipids, and nucleic acids. Moderate oxidative stress may cause cell dysfunction and altered behavior (e.g., accelerated senescence, abnormal proliferation, dysregulated inflammatory responses, and cell tu-

morigenesis), whereas overt oxidative stress usually causes cell death (e.g., oncosis, apoptosis, autophagy, and ferroptosis).

Oxidative stress is a significant contributor to various pathophysiological processes, including aging [1–3]. **Figure 3.1** illustrates the concept of oxidative stress in free radical biology and medicine. It should be borne in mind that not any increases in ROS levels in a biological system are associated with injury. Under certain circumstances, small transient increases in ROS levels can be employed as a signaling mechanism, leading to physiological cellular responses (see Section 3).

2.2. Nitrative Stress

Analogous terms have been coined to describe the conditions associated with increased levels of RNS. For example, the term nitrative stress is defined as a condition under which the levels of RNS significantly overwhelm the capacity of RNS-detoxification mechanisms in a biological system. Nitrative stress

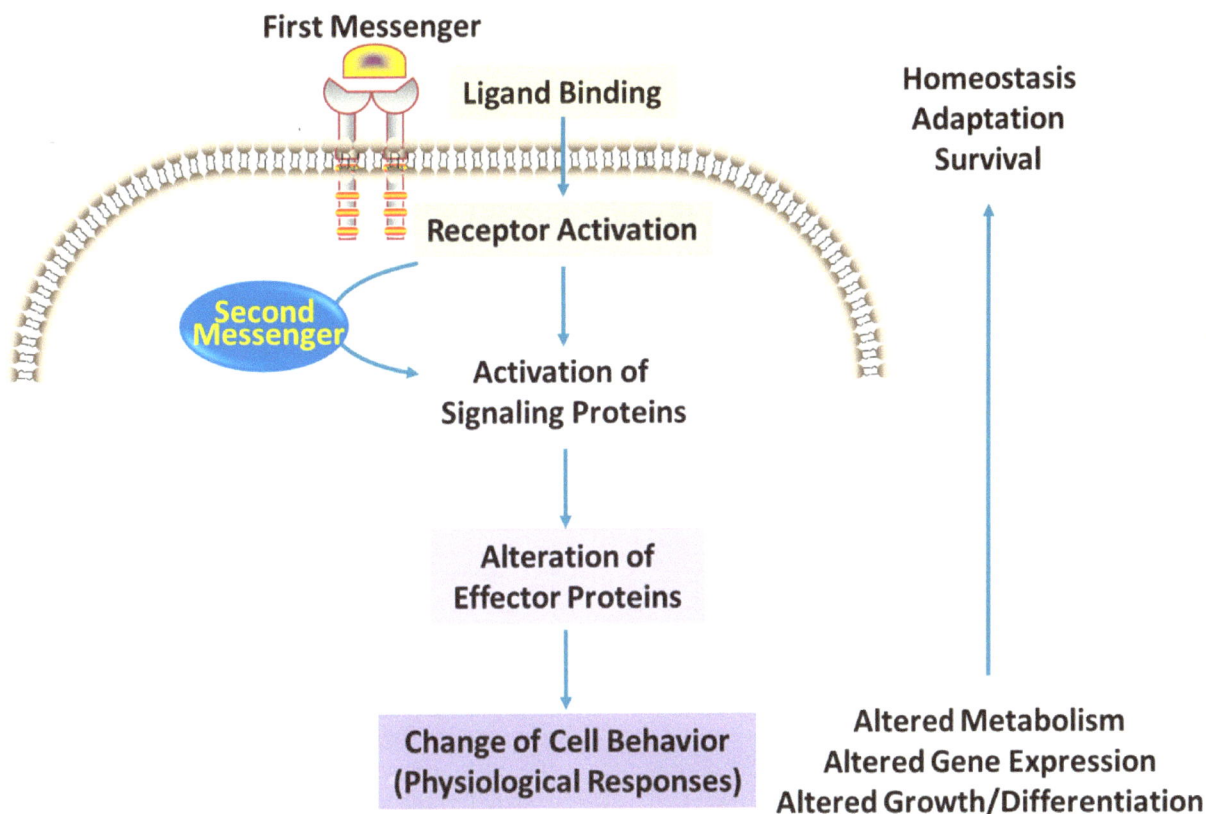

FIGURE 3.2. The three major steps of cell signaling. This scheme illustrates the three major steps involved in cell signal transduction upon extracellular stimulation. The extracellular stimulus (signaling molecule) can be a growth factor that acts on the target cell to cause a physiological cellular response (e.g., cell proliferation). The entire signal transduction process consists of three major steps: (1) binding of the extracellular signaling molecule to its receptor embedded in the plasma membrane of the target cell, leading to receptor activation; (2) the activated receptor in turn either directly or indirectly (via formation of second messengers, such as cyclic AMP) causes activation of the signaling molecules (typically proteins) of one or more of the signal transduction pathways; and finally (3) one or more of the activated signaling proteins alter the activity of effector proteins that reside at the end of signaling pathways and thereby the behavior of the cell.

condition is associated with nitration of biomolecules, leading to cell and tissue injury. Nitration refers to addition of a nitro ($-NO_2$) group to a compound. The RNS peroxynitrite readily causes nitrative stress in biological systems [4, 5].

2.3. Nitrosative Stress

Nitrosative stress is defined as a condition induced by nitric oxide (NO˙) or related species, leading to the formation of nitrosation/nitrosylation of critical protein cysteine thiols and metallocofactors of proteins. Nitrosation and nitrosylation refer to the addition of a nitroso ($-NO$) and nitrosyl (NO bound to a metal) to a thiol group and a redox active metal ion center of a protein, respectively. The most common form of nitrosation is S-nitrosation (more commonly called S-nitrosylation). S-Nitrosylation is now recognized as one of the post-translational modification of proteins by nitric oxide and nitric oxide-derived species. S-Nitrosylation can significantly impact protein function, stability, and localization/trafficking. While dysregulation of S-nitrosylation is associated with a number of pathophysiological conditions [6–8], well-controlled S-nitrosylation plays an important role in cell signal transduction and provides a mechanism of redox-based physiological regulation in both animals and plants [9–11].

3. REDOX SIGNALING AND RELATED CONCEPTS

3.1. General Considerations

A number of terminologies of basic chemistry are also frequently used in free radical biology and medicine. These include oxidation, reduction, redox, as well as oxidant and reductant. Oxidation refers to loss of one or more electrons by an atom or a molecule. Reduction refers to gain of one or more electrons by an atom or a molecule. The term redox refers to reduction-oxidation. Redox biology is the study of oxidation-reduction processes associated with living things.

In a chemical reaction, if chemical A oxidizes chemical B (another way of saying this is that chemical B reduces chemical A), then chemical A is an oxidant, chemical B a reductant for that particular reaction. In biological systems, many reductants act as antioxidants to detoxify ROS via either directly scavenging ROS or serving as electron donors for antioxidant enzymes. As described next, some of the cellular reductants also constitute redox metabolome, which interacts with redox proteome to impact cellular redox signaling and the consequent responses to environmental stimuli.

3.2. Redox Proteome and Redox Metabolome

The redox proteome is a collective term referring to components of the proteome that undergo reversible redox reactions and those modified irreversibly by ROS or related species [12]. Although many amino acids (e.g., tryptophan, tyrosine, and arginine) and the peptide backbone react with ROS, up to date, only three of the amino acids (cysteine, methionine, and selenocysteine) are known to undergo reversible redox reactions. The redox proteome interacts with the redox metabolome, a redox-active subset of the metabolome, with $NADPH/NADP^+$, $GSH/GSSG$ (reduced form of glutathione/oxidized form of glutathione), and cysteine/cystine being specifically relevant to the redox proteome [12].

As mentioned above, the cellular reductants, such as NADPH, cysteine, and GSH can directly scavenge ROS (in the case of cysteine and GSH) or serve as cofactors and electron donors for antioxidant enzymes (in the case of NADPH and GSH). The intrinsic interactions between redox proteome, redox metabolome, and ROS form the basis of cellular redox signaling, an important concept that has emerged in recent years.

3.3. Redox Signaling

Before defining redox signaling, let's first consider the definition of cell signaling. Cell signaling is also known as cell signal transduction.

3.3.1. Cell Signaling: The Three Steps

Essential to the survival of every cell is to monitor the extracellular (as well as intracellular) environment, process the information it gathers, and respond accordingly. The concept of cell signaling defines the ability of cells to detect changes in their environment to generate an appropriate physiological response upon information processing. Cell signaling upon extracellular stimulation typically involves the following three major steps (**Figure 3.2**): (1) binding of the extracellular stimulus (e.g., a cytokine released by an adjacent cell) to a receptor protein embedded in the plasma membrane of the target cell; (2) the activated receptor in turn results in activation of one or more intracellular signaling pathways involving a series of signaling proteins; and finally (3) one or more of the intracellular signaling proteins distribute the signal to the appropriate intracellular targets. The targets that lie at the end of signaling pathways are known as effector proteins, which are altered in some way by the incoming signal and implement the appropriate changes in cell behavior. The effector proteins can be transcription regulators, ion channels, metabolic enzymes, and cytoskeletal components.

3.3.2. Cell Signaling: Second Messengers and Molecular Switches

Most intracellular signaling molecules are proteins which help relay the signal into the cell by either generating second messengers, or activating the next signaling or effector protein in the pathway. Second messengers are small chemicals [e.g., cyclic adenosine monophosphate (cAMP), Ca^{2+}, and diacylglycerol] that are generated upon receptor activation by the extracellular stimulus (also known as extracellular signaling molecule or first messenger) and diffuse away from their source, spreading the signal to other parts of the cell.

Many of the intracellular signaling proteins behave like molecular switches, which are typically controlled or regulated by phosphorylation and dephosphorylation catalyzed by selective protein kinases and phosphatases, respectively. Although phosphorylation/dephosphorylation plays a predominant role in cell signaling, as described next, substan-

TABLE 3.1. Differences between ROS-mediated redox signaling and redox modulation/regulation

Characteristic	Redox Signaling	Redox Modulation/Regulation
Dependence of ROS formation on "first messengers"	Dependent on "first messengers"; always produced by the target cells through a well-defined cellular mechanism and under tight control	Independent of "first messengers"; may be produced by the target cells or adjacent cells or from environmental sources
ROS as second messengers	Yes	No
ROS targets	Signaling proteins only	Signaling proteins; metabolic enzymes; others
Always involving cell signaling	Yes	No
Nature of cellular responses	Physiological	Physiological or pathophysiological
Oxidative stress as a possible outcome	No	Yes

tial evidence also suggests a critical role for ROS-mediated redox reactions in cell signal transduction under certain conditions.

3.3.3. Redox Signaling: Definitions

As noted earlier, due to the presence of various antioxidant defenses, small transient increases in ROS levels are unlikely to cause significant injury to cells. Instead, such transient increases in ROS levels can fulfill a signaling role, resulting in physiological responses. The term redox signaling refers to the process wherein ROS or related reactive species act as second messengers to cause physiological cellular responses via redox reactions. In this context, ROS can cause redox modulation of signaling proteins, such as protein kinases and transcription factors to lead to physiological cellular responses. These responses may include cell proliferation and differentiation, as well as altered production or expression of cellular products, such as cytokine and adhesion molecules. It is necessary to emphasize the difference between redox signaling and redox modulation. Redox signaling refers to a physiological process, where ROS act as second messengers to mediate responses that are required for proper function and survival of the cell. On the other hand, redox modulation (or redox regulation) refers to a process wherein ROS alter the activity or function of the redox-sensitive molecular targets, including signaling proteins and metabolic enzymes, leading to either physiological or pathophysiological responses. When pathophysiological responses occur it is also known as oxidative stress. Hence, in terms of ROS-mediated redox reactions, redox signaling emphasizes the role of ROS as second messengers (like cAMP or Ca^{2+}) to mediate physiological responses, whereas redox modulation (regulation) stresses the role of ROS in altering the redox sensitive targets and that in the process the ROS involved usually do not act as second messengers (**Table 3.1**).

3.3.4. Redox Signaling: The Three Components and an Established Case

Cellular redox reactions and their regulation rely on an extensive array of biomolecules or cellular processes to: (1) generate the ROS in a regulated manner; (2) scavenge or inactivate the ROS; and (3) sense the cellular redox milieu chemically by undergoing oxidation and reduction reactions [13–15]. **Figure 3.3** illustrates the concept of cellular redox signaling. Notably, a number of cellular processes are known to produce ROS under both physiological and pathophysiological conditions.

The emerging role of ROS as second messengers in cell signal transduction has broadened the concept of cell signaling by providing a novel mechanism for cells to respond to their environment. While the area of redox signaling has been rapidly evolving over the past few years, the concept that ROS acting as second messengers in cell signaling originated from the early work on nitric oxide. In this regard, the role of nitric oxide (a free radical), acting as a second messenger, in cell signal transduction is a well-established concept [16–18]. In fact, the Nobel Prize in Physiology or Medicine for 1998 was awarded to Robert F. Furchgott, Louis J. Ignarro, and Ferid

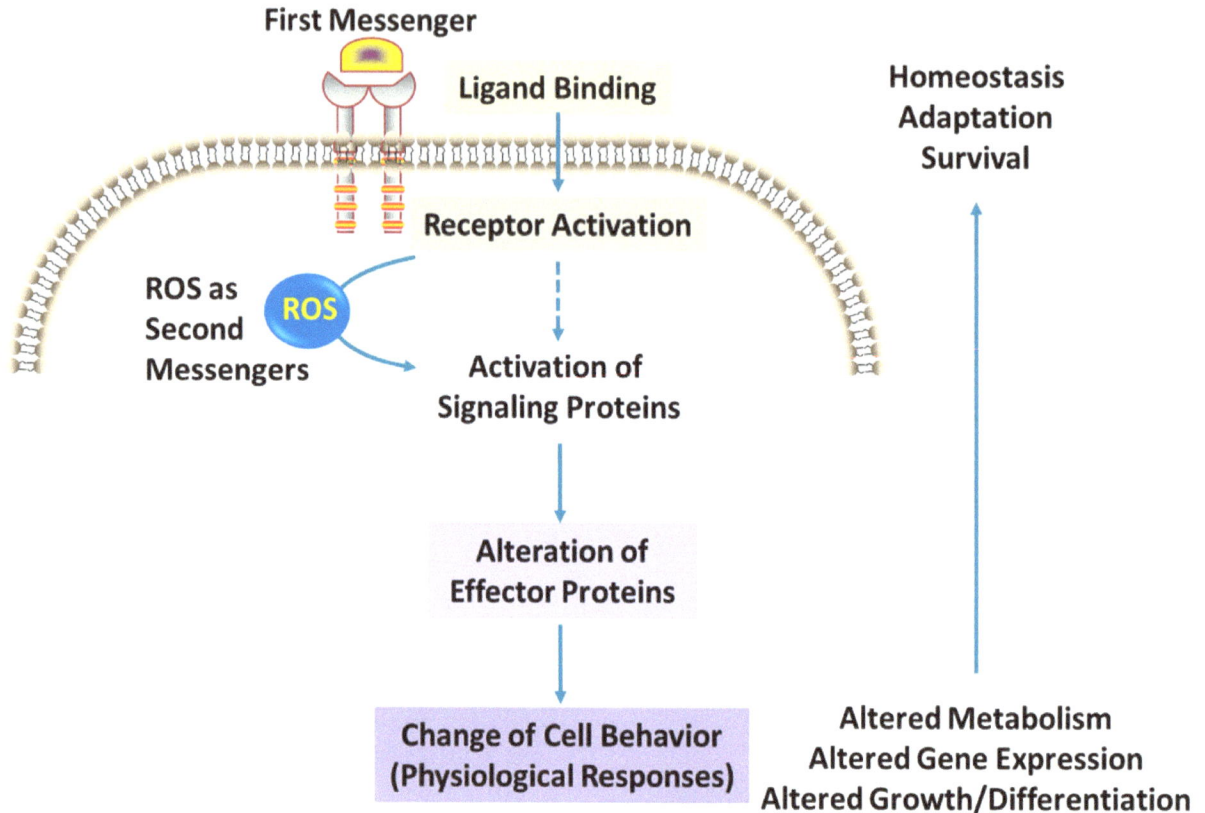

FIGURE 3.3. Components of reactive oxygen species (ROS)-mediated redox signaling. ROS-mediated cellular redox signaling involves multiple components. The generators are cellular processes (e.g., mitochondrial respiration and activation of NAD(P)H oxidases) responsible for the controlled production of the ROS, whereas the terminators (e.g., antioxidants) act to scavenge or inactivate the ROS so that the formation and disappearance of the ROS occur in a regulated manner. The sensor molecules (e.g., protein kinases, transcription factors, or other proteins) sense the ROS-induced changes of the cellular redox milieu chemically by undergoing oxidation and reduction reactions. Such redox reactions modulate the functions or conformations of the sensors, altering activities of downstream effectors, leading to cellular responses. Also see text (Section 3.3) for additional description.

Murad for their discoveries made in the 1980s, concerning nitric oxide as a signaling molecule in the cardiovascular system [19–21].

4. SUMMARY OF CHAPTER KEY POINTS

- Under physiological conditions, cellular ROS and antioxidants are in balance, thereby ensuring physiological homeostasis. Oxidative stress refers to a condition where the levels of ROS significantly overwhelm the capacity of normal antioxidant defenses in a biological system, leading to potential damage.

- Moderate oxidative stress causes cell dysfunction and altered behavior, whereas overt oxidative stress usually induces cell death. Under certain conditions, ROS act as second messengers to participate in cell signal transduction.

- The concept of cell signaling defines the ability of cells to detect changes in their environment to generate an appropriate physiological response upon information processing. The term cellular redox signaling refers to the process wherein ROS or related reactive species act as second messengers to cause cellular responses via redox reactions between ROS and signaling proteins. Redox signaling is considered as a physiological process.

- It is necessary to distinguish redox signaling from redox modulation/regulation. Redox signaling emphasizes a physiological process, wherein ROS act as second messengers to mediate responses that are required for proper function and survival of the cell. On the other hand, redox modulation/regulation refers to a process, wherein ROS alter the activity/function of the redox-sensitive molecular targets, including signaling proteins and metabolic enzymes, leading to physiological or pathophysiological responses.
- Robert F. Furchgott, Louis J. Ignarro, and Ferid Murad won the Nobel Prize for their discovery of the signaling role of nitric oxide, a free radical.

5. SELF-ASSESSMENT QUESTIONS

5.1. Oxidative stress is one of the most popular concepts in free radical biology and medicine. Which of the following best describes this concept?

A. Oxidative stress can result from decreased antioxidant defenses
B. Oxidative stress is also known as redox proteome or redox metabolome
C. Oxidative stress is also known as redox signaling
D. Oxidative stress is only caused by increased levels of reactive oxygen species
E. Oxidative stress is typically a physiological response in a biological system

5.2. Nitrosylation refers to the addition of which of the following chemical groups to a thiol group or a redox active metal ion center of a protein?

A. –GS
B. –NH$_2$
C. –NO
D. –NO$_2$
E. –OH

5.3. Nitrative stress condition is associated with nitration of biomolecules, leading to cell and tissue injury. Which of the following reactive species is most likely to cause nitrative stress in a biological system?

A. H$_2$O$_2$
B. HO$_2$$^{\cdot}$
C. HOCl
D. ONOO$^-$
E. ROO$^{\cdot}$

5.4. Which of the following pairs constitutes cellular redox metabolome?

A. ATP/ADP
B. cAMP/AMP
C. cGMP/GMP
D. GSH/GSSG
E. mRNA/rRNA

5.5. Redox signaling refers to the process wherein ROS or related reactive species act as second messengers to cause cellular responses via redox reactions. Which of the following species is a free radical that has been firmly established to act as a second messenger in cell signal transduction?

A. 8-Nitroguanosine 3′,5′-cyclic monophosphate
B. Hydrogen peroxide
C. Hydroxyl radical
D. Nitric oxide
E. Ozone

ANSWERS AND EXPLANATIONS

5.1. The answer is A. Oxidative stress is typically a pathophysiological condition that is caused by either increased ROS formation or decreased activity of antioxidants or both in a biological system.

5.2. The answer is C. Nitrosylation refers to the addition of a nitrosyl group (–NO, also known as nitroso group) to a cysteine thiol group or a redox active metal ion center of a protein. Nitrosative stress is caused by nitric oxide (NO$^{\cdot}$) or related species.

5.3. The answer is D. Nitration refers to addition of a nitro group (–NO$_2$) to a compound. The RNS peroxynitrite readily causes nitration and nitrative stress in biological systems

5.4. The answer is D. The redox proteome interacts with the redox metabolome, a redox-active subset of the metabolome, with NADPH/NADP$^+$, GSH/GSSG, and cysteine/cystine being specifically relevant to the redox proteome.

5.5. The answer is D. Among the species listed, nitric oxide (a free radical) is a well-established second messenger involved in cell signal transduction. It is also widely believed that H$_2$O$_2$ may act as a second messenger in biological systems. But H$_2$O$_2$ is not a free radical species.

REFERENCES

1. Finkel T, Holbrook NJ. Oxidants, oxidative stress and the biology of ageing. *Nature* 2000; 408(6809):239–47.
2. Lin MT, Beal MF. Mitochondrial dysfunction and oxidative stress in neurodegenerative diseases. *Nature* 2006; 443(7113):787–95.
3. Kujoth GC, Hiona A, Pugh TD, Someya S, Panzer K, Wohlgemuth SE, Hofer T, Seo AY, Sullivan R, Jobling WA, Morrow JD, Van Remmen H, et al. Mitochondrial DNA mutations, oxidative stress, and apoptosis in mammalian aging. *Science* 2005; 309(5733):481–4.
4. Radi R. Peroxynitrite, a stealthy biological oxidant. *J Biol Chem* 2013; 288(37):26464–72.
5. Szabo C, Ischiropoulos H, Radi R. Peroxynitrite: biochemistry, pathophysiology and development of therapeutics. *Nat Rev Drug Discov* 2007; 6(8):662–80.
6. Yang L, Calay ES, Fan J, Arduini A, Kunz RC, Gygi SP, Yalcin A, Fu S, Hotamisligil GS. (METABOLISM) S-Nitrosylation links obesity-associated inflammation to endoplasmic reticulum dysfunction. *Science* 2015; 349(6247):500–6.
7. Nakamura T, Tu S, Akhtar MW, Sunico CR, Okamoto S, Lipton SA. Aberrant protein S-nitrosylation in neurodegenerative diseases. *Neuron* 2013; 78(4):596–614.
8. Akhtar MW, Sanz-Blasco S, Dolatabadi N, Parker J, Chon K, Lee MS, Soussou W, McKercher SR, Ambasudhan R, Nakamura T, Lipton SA. Elevated glucose and oligomeric beta-amyloid disrupt synapses via a common pathway of aberrant protein S-nitrosylation. *Nat Commun* 2016; 7:10242.
9. Hess DT, Matsumoto A, Kim SO, Marshall HE, Stamler JS. Protein S-nitrosylation: purview and parameters. *Nat Rev Mol Cell Biol* 2005; 6(2):150–66.
10. Yun BW, Feechan A, Yin M, Saidi NB, Le Bihan T, Yu M, Moore JW, Kang JG, Kwon E, Spoel SH, Pallas JA, Loake GJ. S-nitrosylation of NADPH oxidase regulates cell death in plant immunity. *Nature* 2011; 478(7368):264–8.
11. Huang ZM, Gao E, Fonseca FV, Hayashi H, Shang X, Hoffman NE, Chuprun JK, Tian X, Tilley DG, Madesh M, Lefer DJ, Stamler JS, et al. Convergence of G protein-coupled receptor and S-nitrosylation signaling determines the outcome to cardiac ischemic injury. *Sci Signal* 2013; 6(299):ra95.
12. Go YM, Jones DP. The redox proteome. *J Biol Chem* 2013; 288(37):26512–20.
13. Rudolph TK, Freeman BA. Transduction of redox signaling by electrophile-protein reactions. *Sci Signal* 2009; 2(90):re7.
14. Kawagishi H, Finkel T. Unraveling the truth about antioxidants: ROS and disease: finding the right balance. *Nat Med* 2014; 20(7):711–3.
15. Willems PH, Rossignol R, Dieteren CE, Murphy MP, Koopman WJ. Redox homeostasis and mitochondrial dynamics. *Cell Metab* 2015; 22(2):207–18.
16. Murad F. Shattuck Lecture. Nitric oxide and cyclic GMP in cell signaling and drug development. *N Engl J Med* 2006; 355(19):2003–11.
17. Moncada S, Palmer RM, Higgs EA. Nitric oxide: physiology, pathophysiology, and pharmacology. *Pharmacol Rev* 1991; 43(2):109–42.
18. Bredt DS, Snyder SH. Nitric oxide: a physiologic messenger molecule. *Annu Rev Biochem* 1994; 63:175–95.
19. Furchgott RF. Endothelium-derived relaxing factor: discovery, early studies, and identification as nitric oxide (Nobel lecture). *Biosci Rep* 1999; 19(4):235–51.
20. Murad F. Discovery of some of the biological effects of nitric oxide and its role in cell signaling (Nobel lecture). *Biosci Rep* 2004; 24(4–5):452–74.
21. Ignarro LJ. Nitric oxide: a unique endogenous signaling molecule in vascular biology (Nobel lecture). *Biosci Rep* 1999; 19(2):51–71.

Chapter 4

Free Radical Paradigm

ABSTRACT | Central dogma is the key to understanding a scientific discipline. Free radical paradigm is the central dogma of free radical biology and medicine, and provides a foundation for this rapidly evolving field. Free radical paradigm addresses five major areas, including: (1) sources of free radicals and related reactive species (FRRS); (2) molecular interactions between FRRS and the biological targets; (3) pathophysiological consequences; (4) physiological responses; and (5) antioxidants and antioxidant-based intervention. Free radical paradigm defines the scope of free radical biology and medicine and offers a framework for understanding the basic biology of FRRS and antioxidants as well as their roles in human health and disease.

KEYWORDS | Antioxidant intervention; Causal relationship; Disease process; Free radicals and related reactive species; Free radical paradigm; Reactive oxygen species

CITATION | Hopkins RZ and Li YR. *Essentials of Free Radical Biology and Medicine. Cell Med Press, Raleigh, NC, USA. 2017. http://dx.doi.org/10.20455/efrbm.2017.04*

ABBREVIATIONS | FRRS, free radicals and related reactive species; GSH, reduced form of glutathione; Nrf2, nuclear factor E2-related factor 2; ROS, reactive oxygen species

CHAPTER AT A GLANCE

1. OVERVIEW

The past two to three decades have witnessed the rapid development of the field of free radical biology and medicine. As new terminologies and concepts keep emerging as a result of ongoing active research, free radical biology and medicine has become an increasingly important subject that impacts both basic bioscience and clinical medicine. The rapidly evolving nature of this field makes it necessary to clearly define the scope of free radical biology and medicine and emphasize the essence of this scientific discipline. To this end, this chapter introduces the concept of free radical paradigm and outlines its scope. The chapter also discusses the implications of this paradigm in understanding the involvement of FRRS in disease process and strategies for the intervention of FRRS-induced tissue injury and disease process.

2. SCOPE OF FREE RADICAL PARADIGM

Free radical paradigm addresses the following aspects: (1) sources (generation) of free radicals and related species, especially reactive oxygen species (ROS); (2) molecular interactions between FRRS and cellular targets in the biological systems; (3) the resulting pathophysiological consequences; and (4) the resulting physiological responses. This paradigm also emphasizes the impact of antioxidants on the above processes and provides a framework for guiding antioxidant-based intervention of human diseases (**Figure 4.1**).

2.1. Sources of FRRS

FRRS are formed from various endogenous sources, including mitochondrial electron transport chain, NAD(P)H oxidases, xanthine oxidase, cytochrome P450 system, and uncoupled nitric oxide synthase, among others. Among the various cellular sources, mitochondrion is widely considered as a major source of cellular ROS under both physiological and pathophysiological conditions [1–5].

FRRS are also derived from exogenous sources, such as radiation, air pollutants, and certain xenobiotics that undergo continuous reduction and oxidation cycles (i.e., redox cycling) [6]. The levels of ROS in a biological system are determined not only by the rates of their production, but also by the presence and activities of cellular antioxidant defenses. Chemicals, including electrophiles (see Section 3.7 of Chapter 2) that deplete cellular GSH (reduced form of glutathione) can lead to secondary oxidative stress [7]. In this regard, a number of environmental chemicals as well as drugs are metabolized to form electrophilic metabolites [6].

2.2. Molecular Interactions between FRRS and Cellular Targets

FRRS are reactive species that cause oxidative damage to cellular biomolecules, including proteins, lipids, and nucleic acids. As such, mammalian cells are equipped with a wide variety of antioxidants and other cytoprotective factors to protect them from

damage by FRRS (see Appendix B). On the other hand, due to their ability to react with redox sensitive signaling proteins, under physiological conditions, FRRS, especially certain ROS can also act as second messengers to participate in cell signal transduction, a process known as redox signaling (see Chapter 3). The coordination between ROS generation and antioxidant-mediated decomposition ensures that ROS levels are tightly controlled and fine-tuned so as to act as second messengers for cell signaling. In this context, mitochondrion, a major source of cellular ROS, has recently been suggested to also act as a signaling organelle via its ROS-mediated redox reactions [2, 8–10].

2.3. Pathophysiological Consequences

When FRRS overwhelm the normal cellular or tissue defenses, oxidative stress ensures, leading to pathophysiological processes (see Chapter 3). Indeed, oxidative stress is an important pathophysiological mechanism underlying various human diseases. In this regard, it is conceivable that decreasing the levels of FRRS or inhibiting the oxidative damage through using antioxidant-based strategies may provide significant beneficial effects.

2.4. Physiological Roles

FRRS, particularly ROS also play important physiological roles. One most widely known scenario in this regard is the production of ROS from phagocytic cells in killing invading pathogenic microorganisms. Production of ROS by phagocytic cell's NADPH oxidase is recognized as an important part of the innate immunity. It has recently become clear that ROS derived from mitochondria in immune cells also play a role in innate as well as adaptive immunity [9, 11–13].

As described in Chapter 3, ROS can act as second messengers to mediate cell redox signaling, leading to physiological responses. Hence, in addition to immunity, ROS also fulfill other important physiological functions. It is conceivable that interference with the above physiological functions of ROS by antioxidants may cause undesired effects in biological systems. In this regard, uncontrolled overexpression of nuclear factor E2-related factor 2 (Nrf2), a master regulator of antioxidant gene expression, promotes tumorigenesis [14, 15]. In addition, FRRS are also involved in drug action. For example, metabolism of certain anticancer drugs leads to the formation of FRRS, which in turn mediates cancer cell

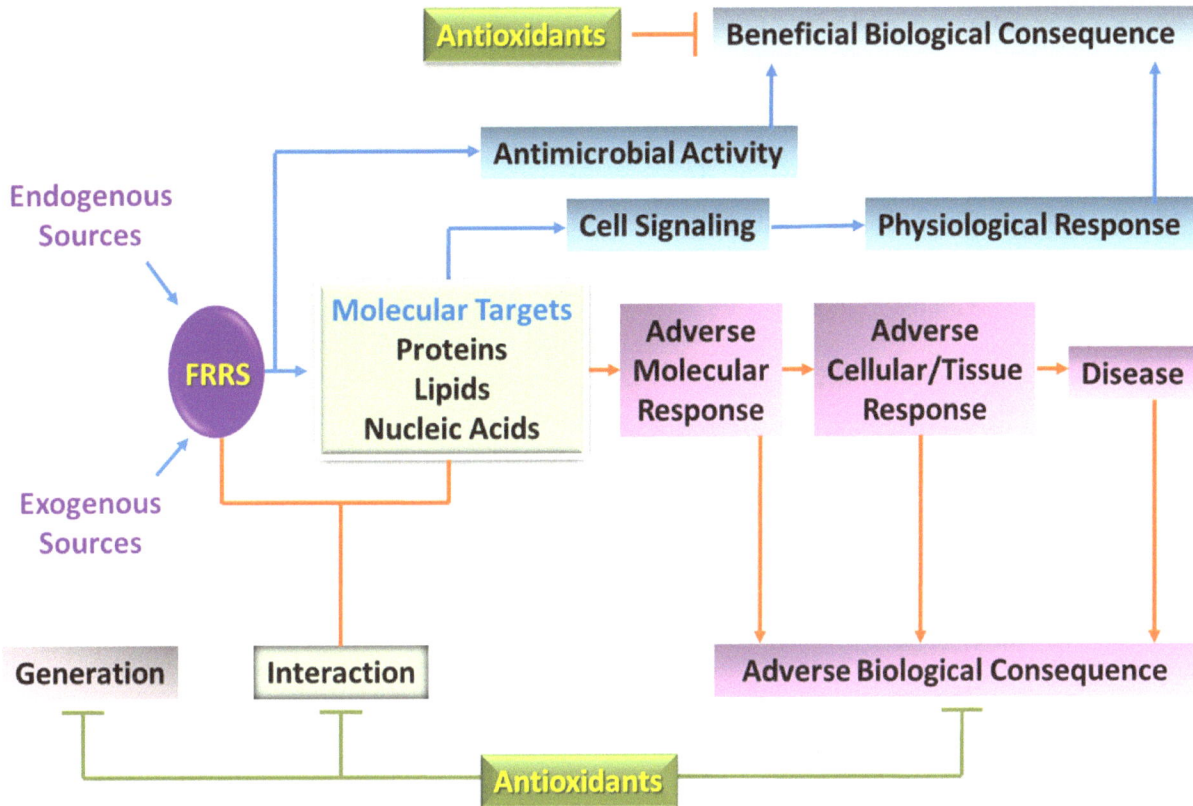

FIGURE 4.1. The free radical paradigm. This paradigm defines the scope of free radical biology and medicine which includes generation of FRRS, the interactions of these reactive species with target biomolecules, and the resulting biological consequences (adverse or beneficial). This paradigm also depicts the antioxidant-based intervention of diseases associated with FRRS, emphasizing the importance of selectively controlling FRRS-mediated adverse effects without compromising the physiological functions of these species.

killing [16–18]. Recently, targeting FRRS to cancer cells has been developed as a potentially promising strategy for cancer therapy [19, 20]. Taken together, FRRS can be either harmful or beneficial in biological systems.

2.5. Antioxidants and Antioxidant-Based Intervention

When examining the biological effects of FRRS, both detrimental and beneficial effects of these species should be taken into consideration. The free radical paradigm defines the scope of free radical biology and medicine. The goals of free radical biology and medicine should include not only determination of the pathophysiological roles of FRRS in disease process, but also investigation of the physiological functions of these reactive species in biological systems. Likewise, antioxidant-based strategies

for disease intervention should be devised to selectively control the adverse effects caused by pathophysiological levels of FRRS without compromising the beneficial effects of these reactive species at physiological levels. Thus, one should be cautious about the overuse of antioxidants or antioxidant supplements, which appear to be overly consumed by many people.

3. FREE RADICAL PARADIGM AND DISEASE PROCESS

Free radical paradigm states that it is the molecular interactions between the FRRS and the molecular targets that result in the oxidative tissue injury and disease development. The paradigm thus emphasizes the causal role for FRRS in disease process and provides the rationale for applying diverse approaches to controlling and preventing FRRS-induced tissue injury and disease development. Accordingly, to conclude a FRRS etiology of a disease process, the relationship between FRRS and the disease state needs to be carefully examined. Accordingly, this section first describes the epidemiological principles of establishment of causal relationships. It then considers the various scenarios regarding the relationships between FRRS and disease process. This section ends with a discussion of the implications of free radical paradigm in devising strategies to control and prevent FRRS-induced tissue injury and disease process.

3.1. Establishment of Causal Relationships

3.1.1. The Three Fundamental Types of Causal Relationships

Most scientific research seeks to identify causal relationships. Indeed, investigation of the causal relationships is one of the most important and challenging tasks of both basic and applied research. Outlined below are the three fundamental types of causal relationships.

3.1.1.1. SUFFICIENT CAUSE

If the factor (cause) is present, the effect (disease) will always occur. For example, homozygous hexosaminidase A deficiency inevitably leads to Tay–Sachs disease. As such, homozygous hexosaminidase A deficiency is the sufficient cause of Tay–Sachs disease.

3.1.1.2. NECESSARY CAUSE

The factor (cause) must be present for the effect (disease) to occur. A necessary cause may be present without the disease occurring. For instance, without the presence of *M. tuberculosis*, the disease tuberculosis cannot occur. However, people may have the *M. tuberculosis* bacteria in their bodies but do not develop tuberculosis.

3.1.1.3. RISK FACTOR

A risk factor is an exposure, behavior, or attribute that, if present and active, clearly increases the probability of a particular disease in a group of people who have the risk factor compared with an otherwise similar group of people who do not. For example, cigarette smoking is a risk factor for lung cancer; hypercholesterolemia is a risk factor for coronary artery disease.

3.1.2. Epidemiological Principles

Establishment of a role for FRRS in a particular disease process is the basis for understanding oxidative mechanism of a disease process and devising strategies to control and prevent that particular disease. The guidelines in modern epidemiology textbook for judging whether an association is causal are also applicable to free radical biology and medicine. These guidelines as applied to free radical biology and medicine are summarized below.

3.1.2.1. TEMPORAL RELATIONSHIP

If a factor is the cause of a disease, exposure to the factor must occur before disease develops. For example, for *M. tuberculosis* to be the cause of tuberculosis, exposure to the bacteria must occur before the development of tuberculosis. Likewise, If FRRS are the cause of a disease, exposure to FRRS must have occurred before the disease developed.

3.1.2.2. STRENGTH OF THE ASSOCIATION

The strength of an association is measured by the relative risk (or odds ratio). The stronger the association, the more likely it is that the relationship is causal. Here the term odds is defined as the ratio of the probability of occurrence of an event to that of non-occurrence, or the ratio of the probability that something is so, to the probability that it is not so. The term odds ratio is defined as the ratio of the odds of an event in one group to the odds of an event in another group. An odds ratio of 1.0 indicates no difference between comparison groups. For undesirable outcomes an odds ratio that is <1.0 indicates that the intervention was effective in reducing the risk of that outcome. With regard to FRRS as a potential cause of a disease, the stronger the association between FRRS and the disease, the more likely it is that the relationship is causal.

3.1.2.3. DOSE-RESPONSE RELATIONSHIP

Dose-response relationship describes the change in effect on, or response of, an organism caused by differing levels of exposure (or doses) to a factor (usually a chemical, a drug, or a pathogen) after a certain exposure time. If a dose-response relationship is present, it is a strong evidence for a causal relationship.

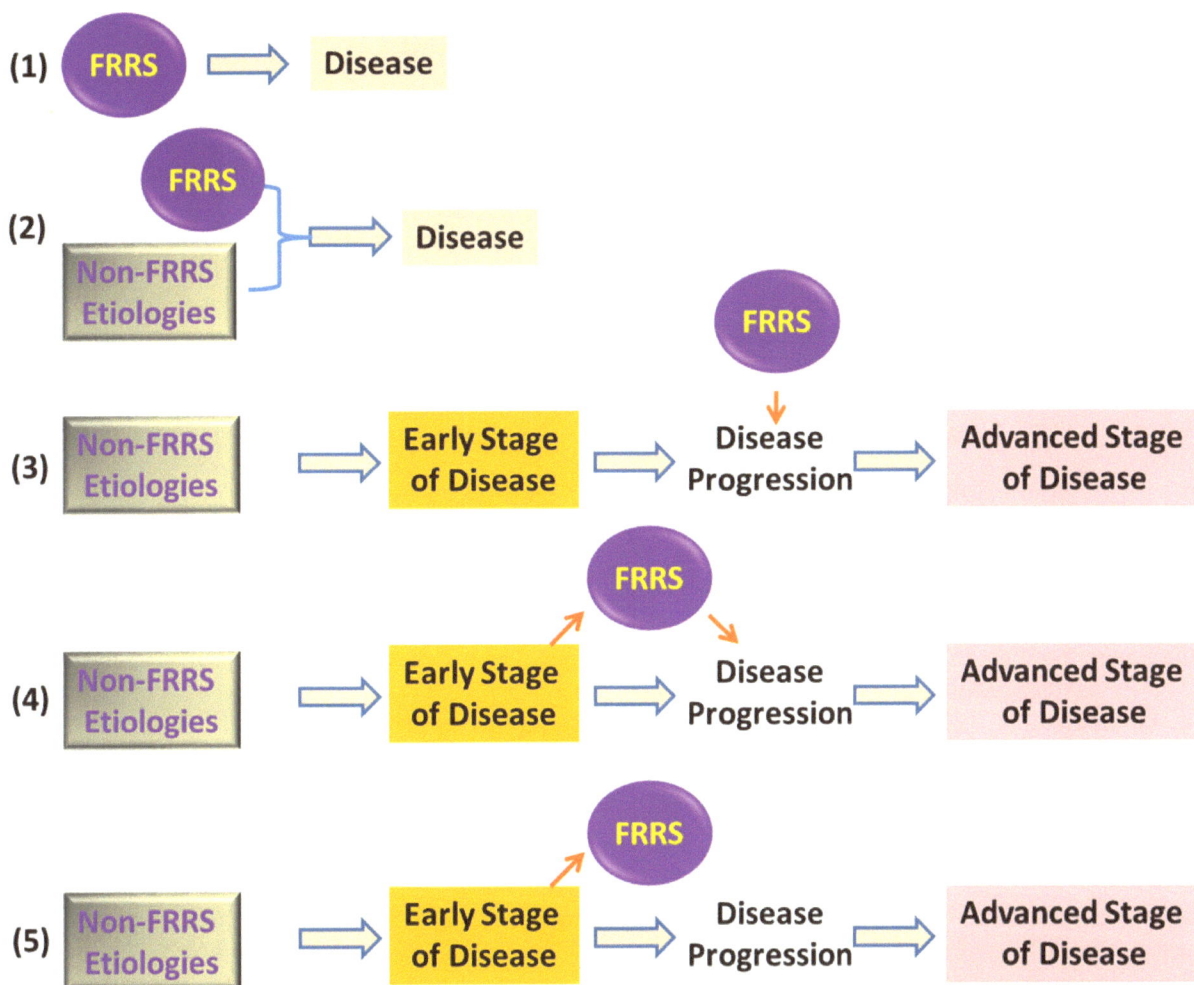

FIGURE 4.2. Potential relationships between FRRS and disease process. This scheme depicts the potential involvement of free radicals and related reactive species (FRRS) in disease process. Identifying these different scenarios represents an important, yet challenging, task of research in free radical biology and medicine. In this context, establishment of a causal relationship between FRRS and a disease process is crucial for the advancement of the field. See text (Section 3.2) for detailed description.

However, the absence of a dose-response relationship does not necessarily rule out a causal relationship. For a FRRS-induced disease process, as the dose of exposure to FRRS increases, the risk or incidence of the disease also increases.

3.1.2.4. REPLICATION OF THE FINDINGS

If the relationship between a factor and a disease is causal, this same relationship would be expected to be found consistently in different studies and in different populations. Likewise, if the relationship between FRRS and a disease is causal, we would

expect to find this relationship consistently in studies carried out by others and in studies involving different populations.

3.1.2.5. BIOLOGICAL PLAUSIBILITY

Biological plausibility refers to coherence with the current body of biological knowledge. A causal relationship between two variables would be explained by or consistent with existing biological knowledge. The causal role of FRRS in a disease process should be coherent with the current body of biological knowledge. In this context, as discussed in Chapter 7,

FRRS are reactive species capable of eliciting various types of cell and tissue injury.

3.1.2.6. CESSATION OF EXPOSURE

If a factor is a cause of a disease, it would be expected that the risk or incidence of the disease declines as the exposure to the risk factor is reduced or eliminated. Similarly, if FRRS are a cause of a disease, we would expect the risk of the disease to decline when exposure to the FRRS is reduced, or at the individual level the intensity of the disease pathophysiology to abate and clinical conditions to improve as the FRRS levels are reduced.

3.1.2.7. CONSIDERATION OF ALTERNATE EXPLANATIONS

In judging whether a reported association between FRRS and a disease process is causal, the extent to which the investigators have taken other possible explanations into account and the extent to which they have ruled out such explanations are important considerations.

3.2. Different Roles of FRRS in the Disease Process

As noted earlier, identifying the causal relationships is both important and challenging in scientific research. Research in free radical biology and medicine is without exception. Continued efforts in determining the relationships between FRRS and disease process will certainly enrich free radical paradigm and advance the field of free radical biology and medicine as a whole. Considering the above epidemiological principles in judging causal relationships, the potential involvement of FRRS in disease process is summarized as following, and also illustrated in **Figure 4.2**.

3.2.1. FRRS as the Only Initial Cause of the Disease Process

FRRS act as the only initial cause of the disease. Control of the FRRS will prevent or stop the disease development.

3.2.2. FRRS as One of the Initial Causes of the Disease Process

FRRS act as one of the causes of the disease. Control of the FRRS will mitigate the disease development.

3.2.3. FRRS as a Contributing Factor in the Disease Process

FRRS act as a contributing factor in the disease progression. Control of the FRRS will slow the disease progression.

3.2.4. FRRS as a Consequence of and Also a Contributor to the Disease Process

FRRS are formed as a consequence of the disease pathophysiology and contribute to the progression of the disease. Control of the FRRS will slow the disease progression.

3.2.5. FRRS as a Consequence of, but not a Contributor to the Disease Process

FRRS are formed as a consequence of the disease and play no role in disease development and progression. Control of the FRRS will have no effects on the disease process.

3.2.6. Other Considerations

Based on extensive investigations in animal models of human diseases as well as studies in human subjects over the last several decades, it has been widely recognized that FRRS are involved in a number of diverse diseases, including cardiovascular diseases, diabetes, neurodegeneration, and cancer, to name a few. For certain diseases, such as cardiovascular disorders, diabetes, and neurodegenerative disorders, there is substantial evidence supporting a causal role for FRRS in disease pathophysiology, especially in animal models [21–23]. For many others, the exact roles of FRRS in disease pathophysiology and development remain to be established. Moreover, as noted earlier, FRRS may also play important physiological roles. Hence, the beneficial effects of FRRS should be taken into consideration when one designs strategies for the intervention of FRRS-induced disease process (see Section 3.3.2).

3.3. Control and Prevention of FRRS-Induced Disease Process

3.3.1. Overall Approaches

In view of the potential causal role of FRRS in various diseases, it is important to devise strategies to mitigate FRRS-induced tissue injury and disease process. Intervention of FRRS-associated tissue injury and disease process could be potentially achieved by various approaches that address the key events depicted in free radical paradigm (**Figure 4.1**). Effectiveness of these approaches would in turn confirm the causal involvement of FRRS in the disease process. Summarized below are the potential approaches to controlling and preventing FRRS-induced disease process.

3.3.1.1. AVOIDANCE OF EXOGENOUS FRRS

This could be achieved by avoiding exposure to FRRS (e.g., the air pollutants ozone and nitrogen oxides) or FRRS-generating agents (e.g., xenobiotics capable of undergoing redox cycling). Avoidance of exposure to FRRS is the most effective way to prevent FRRS-induced tissue injury and disease process. This is, however, not always practicable. For example, exposure to FRRS or FRRS-generating chemicals in air pollution may be inevitable for those who live in polluted areas.

3.3.1.2. SCAVENGING OF FRRS

This could be achieved by administration of exogenous compounds with FRRS-scavenging capacities. In this context, many natural compounds derived from diet possess antioxidative properties (e.g., vitamin E, polyphenols, and carotenoids), which have been investigated for the sake of intervention of human diseases that are believed to involve an oxidative stress mechanism [24, 25].

3.3.1.3. INHIBITION OF ENDOGENOUS FRRS FORMATION

This could be achieved by administration of chemicals or pharmacological agents that inhibit FRRS formation from cellular sources, such as NADPH oxidases and xanthine oxidase. For example, apocynin (a selective inhibitor of NADPH oxidases) and allopurinol (a specific inhibitor of xanthine oxidase) have been used in experimental models for protecting against disease processes involving oxidative stress [26–28].

3.3.1.4. INCREASE OF ENDOGENOUS ANTIOXIDANT ENZYME DEFENSES BY PHARMACOLOGICAL AGENTS

This could be achieved by administration of chemicals or pharmacological agents that induce cellular antioxidants and other cytoprotective enzymes. In this regard, pharmacological activators of Nrf2, a master regulator of antioxidant genes, have been extensively studied for their efficacy in protecting against oxidative tissue injury in animal models as well as in clinical trials [29, 30].

3.3.1.5. ANTIOXIDANT GENE THERAPY

Transgenic overexpression of antioxidant genes has been demonstrated to protect against oxidative stress-associated tissue injury and disease process in a wide variety of animal models (see Unit III). Indeed, this approach along with gene knockout models has greatly contributed to our current understanding of the oxidative stress mechanism of human diseases. Antioxidant gene therapy has been investigated in a number of animal models of human disorders [31–33]. However, at the present time, antioxidant gene therapy is not practicable in human subjects due, largely, to regulatory concerns.

3.3.1.6. AUGMENTATION OF REPAIRING MECHANISMS

This could be achieved by administration of chemicals or pharmacological agents that upregulate cellular repairing mechanisms for damage caused by FRRS. For example, the cellular antioxidant enzymes glutathione peroxidase 4 and methionine sulfoxide reductase can repair oxidized lipids and proteins, respectively (see Unit III). Pharmacological upregulation of these enzymes would augment the endogenous repairing mechanisms of oxidatively damaged cellular targets that are vital for cell function and survival.

3.3.2. The Two Faces of FRRS

When applying the above approaches to the intervention of diseases involving FRRS mechanisms, it is important to bear in mind that although overproduction of FRRS causes tissue injury, complete elimination of these species might also have adverse consequences. As discussed above, under certain conditions FRRS act as useful molecules, participating in physiological processes. Therefore, a rational approach to the intervention of a disease process caused by elevated levels of FRRS is to bring the FRRS levels under control instead of completely eliminating them. This would ensure that the adverse effects caused by pathophysiological levels of FRRS are controlled without compromising the normal functions carried out by physiological levels of FRRS.

3.3.3. Application to Disease Intervention in Humans

The above potential approaches may be applied to the management of human diseases that involve FRRS mechanisms. Indeed, as noted earlier, administration of compounds with antioxidant properties, such as vitamins E and C, and polyphenols has been employed for the intervention of human degenerative diseases, including cardiovascular diseases, cancer, and neurodegenerative disorders. Induction of antioxidants and phase 2 enzymes by chemoprotective agents, including oltipraz and sulforaphane has also been investigated in humans as a potentially effective strategy for protecting against carcinogenesis and other disorders although the efficacy of such a strategy remains to be established [30, 34].

In general, management of human diseases includes the use of strategies to prevent and treat the diseases. Observational epidemiological studies support the effectiveness of various antioxidant compounds in preventing certain human diseases. However, the use of antioxidant compounds vitamins E and C in randomized controlled clinical trials for the intervention of such diseases as cardiovascular disorders and cancer has yielded inconsistent results (frequently with no benefits, and sometimes causing harms) [35, 36]. It is reasoned that the effectiveness of antioxidant-based strategies for human disease intervention is influenced by multiple factors. These include: (1) the types of antioxidant compounds used, the chemical and biological activities of these compounds in vivo, as well as the dosage and time window of treatment; (2) the populations of the patients, the status of oxidative stress in these patients, as well as the disease stage; and (3) the availability of sensitive and reliable biomarkers to assess both the oxidative stress status and the tissue antioxidant defenses in the patient populations. Indeed, many small scale clinical studies in subpopulations of patients with overt oxidative stress have shown an efficacy of antioxidant therapy.

Obviously, development of effective mechanistically-based strategies, including the use of antioxidant compounds for the management of human diseases continues to be an important objective of free radical biology and medicine. A thorough understanding of both the role of FRRS in disease process and the biological activities of antioxidants is instrumental in achieving the above objective. Units II and III provide a detailed discussion of common FRRS and antioxidants, respectively, in biology and medicine.

4. SUMMARY OF CHAPTER KEY POINTS

- Free radical paradigm defines the scope of free radical biology and medicine, and thereby provides a framework for understanding the involvement of FRRS in health and disease.
- Free radical paradigm states that it is the molecular interactions between the FRRS and the molecular targets that result in the tissue injury and disease development.
- The paradigm thus emphasizes the causal role for FRRS in disease process and provides the rationale for applying diverse approaches to controlling and preventing FRRS-induced tissue injury and disease development.
- Free radical paradigm considers the two faces of FRRS and also provides a frame work for guiding antioxidant-based strategies to selectively control FRRS-induced damage without compromising the physiological functions of these species.
- Identifying the causal relationships between FRRS and disease process and devising effective strategies to control and prevent FRRS-induced tissue injury and disease process continue to be among the top priorities of research in free radical biology and medicine.

5. SELF-ASSESSMENT QUESTIONS

5.1. Free radical paradigm is considered the central dogma of free radical biology and medicine. This paradigm emphasizes which of the following?

A. FRRS are always beneficial in aerobic organisms, including humans
B. FRRS are always harmful in biological systems
C. FRRS are not affected by exogenous antioxidant compounds
D. FRRS are the only cause of a large majority of human diseases
E. FRRS can be either harmful or beneficial

5.2. FRRS can be produced from various cellular sources. Which of the following sources is considered to produce both FRRS and adenosine triphosphate (ATP)?

A. Drug redox cycling
B. Mitochondrion
C. NADPH oxidase
D. Uncoupled nitric oxide synthase
E. Xanthine oxidase

5.3. Which of the following is a typical example of a physiological role played by FRRS?

A. Apoptosis
B. Killing of invading pathogens
C. Mitochondrial damage
D. Oxidation of protein kinases
E. Tissue necrosis

5.4. Free radical paradigm dictates the strategies for controlling and preventing FRRS-induced tissue injury and disease process. Which of the following approaches is considered the most effective one in preventing FRRS-induced tissue injury?

A. Antioxidant gene therapy
B. Avoidance of exposure to FRRS
C. Boosting the repairing mechanisms of oxidative damage
D. Intake of exogenous antioxidant compounds
E. Pharmacological induction of antioxidant genes

5.5. FRRS may be risk factors for certain human diseases. Which of the following defines a risk factor?

A. It is a necessary cause of a disease
B. It is a sufficient cause of a disease
C. It occurs before the development of a disease
D. It results from a disease process
E. Its presence increases the probability of a disease

ANSWERS AND EXPLANATIONS

5.1. The answer is E. Free radical paradigm emphasizes the two faces of FRRS: FRRS can cause tissue injury, leading to disease process. On the other hand, under certain conditions, FRRS play important physiological roles.

5.2. The answer is B. Among the souces listed, only mitochondrion produces both FRRS and ATP. In fact, mitochondrion is widely considered as the major source of cellular ROS.

5.3. The answer is B. Under certain conditions well-controlled production of ROS may play important physiological roles. One most widely known scenario in this regard is the production of ROS from phagocytic cells in killing invading pathogenic microorganisms. In fact, production of ROS by phagocytic cells is recognized as an essential part of the innate immunity.

5.4. The answer is B. Avoidance of exposure to FRRS or FRRS-generating machineries is the most effective way to prevent FRRS-induced tissue injury and disease process. However, this is not always practicable.

5.5. The answer is E. Risk factor is one of the three fundamental causal relationships. It is defined as an exposure, behavior, or attribute that, if present and active, clearly increases the probability of a particular disease in a group of people who have the risk factor compared with an otherwise similar group of people who do not.

REFERENCES

1. Sena LA, Chandel NS. Physiological roles of mitochondrial reactive oxygen species. *Mol Cell* 2012; 48(2):158–67.
2. Shadel GS, Horvath TL. Mitochondrial ROS signaling in organismal homeostasis. *Cell* 2015; 163(3):560–9.
3. Chouchani ET, Pell VR, Gaude E, Aksentijevic D, Sundier SY, Robb EL, Logan A, Nadtochiy SM, Ord EN, Smith AC, Eyassu F, Shirley R, et al. Ischaemic accumulation of succinate controls reperfusion injury through mitochondrial ROS. *Nature* 2014; 515(7527):431–5.
4. Chouchani ET, Pell VR, James AM, Work LM, Saeb-Parsy K, Frezza C, Krieg T, Murphy MP. A unifying mechanism for mitochondrial superoxide production during ischemia-reperfusion injury. *Cell Metab* 2016; 23(2):254–63.
5. Wang Y, Hekimi S. Mitochondrial dysfunction and longevity in animals: untangling the knot. *Science* 2015; 350(6265):1204–7.
6. Bolton JL, Trush MA, Penning TM, Dryhurst G, Monks TJ. Role of quinones in toxicology. *Chem Res Toxicol* 2000; 13(3):135–60.
7. Martensson J, Jain A, Stole E, Frayer W, Auld PA, Meister A. Inhibition of glutathione synthesis in the newborn rat: a model for endogenously produced oxidative stress. *Proc Natl Acad Sci USA* 1991; 88(20):9360–4.
8. Mills EL, Kelly B, Logan A, Costa AS, Varma M, Bryant CE, Tourlomousis P, Dabritz JH, Gottlieb E, Latorre I, Corr SC, McManus G, et al. Succinate dehydrogenase supports metabolic repurposing of mitochondria to drive inflammatory macrophages. *Cell* 2016; 167(2):457–70 e13.

9. West AP, Brodsky IE, Rahner C, Woo DK, Erdjument-Bromage H, Tempst P, Walsh MC, Choi Y, Shadel GS, Ghosh S. TLR signalling augments macrophage bactericidal activity through mitochondrial ROS. *Nature* 2011; 472(7344):476–80.

10. Chouchani ET, Kazak L, Jedrychowski MP, Lu GZ, Erickson BK, Szpyt J, Pierce KA, Laznik-Bogoslavski D, Vetrivelan R, Clish CB, Robinson AJ, Gygi SP, et al. Mitochondrial ROS regulate thermogenic energy expenditure and sulfenylation of UCP1. *Nature* 2016; 532(7597):112–6.

11. Hall CJ, Boyle RH, Astin JW, Flores MV, Oehlers SH, Sanderson LE, Ellett F, Lieschke GJ, Crosier KE, Crosier PS. Immunoresponsive gene 1 augments bactericidal activity of macrophage-lineage cells by regulating beta-oxidation-dependent mitochondrial ROS production. *Cell Metab* 2013; 18(2):265–78.

12. Geng J, Sun X, Wang P, Zhang S, Wang X, Wu H, Hong L, Xie C, Li X, Zhao H, Liu Q, Jiang M, et al. Kinases Mst1 and Mst2 positively regulate phagocytic induction of reactive oxygen species and bactericidal activity. *Nat Immunol* 2015; 16(11):1142–52.

13. Sena LA, Li S, Jairaman A, Prakriya M, Ezponda T, Hildeman DA, Wang CR, Schumacker PT, Licht JD, Perlman H, Bryce PJ, Chandel NS. Mitochondria are required for antigen-specific T cell activation through reactive oxygen species signaling. *Immunity* 2013; 38(2):225–36.

14. DeNicola GM, Karreth FA, Humpton TJ, Gopinathan A, Wei C, Frese K, Mangal D, Yu KH, Yeo CJ, Calhoun ES, Scrimieri F, Winter JM, et al. Oncogene-induced Nrf2 transcription promotes ROS detoxification and tumorigenesis. *Nature* 2011; 475(7354):106–9.

15. Chio, II, Jafarnejad SM, Ponz-Sarvise M, Park Y, Rivera K, Palm W, Wilson J, Sangar V, Hao Y, Ohlund D, Wright K, Filippini D, et al. NRF2 promotes tumor maintenance by modulating mrna translation in pancreatic cancer. *Cell* 2016; 166(4):963–76.

16. Trush MA, Mimnaugh EG, Gram TE. Activation of pharmacologic agents to radical intermediates. Implications for the role of free radicals in drug action and toxicity. *Biochem Pharmacol* 1982; 31(21):3335–46.

17. Noh J, Kwon B, Han E, Park M, Yang W, Cho W, Yoo W, Khang G, Lee D. Amplification of oxidative stress by a dual stimuli-responsive hybrid drug enhances cancer cell death. *Nat Commun* 2015; 6:6907.

18. Li JZ, Ke Y, Misra HP, Trush MA, Li YR, Zhu H, Jia Z. Mechanistic studies of cancer cell mitochondria- and NQO1-mediated redox activation of beta-lapachone, a potentially novel anticancer agent. *Toxicol Appl Pharmacol* 2014; 281(3):285–93.

19. Trachootham D, Alexandre J, Huang P. Targeting cancer cells by ROS-mediated mechanisms: a radical therapeutic approach? *Nat Rev Drug Discov* 2009; 8(7):579–91.

20. Kasiappan R, Safe SH. ROS-inducing agents for cancer chemotherapy. *Reactive Oxygen Species* 2016; 1(1):22–37.

21. Griendling KK, Touyz RM, Zweier JL, Dikalov S, Chilian W, Chen YR, Harrison DG, Bhatnagar A, American Heart Association Council on Basic Cardiovascular S. Measurement of reactive oxygen species, reactive nitrogen species, and redox-dependent signaling in the cardiovascular system: a scientific statement from the American Heart Association. *Circ Res* 2016; 119(5):e39–75.

22. Lin MT, Beal MF. Mitochondrial dysfunction and oxidative stress in neurodegenerative diseases. *Nature* 2006; 443(7113):787–95.

23. Shah MS, Brownlee M. Molecular and cellular mechanisms of cardiovascular disorders in diabetes. *Circ Res* 2016; 118(11):1808–29.

24. Taubert D, Roesen R, Lehmann C, Jung N, Schomig E. Effects of low habitual cocoa intake on blood pressure and bioactive nitric oxide: a randomized controlled trial. *JAMA* 2007; 298(1):49–60.

25. Sanyal AJ, Chalasani N, Kowdley KV, McCullough A, Diehl AM, Bass NM, Neuschwander-Tetri BA, Lavine JE, Tonascia J, Unalp A, Van Natta M, Clark J, et al. Pioglitazone, vitamin E, or placebo for nonalcoholic steatohepatitis. *N Engl J Med* 2010; 362(18):1675–85.

26. Han BH, Zhou ML, Johnson AW, Singh I, Liao F, Vellimana AK, Nelson JW, Milner E, Cirrito JR, Basak J, Yoo M, Dietrich HH, et al. Contribution of reactive oxygen species to cerebral amyloid angiopathy, vasomotor dysfunction, and microhemorrhage in aged Tg2576 mice. *Proc Natl Acad Sci USA* 2015; 112(8):E881–90.

27. Cutler MJ, Plummer BN, Wan X, Sun QA, Hess D, Liu H, Deschenes I, Rosenbaum DS, Stamler JS, Laurita KR. Aberrant S-nitrosylation

mediates calcium-triggered ventricular arrhythmia in the intact heart. *Proc Natl Acad Sci USA* 2012; 109(44):18186–91.

28. George J, Carr E, Davies J, Belch JJ, Struthers A. High-dose allopurinol improves endothelial function by profoundly reducing vascular oxidative stress and not by lowering uric acid. *Circulation* 2006; 114(23):2508–16.

29. Keleku-Lukwete N, Suzuki M, Otsuki A, Tsuchida K, Katayama S, Hayashi M, Naganuma E, Moriguchi T, Tanabe O, Engel JD, Imaizumi M, Yamamoto M. Amelioration of inflammation and tissue damage in sickle cell model mice by Nrf2 activation. *Proc Natl Acad Sci USA* 2015; 112(39):12169–74.

30. Singh K, Connors SL, Macklin EA, Smith KD, Fahey JW, Talalay P, Zimmerman AW. Sulforaphane treatment of autism spectrum disorder (ASD). *Proc Natl Acad Sci USA* 2014; 111(43):15550–5.

31. Kawamoto K, Sha SH, Minoda R, Izumikawa M, Kuriyama H, Schacht J, Raphael Y. Antioxidant gene therapy can protect hearing and hair cells from ototoxicity. *Mol Ther* 2004; 9(2):173–81.

32. Levonen AL, Vahakangas E, Koponen JK, Yla-Herttuala S. Antioxidant gene therapy for cardiovascular disease: current status and future perspectives. *Circulation* 2008; 117(16):2142–50.

33. Nanou A, Higginbottom A, Valori CF, Wyles M, Ning K, Shaw P, Azzouz M. Viral delivery of antioxidant genes as a therapeutic strategy in experimental models of amyotrophic lateral sclerosis. *Mol Ther* 2013; 21(8):1486–96.

34. Wise RA, Holbrook JT, Criner G, Sethi S, Rayapudi S, Sudini KR, Sugar EA, Burke A, Thimmulappa R, Singh A, Talalay P, Fahey JW, et al. Lack of effect of oral sulforaphane administration on Nrf2 expression in COPD: a randomized, double-blind, placebo controlled trial. *PLoS One* 2016; 11(11):e0163716.

35. Willcox BJ, Curb JD, Rodriguez BL. Antioxidants in cardiovascular health and disease: key lessons from epidemiologic studies. *Am J Cardiol* 2008; 101(10A):75D–86D.

36. Gaziano JM, Glynn RJ, Christen WG, Kurth T, Belanger C, MacFadyen J, Bubes V, Manson JE, Sesso HD, Buring JE. Vitamins E and C in the prevention of prostate and total cancer in men: the Physicians' Health Study II randomized controlled trial. *JAMA* 2009; 301(1):52–62.

UNIT II

CHEMICAL AND BIOLOGICAL PRINCIPLES

Chapter 5

Basic Chemistry of Free Radicals and Related Reactive Species

ABSTRACT | The biological effects of free radicals and related reactive species (FRRS) are determined by their chemical properties. Due to the unpaired electrons in free radicals, these species can bring about three general types of reactions in biological systems. They are atom abstraction, free radical addition, and electron transfer. A key chemical determinant of FRRS-induced biological effects is the reaction rate constant for a reaction between a FRRS and a particular biological target. Likewise, reduction potential is also an important chemical property that affects the reactions mediated by FRRS and thereby their biological effects.

KEYWORDS | Atom abstraction; Electron transfer; Free radical addition; Free radicals and related reactive species; Reaction rate constant; Reduction potential

CITATION | Hopkins RZ and Li YR. *Essentials of Free Radical Biology and Medicine. Cell Med Press, Raleigh, NC, USA. 2017. http://dx.doi.org/10.20455/efrbm.2017.05*

ABBREVIATIONS | DEPMPO, 5-(diethoxyphosphoryl)-5-methyl-1-pyrroline *N*-oxide; EPR, electron paramagnetic resonance; FRRS, free radicals and related reactive species; 8-OH-dG, 8-hydroxy-2'-deoxyguanosine; 8-oxo-dG, 8-oxo-2'-deoxyguanosine

CHAPTER AT A GLANCE

1. OVERVIEW

As described in Chapter 4, it is the direct molecular interaction between free radical and related reactive species (FRRS) and the cellular targets that dictates the subsequent biological consequences (either pathophysiological or physiological). The direct molecular interaction between FRRS and cellular targets is in turn determined largely by the chemical reactivity between the reactive species and their molecular targets. Hence, the chemical properties of FRRS are critical determinants of their biological effects. To understand the basic chemistry of FRRS, three aspects are discussed in this chapter. They are (1) free

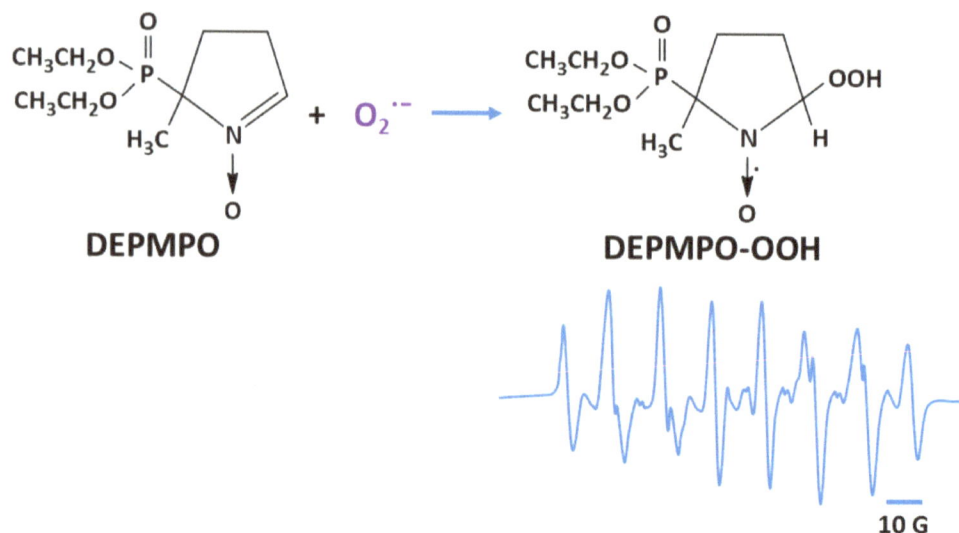

FIGURE 5.1. The reaction between superoxide anion radical and the spin trap 5-(diethoxyphosphoryl)-5-methyl-1-pyrroline *N*-oxide (DEPMPO). As illustrated in the scheme, the resulting spin adduct of DEPMPO-superoxide ([DEPMPO-OOH]') is still a radical species that can be detected by electron paramagnetic resonance spectrometry.

radical reactions, (2) reaction rate constant, and (3) reduction potential.

2. FREE RADICAL REACTIONS

Many FRRS are either free radicals or derived from free radical reactions. Free radical reactions are crucially involved in FRRS-mediated biological effects. Thus, it is imperative to understand the basic chemistry of free radical reactions. Free radicals usually do not react with great selectivity. The inherent chemical complexity of the biological systems further complicates the study of free radical-mediated biological reactions. Nevertheless, three general classes of free radical reactions are recognized. They are (1) hydrogen atom abstraction, (2) free radical addition, and (3) electron transfer.

2.1. Hydrogen Atom Abstraction

A free radical may abstract a hydrogen atom (H) from a C-H bond of a biomolecule such as a polyunsaturated fatty acid (LH). As the hydrogen atom has only one electron, an unpaired electron must be left on the carbon after removal of the hydrogen atom. This gives rise to the carbon-centered radical (L'). For example, hydroxyl radical (OH') is able to ab-

stract a hydrogen atom from a hydrocarbon side chain of a polyunsaturated fatty acid (Reaction 1).

$$OH^{\cdot} + LH \rightarrow H_2O + L^{\cdot} \quad (1)$$

In the above reaction, the hydroxyl radical combines with the hydrogen atom to form water, and the fatty acid is converted to a carbon-centered radical. The carbon-centered radical can then react with molecular oxygen (O_2) to form a lipid peroxyl radical (LOO') [1]. As discussed in Chapter 7, hydrogen atom abstraction by hydroxyl radical initiates lipid peroxidation in biological systems. Hydroxyl radicals can also cause hydrogen atom abstraction from a DNA deoxyribose carbon, resulting in DNA strand breakage [2].

2.2. Free Radical Addition

There are two types of free radical addition reactions. One occurs between a free radical and a non-free radical. The other occurs between two free radicals.

2.2.1. Free Radical Addition between a Free Radical and a Non-Free Radical

A free radical (A') adds onto a non-free radical molecule (B) to form an adduct species. Such an adduct species still has an unpaired electron initially associated with the free radical. The reaction is depicted as following: $A^· + B → [A-B]^·$. For example, a superoxide anion radical ($O_2^{·-}$) reacts with the spin-trap 5-(diethoxyphosphoryl)-5-methyl-1-pyrroline N-oxide (DEPMPO) to form a DEPMPO-superoxide adduct ([DEPMPO-OOH]$^·$) [3, 4] (**Figure 5.1**). This adduct still possesses an unpaired electron, and is thus a free radical species.

The DEPMPO-superoxide adduct has a much longer half-life (~15 min) than does the free superoxide anion radical (microseconds), and as such, can be readily detected by electron paramagnetic resonance (EPR) technique. Free radical addition is the basis for EPR spin-trapping detection of short-lived free radicals, including superoxide anion radical, hydroxyl radical, and other free radical species.

Another example of free radical addition is the reaction between hydroxyl radical and DNA bases. Hydroxyl radicals react with DNA bases via addition to the electron-rich pi bonds, which are located between C5 and C6 of pyrimidines, and N7 and C8 in purines [5]. During the reaction with a guanine base, the hydroxyl radical is added to the pi bond between N7 and C8 of guanine forming an unstable intermediate free radical adduct, which is subsequently converted to 8-hydroxy-2'-deoxyguanosine (8-OH-dG) (**Figure 5.2**). The oxidized guanine base may also exist as a keto form, which is known as 8-oxo-2'-deoxyguanosine (8-oxo-dG). 8-OH-dG or 8-oxo-dG is a commonly used biomarker for oxidative DNA damage [6, 7].

2.2.2. Free Radical Addition between Two Free Radicals

A free radical ($A^·$) is added onto another free radical ($B^·$) or the same radical ($A^·$) to form a non-free radical product. The reaction is depicted as: $A^· + B^· →$ AB, or $A^· + A^· →$ AA. In the reactions, the unpaired electrons from the two free radical substrates are paired in the resulting product, thus leading to the termination of the free radicals. For example, the free radical nitric oxide ($NO^·$) reacts with superoxide anion radical ($O_2^{·-}$) to form the non-free radical species, known as peroxynitrite anion ($ONOO^-$) (Reaction 2) [8].

$$NO^· + O_2^{·-} → ONOO^- (2)$$

As described in Chapter 11, peroxynitrite anion is a potent oxidant capable of inducing damage to various biomolecules [9].

2.3. Electron Transfer

In electron transfer, a free radical ($A^·$) acts as a reducing agent, donating a single electron to a non-free radical species (B). After receiving the single electron, the non-free radical species then becomes a free radical ($B^·$). The reaction is depicted as the following: $A^· + B → A + B^·$. For example, a superoxide anion radical can donate one electron to a molecule of hydrogen peroxide leading to the formation of one molecule of molecular oxygen, a hydroxyl radical, and a hydroxide ion: $O_2^{·-} + H_2O_2 → O_2 + OH^· + OH^-$. This is also known as the Haber–Weiss reaction or Haber–Weiss cycle [10] (see Chapter 8). In the absence of iron ion (Fe^{3+}), the above reaction proceeds very slowly. However, the presence of Fe^{3+} markedly accelerates the reaction to produce hydroxyl radical, thereby causing oxidative biological damage. In this context, hydroxyl radical is considered the most potent oxidizing species formed in biological systems.

3. REACTION RATE CONSTANT

3.1. Chemical Reactions

The chemical reactivity is an important factor involved in FRRS-induced biological effects. The chemical reactions in free radical biology and medicine include: (1) the reaction between a FRRS and a critical cellular target, such as a DNA molecule; (2) the reaction between a FRRS (e.g., H_2O_2) and a cellular antioxidant (e.g., glutathione); (3) the reaction between a FRRS (e.g., $O_2^{·-}$) and another FRRS (e.g., H_2O_2); and (4) the reaction between two molecules of the same FRRS (e.g., $O_2^{·-}$). Regardless of the above different types of possible reactions, the readiness for a reaction to occur can be described by the reaction rate constant.

3.2. Reaction Rate Constant

To understand the concept of reaction rate constant, let's first look at the rate of a chemical reaction. The rate of a chemical reaction can be measured either by following the loss of the starting reactants or the formation of the products. The term reaction rate refers to the amount of product formed per unit time, or the amount of reactant used up per unit time. Both temperature and concentrations of the reactants affect the reaction rate. The mathematical relationship between the rate (R) of a reaction and the concentra-

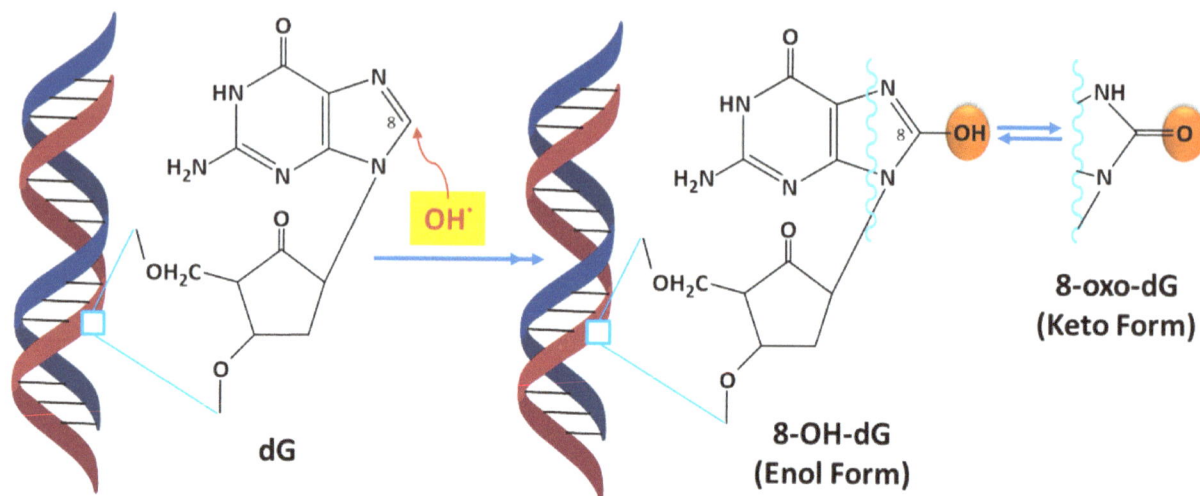

FIGURE 5.2. Reaction between hydroxyl radical (OH⁺) and the DNA guanine base. As illustrated in the scheme, hydroxyl radical reacts with the DNA guanine base via addition to the electron-rich, pi bond located between N7 and C8 of the purine, leading to the formation of 8-OH-dG or 8-oxo-dG.

tions of the reactants is known as the rate law. For example, two reactive species A and B react together to form a product or more than one product: A + B → Product(s). Then R = k [A][B], where R is the reaction rate, and k is the reaction rate constant with the unit being $M^{-1}s^{-1}$ (or $M^{-1}min^{-1}$), and [A] and [B] represent the concentrations of the reactive species A and B, respectively. The larger the k is, the faster the reaction between A and B will take place. In this example, the reaction rate constant k for the above reaction is a second-order rate constant.

Here it is necessary to define the order of reactions. A zero-order reaction has a constant rate that is independent of the reactant's concentrations (i.e., R = k, where k has the unit of $M\ s^{-1}$). A first-order reaction has a rate proportional to the concentration of one reactant (i.e., R = k[A] or R = k[B], where the unit of k is s^{-1}). A second-order reaction has a rate proportional to the product of the concentrations of two reactants (i.e., R = k[A][B]), as indicated earlier, where k has the unit of $M^{-1}s^{-1}$. Second order reactions are the most commonly encountered reactions in free radical biology and medicine.

Below are examples showing the reaction rate constants for two different reactions between two chemical species (Reactions 3 and 4).

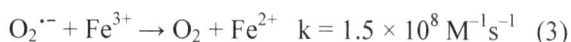

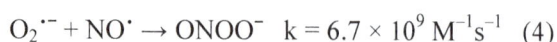

$$O_2^{\cdot -} + Fe^{3+} \rightarrow O_2 + Fe^{2+} \quad k = 1.5 \times 10^8\ M^{-1}s^{-1} \quad (3)$$

$$O_2^{\cdot -} + NO^{\cdot} \rightarrow ONOO^- \quad k = 6.7 \times 10^9\ M^{-1}s^{-1} \quad (4)$$

As indicated by the reaction rate constants, the reaction between $O_2^{\cdot -}$ and $NO^{\cdot}$ is much faster than that between $O_2^{\cdot -}$ and Fe^{3+}. In fact, the reaction between $O_2^{\cdot -}$ and $NO^{\cdot}$ occurs at a near diffusion-limited rate to give rise to peroxynitrite anion [8].

4. REDUCTION POTENTIAL

Reduction potential is also an important chemical property affecting the reactions mediated by FRRS and thereby their biological effects. Reduction potential is also known as redox potential. It is a measure (in volts) of the tendency of a chemical species to acquire electrons and thereby be reduced during the redox reaction. Each chemical species (including FRRS) has its own intrinsic reduction potential; the more positive the reduction potential of a chemical species is, the more likely it will be reduced and thereby more likely to act as an oxidizing species in a biological system.

Table 5.1 lists the standard reduction potentials for some common redox couples encountered in free radical biology and medicine, with the most oxidizing ones at the top and the most reducing ones at the bottom. A lower reduction potential for a redox couple indicates a higher potential to give away electrons, and thus to cause reduction. On the other hand, a higher reduction potential indicates a higher potential to accept electrons, and thus to cause oxidation.

TABLE 5.1. Standard reduction potential (E_o) of common redox couples

Redox Couple	E_o (mV)
$OH^{\cdot}, H^+/H_2O$	+2310
$CO_3^{\cdot-}, H^+/HCO_3^-$	+1780
$LO^{\cdot}, H^+/LOH$	+1600
$ONOO^-, 2H^+/NO_2, H_2O$	+1400
$ONOO^-, 2H^+/NO_2^-, H_2O$	+1200
$LOO^{\cdot}, H^+/LOOH$	+1000
$GS^{\cdot}/GS^-$	+920
Fe^{3+}/Fe^{2+}	+770
$PUFA^{\cdot}, H^+/PUFA\text{-}H$	+600
$TO^{\cdot}, H^+/TOH$	+480
$H_2O_2, H^+/H_2O, OH^{\cdot}$	+320
$Ascorbate^{\cdot-}, H^+/ascorbate^-$	+282
Ce^{4+}/Ce^{3+}	+160
Cu^{2+}/Cu^{1+}	+150
$Fe^{3+}EDTA/Fe^{2+}EDTA$	+120
$Dehydroascorbate/ascorbate^{\cdot-}$	−170
$O_2/O_2^{\cdot-}$	−330
$Paraquat^{++}/Paraquat^{\cdot+}$	−448
$NO^{\cdot}/NO^-$	−800
$H_2O/hydrated\ electron\ (e^-_{aq})$	−2870

Note: For each redox couple, the oxidizing species is on the left and the reducing species on the right. OH`, hydroxyl radical; CO₃·⁻, carbonate radical; LO`, alkoxyl radical; LOH, lipid alcohol; ONOO⁻, peroxynitrite anion; NO₂, nitrogen dioxide (also called nitrogen dioxide radical); NO₂⁻, nitrite; LOO`, peroxyl radical; LOOH, lipid hydroperoxide; GS`, glutathione radical; GS⁻, glutathione anion; PUFA`, polyunsaturated fatty acid radical (or carbon-centered radical); PUFA, polyunsaturated fatty acid; TO`, α-tocopherol radical; TOH, α-tocopherol; O₂·⁻, superoxide anion radical; NO`, nitric oxide; NO⁻, nitroxyl anion; Hydrated electron (e⁻ₐq) is the most reducing species. Based partly on "B Halliwell and GMC Gutteridge. Free Radicals in Biology and Medicine, 4th edition. Oxford University Press, London, UK. 2007".

As shown in the table, the redox couple ($OH^{\cdot}$ + H^+/H_2O) has the highest reduction potential among the redox couples listed, and indeed hydroxyl radical is the most reactive oxygen free radical known. Hydroxyl radical can readily oxidize biomolecules, including lipids, proteins, and nucleic acids at an almost diffusion-limited rate (see Chapter 10).

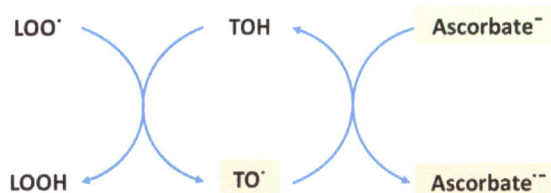

**FIGURE 5.3. Reduction potential-dictated redox reactions between lipid peroxyl radical (LOO`) and α-tocopheral and ascorbate.** Based on the pecking order of the redox couples, LOO` oxidizes α-tocopherol (TOH) resulting in the formation of lipid hydroperoxide (LOOH) and α-tocopherol radical (TO`). The resulting TO` can then be reduced by ascorbate to form the original α-tocopheral, and the ascorbate is oxidized to ascorbate radical.

The pecking order of the redox couples predicts the flow of electrons and which species might react with each other [11]. In general, the reactive species higher in the pecking order steal electrons from the reduced species lower in the pecking order. For example, the pecking order predicts that peroxyl radical (LOO`) can oxidize α-tocopherol (TOH) to α-tocopherol radical (TO`). This is because the reduction potential for the [LOO`, $H^+$/LOOH] redox couple is higher than that for the [TO`, H^+/TOH] redox couple. The α-tocopherol radical formed can then be reduced to α-tocopherol by ascorbate, because the reduction potential for [ascorbate`⁻, $H^+$/ascorbate⁻] is lower than that for the [TO`, H^+/TOH] redox couple. The above reactions are shown in **Figure 5.3**.

5. SUMMARY OF CHAPTER KEY POINTS

- The direct molecular interaction between FRRS and cellular targets is dictated by the chemical reactivity between the reactive species and their molecular targets.
- Three general classes of free radical reactions are recognized. They are hydrogen atom abstraction, free radical addition, and electron transfer. Free radical reactions may be considered the chemical basis of FRRS-mediated biological effects.
- The readiness of the chemical reactions between FRRS and biological targets or between FRRS themselves is determined by the reaction rate constant (k). The larger the k is, the faster the reaction between the reactants will take place.

- Reduction potential, also known as redox potential, is an important chemical property affecting the redox reactions mediated by FRRS and thereby their biological effects.
- Reduction potential is a measure (in volts) of the tendency of a chemical species to acquire electrons and thereby be reduced (or cause oxidation) during the redox reaction.
- The pecking order of the redox couples predicts the flow of electrons and which species might react with each other.
- A higher reduction potential indicates a higher potential for a chemical species to accept electrons, and thus to cause oxidation.
- On the other hand, a lower reduction potential indicates a lower potential to accept electrons or a higher potential to give away electron, and thus to cause reduction.

6. SELF-ASSESSMENT QUESTIONS

6.1. The reaction of $OH^\bullet + LH \rightarrow H_2O + L^\bullet$ is best known as an example of which of the following reactions involving free radicals?

A. Dismutation
B. Electron transfer
C. Free radical addition
D. Free radical reduction
E. Hydrogen atom abstraction

6.2. Superoxide anion radical ($O_2^{\bullet-}$) reacts with 5-(diethoxyphosphoryl)-5-methyl-1-pyrroline *N*-oxide (DEPMPO), a spin trap, to form a DEPMPO-superoxide adduct ([DEPMPO-OOH]$^\bullet$). This is an example of which of the following?

A. Free radical addition
B. Free radical oxidation
C. Hydrogen atom abstraction
D. Lipid peroxidation
E. Redox reaction

6.3. Hydroxyl radicals attack DNA bases, leading to the formation of 8-OH-dG. Which of the following best describes the above reaction?

A. Dismutation
B. Free radical addition
C. Hydrogen atom abstraction
D. Monooxygenation
E. Reduction

6.4. Which of the following best describes the reaction of $O_2^{\bullet-} + NO^\bullet \rightarrow ONOO^-$ $k = 6.7 \times 10^9$ $M^{-1}s^{-1}$ in a biological system?

A. A dismutation reaction
B. A first order reaction
C. A hydroxylation reaction
D. A second order reaction
E. A zero order reaction

6.5. Reduction potential is also known as redox potential. It is a measure of the tendency of a chemical species to acquire electrons and thereby be reduced during the redox reaction. Which of the following is the unit of standard reduction potential for the redox couple [$OH^\bullet + H^+/H_2O$]?

A. Amperes
B. $M s^{-1}$
C. $M^{-1}min^{-1}$
D. s^{-1}
E. Volts

ANSWERS AND EXPLANATIONS

6.1. The answer is E. This is a typical example of hydroxyl radical-caused hydrogen atom abstraction. Hydrogen atom abstraction by hydroxyl radical is an important mechanism underlying lipid peroxidation in biological systems.

6.2. The answer is A. This is an example of free radical addition between a free radical ($O_2^{\bullet-}$) and a non-free radical (DEPMPO). The resulting DEPMPO-superoxide adduct ([DEPMPO-OOH]$^\bullet$) still possesses an unpaired electron, and is thus a free radical species. This free radical adduct has a much longer half-life (~15 min) than does $O_2^{\bullet-}$ (microseconds), and as such, can be readily detected by electron paramagnetic resonance technique.

6.3. The answer is B. Hydroxyl radicals react with DNA bases via addition to the electron-rich, pi bonds, which are located between N7-C8 in guanine, resulting in the formation of 8-OH-dG.

6.4. The answer is D. A second-order reaction has a rate proportional to the product of the concentrations of two reactants (i.e., R = k[A][B]), where k has the unit of $M^{-1}s^{-1}$. Second order reactions are the most commonly encountered reactions in free radical biology and medicine.

6.5. The answer is E. Reduction potential is a measure in volts of the tendency of a chemical species to acquire electrons and thereby be reduced during the redox reaction. Reduction potential is an intrinsic property of a particular chemical species, including both free radical and non-free radical species.

REFERENCES

1. Tejero I, Gonzalez-Lafont A, Lluch JM, Eriksson LA. Theoretical modeling of hydroxyl-radical-induced lipid peroxidation reactions. *J Phys Chem B* 2007; 111(20):5684–93.
2. Balasubramanian B, Pogozelski WK, Tullius TD. DNA strand breaking by the hydroxyl radical is governed by the accessible surface areas of the hydrogen atoms of the DNA backbone. *Proc Natl Acad Sci USA* 1998; 95(17):9738–43.
3. Li Y, Zhu H, Kuppusamy P, Roubaud V, Zweier JL, Trush MA. Validation of lucigenin (bis-*N*-methylacridinium) as a chemilumigenic probe for detecting superoxide anion radical production by enzymatic and cellular systems. *J Biol Chem* 1998; 273(4):2015–23.
4. Zhu H. Assays for detecting biological superoxide. *Reactive Oxygen Species* 2016; 1(1):65–80.
5. Steenken S. Purine bases, nucleosides, and nucleotides: aqueous solution redox chemistry and transformation reactions of their radical cations and e-and OH adducts. *Chem Rev* 1989; 89(3):503–20.
6. Shigenaga MK, Gimeno CJ, Ames BN. Urinary 8-hydroxy-2'-deoxyguanosine as a biological marker of in vivo oxidative DNA damage. *Proc Natl Acad Sci USA* 1989; 86(24):9697–701.
7. Helbock HJ, Beckman KB, Shigenaga MK, Walter PB, Woodall AA, Yeo HC, Ames BN. DNA oxidation matters: the HPLC-electrochemical detection assay of 8-oxo-deoxyguanosine and 8-oxo-guanine. *Proc Natl Acad Sci USA* 1998; 95(1):288–93.
8. Mukhopadhyay R. When the good and the bad make the ugly: the discovery of peroxynitrite. *J Biol Chem* 2015; 290(52):30726–7.
9. Radi R. Peroxynitrite, a stealthy biological oxidant. *J Biol Chem* 2013; 288(37):26464–72.
10. Koppenol WH. The Haber–Weiss cycle: 70 years later. *Redox Report* 2001; 6(4):229–34.
11. Buettner GR. The pecking order of free radicals and antioxidants: lipid peroxidation, alpha-tocopherol, and ascorbate. *Arch Biochem Biophys* 1993; 300(2):535–43.

Sources of Free Radicals and Related Reactive Species

ABSTRACT | Utilization of molecular oxygen by aerobic organisms leads to the formation of free radicals and related reactive species (FRRS), especially reactive oxygen species (ROS). FRRS are produced from various cellular sources, including NADPH oxidases and mitochondria, among many others. FRRS are also generated from a variety of exogenous sources, such as physical agents, xenobiotics, and microorganisms. Recent studies also suggest the existence of ROS in oceans and deserts, as well as the universe.

KEYWORDS | Cytochrome P450; DUOX; Free radicals and related reactive species; Mitochondria; NADPH oxidase; NOX; Reactive oxygen species; Redox cycling; Xanthine oxidoreductase

CITATION | *Hopkins RZ and Li YR. Essentials of Free Radical Biology and Medicine. Cell Med Press, Raleigh, NC, USA. 2017. http://dx.doi.org/10.20455/efrbm.2017.06*

ABBREVIATIONS | CYP, cytochrome P450; DUOX, dual oxidase; FRRS, free radicals and related reactive species; NOX, NADPH oxidase; NRROS, negative regulator of ROS; ROS, reactive oxygen species

CHAPTER AT A GLANCE

1. OVERVIEW

The first component of the free radical paradigm introduced in Chapter 4 deals with the sources of free radicals and related reactive species (FRRS). Production of FRRS, especially reactive oxygen species (ROS) from the various sources is the first step that brings about the consequent biological effects, including both detrimental and beneficial effects. This chapter considers the various endogenous and exogenous sources of FRRS with an emphasis on the cellular machineries of FRRS production.

2. ENDOGENOUS SOURCES

The cellular sources of FRRS include NADPH oxidases, mitochondria, cytochrome P450 system, xanthine oxidoreductase, and others. Among them, NADPH oxidases and mitochondria, especially mitochondria are considered the chief sources of cellular ROS.

2.1. NADPH Oxidases

The NADPH oxidase in phagocytic cells produces superoxide during respiratory burst (also see Section 5.6 of Chapter 1). Phagocytic NADPH oxidase is perhaps the best characterized cellular source of ROS. This multicomponent enzyme complex consists of the catalytic subunit gp91^{phox} (also referred to as NOX2; see below for nomenclature), together with the regulatory subunits p22^{phox}, p47^{phox}, p40^{phox}, and p67^{phox}, and the small GTPase Rac (**Figure 6.1**).

ROS produced by phagocytes are essential for host immunity against bacterial and fungal infections. Individuals with defective phagocytic NADPH oxidase develop chronic granulomatous disease manifested as severe recurrent infections [1]. Conversely, excessive ROS can cause collateral tissue damage during inflammatory processes and therefore needs to be tightly regulated. In this regard, Noubade et al. recently show that a protein, known as negative regulator of ROS (NRROS), limits ROS generation by phagocytes during inflammatory responses [2]. They show that NRROS localizes to the endoplasmic reticulum, where it directly interacts with nascent gp91^{phox} and facilitates the degradation of gp91^{phox} through the endoplasmic reticulum-associated degradation pathway. Thus, NRROS provides a unique mechanism for regulating ROS production so that phagocytes can produce adequate amounts of ROS, if required to control invading microorganisms, while minimizing unwanted collateral tissue damage [2]. On the other hand, the polarity protein Scribble positively regulates ROS formation from phagocytic NADPH oxidase. Upon bacterial infection, Scribble localizes to phagosomes in a leucine-rich repeat-dependent manner and promotes ROS production within phagosomes of macrophages to kill phagocytosed bacteria [3].

For many years, NADPH oxidase was thought to exist as a single isoform only in phagocytes and its function restricted to antimicrobial action. This notion changed with the discovery of multiple NOX forms that represent an enzyme family containing at least five members, namely NOX1, NOX2, NOX3,

NOX4, and NOX5. NOX stands for NADPH oxidase. The NOX enzymes are expressed in various types of cells, and constitute an important source of ROS under a wide variety of physiological and pathophysiological conditions [4–6]. The NOX1–5 along with the dual oxidases (DUOX 1 and DUOX 2) are now members of an enzyme family, known as the NOX/DUOX family.

While superoxide is the primary product of most NOX enzymes, NOX4 may predominantly produce hydrogen peroxide (H$_2$O$_2$) rather than superoxide [7, 8]. DUOX1 and DUOX 2 may also primarily generate H$_2$O$_2$ [9]. However, it remains unclear whether these enzymes can directly catalyze the two electron reduction of oxygen to H$_2$O$_2$ or they produce H$_2$O$_2$ via a possible superoxide intermediate that may not be detected by current techniques due to rapid intramolecular dismutation or inaccessibility to the superoxide-detecting probes [9, 10].

2.2. Mitochondria

Another important cellular source of ROS is mitochondria. While the electron transport chain is a well-established site of ROS formation in mitochondria, other sources of mitochondrial ROS have also been identified. Uncontrolled production of mitochondria-derived ROS has been implicated in a number of pathophysiological conditions, including aging, neurodegeneration, and myocardial ischemia-reperfusion injury [11, 12].

2.2.1. Electron Transport Chain

In mammalian cells, mitochondrial respiration usually accounts for 80–90% of the oxygen consumed by the cells. Under physiological conditions, both complexes I and III of the mitochondrial electron transport chain are involved in the univalent reduction of molecular oxygen to superoxide [13] (**Figure 6.2**). It is estimated that about 0.1–1% of the oxygen utilized by mitochondria is converted to superoxide. The superoxide formed in mitochondria undergoes dismutation to yield H$_2$O$_2$ either spontaneously or catalyzed by manganese superoxide dismutase in mitochondrial matrix. The formation of ROS by mitochondrial electron transport chain is increased under various pathophysiological conditions, especially tissue ischemia-reperfusion [12, 14, 15].

Notably, a recent study shows that selective accumulation of the citric acid cycle intermediate succinate is a universal metabolic signature of ischemia in a range of tissues, including myocardium, and is re-

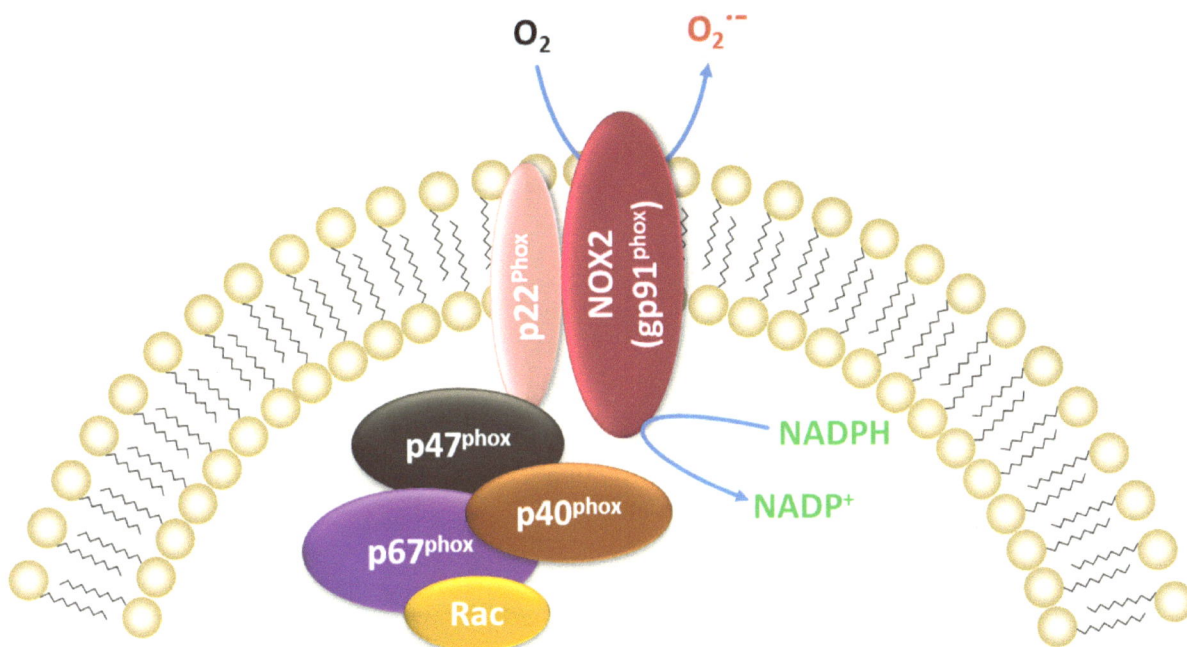

FIGURE 6.1. **Production of ROS by phagocytic NADPH oxidase.** As illustrated in the diagram, the activity of the phagocytic NADPH oxidase requires NOX2 and several regulatory proteins to assemble to form a functional enzyme complex that reduces oxygen to superoxide. The superoxide formed can further be converted to H_2O_2 and other ROS that constitute an important part of the innate immunity. NADPH oxidases are now known to belong to a family of enzymes (NOX1, 2, 3, and 4, and 5, and DUOX1 and 2) that are expressed in various types of tissues and constitute a major source of cellular ROS under physiological and a wide variety of pathophysiological conditions.

sponsible for mitochondrial ROS production during reperfusion [12]. Ischemic succinate accumulation arises from reversal of succinate dehydrogenase-catalyzed reaction, which in turn is driven by fumarate overflow from purine nucleotide breakdown and partial reversal of the malate/aspartate shuttle. After reperfusion, the accumulated succinate is rapidly re-oxidized by succinate dehydrogenase, driving extensive ROS generation by reverse electron transport at mitochondrial complex I [12]. In addition, Millis et al. show that succinate-driven mitochondrial ROS production is also involved in inflammatory responses [16].

Certain xenobiotics, such as quinone compounds undergo redox cycling catalyzed by mitochondrial electron transport chain complexes, leading to increased ROS formation. The ROS formed via the above mechanism may contribute to the cardiotoxicity of doxorubicin, a quinone-containing anticancer drug [17]. The concept of chemical redox cycling is illustrated in **Figure 6.3**.

2.2.2. Other ROS-Generating Enzymes in Mitochondria

In addition to mitochondrial electron transport chain, NOX4 has been recently identified to be present in mitochondria, and may contribute to ROS formation in this organelle [18]. In addition, monoamine oxidase associated with mitochondria is known to produce H_2O_2. Hence, the ROS formed in mitochondria may result from two general pathways: mitochondrial electron transport chain complexes and oxidases present in mitochondria. Nitric oxide is also formed in mitochondria via the action of mitochondrial nitric oxide synthase [19], which may react with superoxide to form the potent oxidant peroxynitrite in the mitochondrial compartment.

The gene SHC1 (Src homology 2 domain containing transforming protein 1) is located on chromosome 1 and encodes 3 protein isoforms: p66[SHC], p52[SHC], and p46[SHC]. p66[SHC] was the first mammalian gene whose mutation was demonstrated to increase

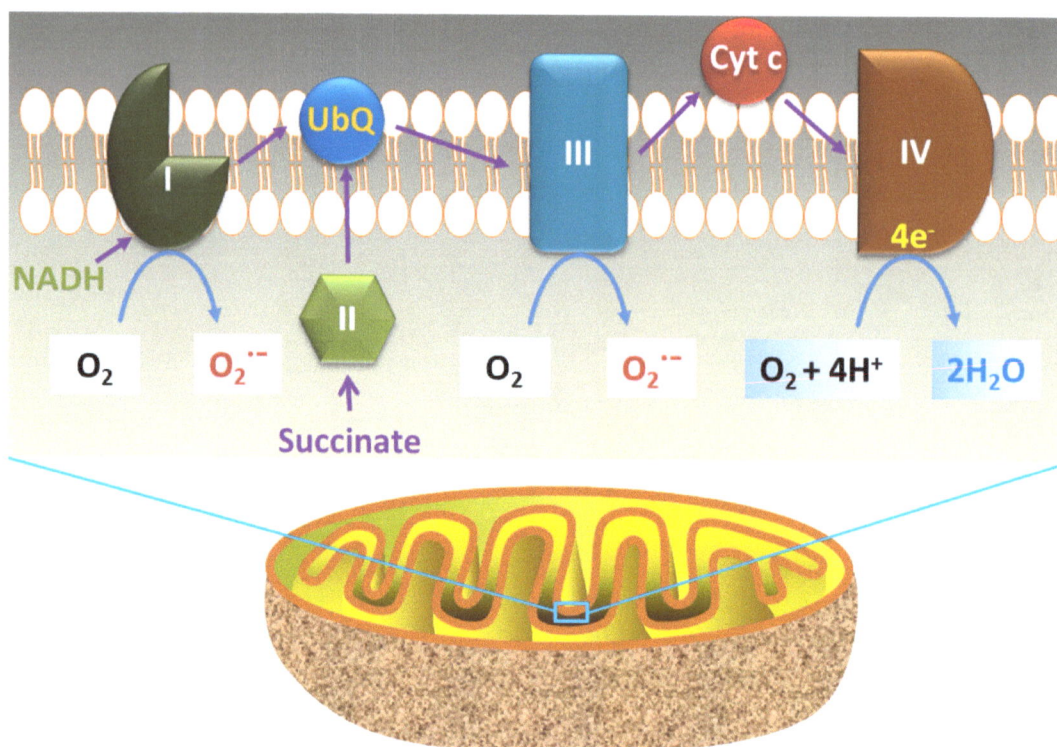

FIGURE 6.2. Formation of ROS by mitochondrial electron transport chain. As shown in the scheme, complexes I and III are believed to be the major sites of electron leakage, resulting in one-electron reduction of molecular oxygen to superoxide. As described in the text, besides the electron transport chain, other enzymes in the mitochondria, including NOX4, monoamine oxidase, and p66[SHC] are also sources of mitochondrial ROS production.

resistance to oxidative stress and to prolong life span [20]. p[66SHC] is located in mitochondria and is a redox enzyme that generates mitochondrial H_2O_2 by accepting electrons from cytochrome c [21].

2.3. Cytochrome P450 and Related Proteins

Cytochrome P450 (CYP) enzyme system, especially CYP2E1, is also a significant source of superoxide formation in cells, particularly under conditions when these enzymes are induced by chemicals (e.g., ethanol) [22]. CYP2E1-derived superoxide/ROS upon ethanol consumption may also be responsible for the upregulation of CYP2A5/2A6 by alcohol [23]. Recently, a redox signaling heme-containing globin, namely, GLB-12, in *Caenorhabditis elegans* has been shown to generate superoxide, and the superoxide produced may play a critical signaling role in regulating apoptosis and controlling the reproduction of the organism [24].

2.4. Other Endogenous Sources

Other cellular sources of ROS include xanthine oxidoreductase, uncoupled nitric oxide synthase, and peroxisomes. Xanthine oxidoreductase has two interconvertible forms: xanthine dehydrogenase and xanthine oxidase. Both forms catalyze the conversion of hypoxanthine to xanthine, and xanthine to uric acid. Both forms also catalyze one- and two-electron reduction of molecular oxygen to form superoxide and H_2O_2, respectively, with xanthine oxidase being more active in generating the above ROS. Xanthine oxidoreductase-derived ROS have been implicated in a number of pathophysiological processes, such as atherosclerosis, inflammation, and tissue ischemia-reperfusion injury in the heart, liver, and kidneys, among others [25].

Nitric oxide synthases normally catalyze the formation of nitric oxide. Under conditions of substrate deficiency, these enzymes can catalyze one-electron

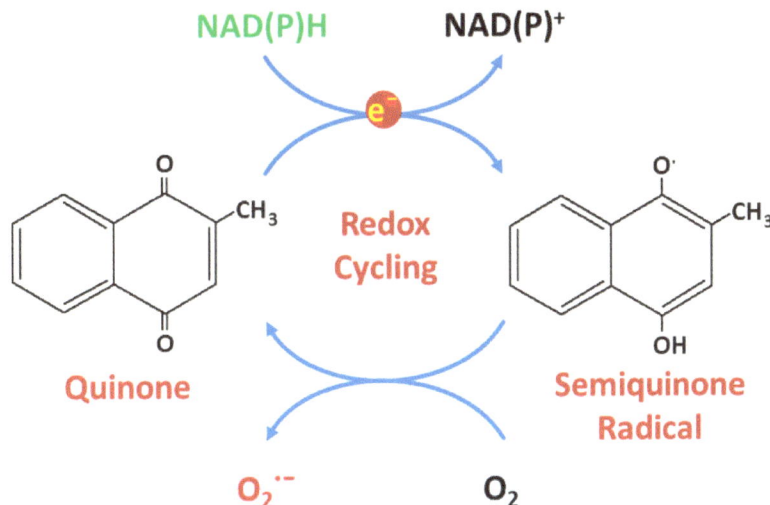

FIGURE 6.3. **Schematic illustration of the concept of chemical redox cycling.** Redox cycling of quinone compounds gives rise to an enormous amount of superoxide via one electron reduction of molecular oxygen by the semiquinone radical intermediate. Shown in the scheme is menadione (2-methyl-1,4-naphthoquinone), a typical redox cycling quinone. It is also known as vitamin K3.

reduction of molecular oxygen to superoxide. The organelle peroxisome contains enzymes, especially the flavoprotein dehydrogenases that produce significant amounts of H_2O_2. Peroxisome also contains large amounts of catalase which decomposes H_2O_2.

In addition to its presence in mitochondria, NOX4 is also found to undergo translocation into the nucleus via a leukotriene C4-dependent mechanism, and its presence in the nucleus contributes to oxidative damage to the nuclear DNA under stress conditions, including inflammatory responses and treatment with cancer chemotherapeutic agents [26]. The presence of NOX4 in cardiac cell nucleus is shown to cause oxidative stress in the nucleus, resulting in oxidation of class II histone deacetylase 4 (HDAC4) and cardiac hypertrophy [27]. The presence of NOX4 and possibly other ROS-generating NOX and non-NOX enzymes in the nucleus explains the existence of antioxidant enzymes (e.g., Cu,Zn superoxide dismutase) in this organelle and the organelle's constitutive production of ROS [28, 29].

3. EXOGENOUS SOURCES

The exogenous sources of FRRS include physical agents, airborne particulate matter, xenobiotics, and pathogenic as well as environmental microorganisms. In addition, FRRS, including superoxide, H_2O_2 and hydroxyl radicals are also found in Earth's deserts as well in the universe.

3.1. Physical Agents

Ionizing radiation causes homolysis of water to form hydroxyl radical, which contributes to radiation-induced tissue injury. Hydroxyl radical is also formed from ultraviolet light-induced homolysis of H_2O_2. Exposure of biological systems to ionizing radiation and ultraviolet light may result in the formation of other ROS as well.

3.2. Particulate Matter

In addition to ionizing radiation and ultraviolet light, exposure to asbestos fibers or silicon dusts leads to the formation of ROS in biological systems. The metal ions associated with the asbestos fibers participate in Fenton- or Fenton-type reaction to yield ROS (see Chapter 8). Similarly, the surface redox chemical properties of silicon dusts play a role in ROS formation. On the other hand, both asbestos fibers and silicon dusts can provoke inflammatory responses, resulting in production of ROS. Various types of nanomaterials, including silicon, gold, and copper nanoparticles as well as CdTe quantum dots have been shown to induce ROS formation in biological systems though the detailed mechanisms remain to be elucidated [30]. In contrast, cerium oxide nano-particles and fullerene-derived nanomaterials exert antioxidant effects via scavenging ROS in biological systems [31, 32].

3.3. Xenobiotics

Many xenobiotic compounds, including drugs are able to cause increased ROS levels in cells and tissues. As outlined below, there are four general mechanisms for xenobiotic-augmented ROS levels in biological systems.

(1) Redox cycling of xenobiotics, such as quinone compounds (**Figure 6.3**)
(2) Interference with the mitochondrial electron transport chain enzyme complexes, causing increased electron leakage and thereby the augmented formation of superoxide
(3) Induction of ROS-producing enzymes, such as CYP2E1
(4) Inhibition of cellular antioxidants

In addition, some ROS, such as ozone and nitrogen oxides exist as air pollutants. Exposure to these ROS air pollutants via inhalation may cause pulmonary inflammation and oxidative injury.

3.4. Microorganisms

Microorganisms, including bacteria and viruses may cause increased levels of ROS in target cells and tissues. As summarized next, there are four potential mechanisms for the increased ROS levels caused by microorganisms, including both pathogenic and commensal bacteria.

(1) Microorganisms cause activation of inflammatory cells, such as phagocytic cells, resulting in ROS formation from NADPH oxidase.
(2) Microorganisms can cause activation of other ROS-producing enzymes, such as inducible nitric oxide synthase to generate large amounts of nitric oxide in inflammatory cells. Nitric oxide reacts with superoxide, generating the highly reactive species peroxynitrite. Bacteria may also interact with epithelia to cause increased release of ROS [33].
(3) Certain bacteria contain ROS-producing enzymes that may release significant amounts of ROS. For instance, Streptococcus pyruvate oxidase (SpxB) is able to synthesize H_2O_2 and the H_2O_2 released by *Streptococcus pneumoniae* is

shown to cause DNA damage and apoptosis in lung cells of the host animals [34].
(4) Some bacteria may downregulate tissue antioxidants. For example, bacteria in the small intestine consume glycine, thereby downregulating the production of glutathione in the intestinal tissue [35]. Viral infections may also decrease the expression of certain antioxidants via modulating cell signal transduction [36–38].

ROS formation stimulated by commensal bacteria in the gut may also play a beneficial role. Recently, Jones et al. show that commensal bacteria, particularly members of the genus Lactobacillus, can stimulate NADPH oxidase-dependent ROS generation and consequent cellular proliferation in intestinal stem cells upon initial ingestion into the murine or Drosophila intestine [39]. The work suggests a potential novel mechanism by which commensal bacteria support gut epithelial turnover and health [40].

3.5. Oceans, Deserts, and the Universe

Superoxide is produced in the oceans. In the photic zone, superoxide is generated via photolysis of organic matter or by biological processes. In coastal waters, corals, macroalgae, and toxic red tide phytoplankton are potential sources of superoxide. In the open ocean, phytoplankton have been considered as the major source of biologically produced superoxide [41]. Recently, Julia M. Diaz and coworkers show that taxonomically and ecologically diverse heterotrophic bacteria from aquatic and terrestrial environments are a vast, unrecognized, and light-independent source of superoxide, and perhaps other ROS derived from superoxide. Production of superoxide by these bacteria might represent a substantial source of ROS in the sea [42]. Bacteria-derived superoxide might also have significant impact on elemental cycles, including carbon and trace metals in the deep ocean [42].

Like oceans, deserts may also be a significant source of FRRS, including ROS and reactive nitrogen species (RNS). The combination of intense solar radiation and soil desiccation creates a short circuit in the biogeochemical carbon cycle, where soils release significant amounts of carbon dioxide and reactive nitrogen oxides by abiotic oxidation. Recently, Georgiou et al. show that desert soils accumulate metal superoxides and peroxides at higher levels than non-desert soils. They also show the photogeneration of equimolar superoxide and hydroxyl radical in desiccated and aqueous soils, respectively, by a photo-induced electron transfer mechanism supported by their mineralogical composition [43]. The findings let Georgiou et al. suspect that processes driven by ultraviolet radiation may be operating in the surface soils on Mars, where ROS are believed to be present. In this context, The Viking Landers were unable to detect evidence of life on Mars but, instead, found a chemically reactive soil capable of decomposing organic molecules. Using EPR spectrometry, Albert S. Yen and coworkers show that superoxide forms directly on Mars-analog mineral surfaces exposed to ultraviolet radiation under a simulated Martian atmosphere. The superoxide can explain the reactive nature of the soil and the apparent absence of organic material at the Martian surface [44]. Moreover, ROS including H_2O_2 and hydroxyl radicals not only exist in Earth's atmosphere [45–47], but also occur in interstellar space [48, 49].

4. SUMMARY OF CHAPTER KEY POINTS

- Knowing the sources of FRRS is the first step in understanding free radical paradigm and the field of free radical biology and medicine as a whole.
- The biologically relevant FRRS can result from both cellular FRRS-generating machineries and exogenous agents.
- The cellular sources of FRRS include NADPH oxidases, mitochondria, cytochrome P450 system; xanthine oxidoreductase, peroxisomes, and nuclei. Among them, NADPH oxidases and mitochondria, especially mitochondria are considered the chief sources of cellular ROS.
- The major exogenous sources of FRRS include physical agents, airborne particulate matter, xenobiotics, and pathogenic as well as environmental microorganisms.
- FRRS, including superoxide, H_2O_2, and/or hydroxyl radicals, are also found in Earth's deserts, interstellar space, and the surface soils on Mars.

5. SELF-ASSESSMENT QUESTIONS

5.1. NADPH oxidases, also known as NOX enzymes belong to the enzyme family of NOX/DUOX. Which of the following NOX/DUOX enzymes is the chief machinery for producing ROS in phagocytic cells during bacteria-caused inflammation?

A. DUOX1
B. DUOX2
C. NOX1
D. NOX2
E. NOX5

5.2. Which of the following is a major intracellular site or source for both oxygen utilization and ROS production in mammalian cells under normal physiological conditions?

A. Cytochrome P450 system
B. Endoplasmic reticulum
C. Mitochondrion
D. Nucleus
E. Peroxisome

5.3. Mitochondrial electron transport chain (METC) is widely considered the chief site of ROS production by this organelle. In addition to METC, which of the following enzymes has recently been demonstrated to be also present in mitochondria and contribute to the generation of ROS by this energy-producing organelle?

A. DUOX1
B. DUOX2
C. NOX1
D. NOX2
E. NOX4

5.4. Cytochrome P450 (CYP) system is known to produce ROS. Among the various CYP enzymes, which of the following is considered the major ROS-generating enzyme, especially following its induction by ethanol?

A. CYP1A1
B. CYP1B1
C. CYP2C9
D. CYP2E1
E. CYP3A4

5.5. A recent study demonstrated that *Streptococcus pneumoniae,* a major etiology of pneumonia, can cause DNA damage and apoptosis in lung cells of the host animals via release of which of the following reactive species that is synthesized by Streptococcus pyruvate oxidase in the bacteria?

A. Hydrogen peroxide
B. Hypochlorous acid
C. Nitric oxide
D. Peroxynitrite
E. Singlet oxygen

ANSWERS AND EXPLANATIONS

5.1. The answer is D. NOX2 is the catalytic subunit gp91^{phox} of the phagocytic NADPH oxidase complex.

5.2. The answer is C. Mitochondrial respiration usually accounts for 80–90% of the oxygen consumed by the cells and is widely considered the chief source of cellular ROS production under physiological as well as many pathophysiological conditions.

5.3. The answer is E. NOX4 is known to exist in mitochondria and contributes to the ROS production capacity of this organelle. This NOX enzyme is also present in the nucleus.

5.4. The answer is D. Among cytochrome P450 (CYP) enzymes, CYP2E1 is the most potent ROS-generating enzyme. CYP2E1 is inducible by ethanol and this markedly augments the ROS production by this enzyme.

5.5. The answer is A. Streptococcus pyruvate oxidase (SpxB) produces H_2O_2 in *Streptococcus pneumoniae*. The H_2O_2 released by the bacteria is shown to cause DNA damage and apoptosis in lung cells of the host animals.

REFERENCES

1. Kuhns DB, Alvord WG, Heller T, Feld JJ, Pike KM, Marciano BE, Uzel G, DeRavin SS, Priel DA, Soule BP, Zarember KA, Malech HL, et al. Residual NADPH oxidase and survival in chronic granulomatous disease. *N Engl J Med* 2010; 363(27):2600–10.
2. Noubade R, Wong K, Ota N, Rutz S, Eidenschenk C, Valdez PA, Ding J, Peng I, Sebrell A, Caplazi P, DeVoss J, Soriano RH, et al. NRROS negatively regulates reactive oxygen species during host defence and autoimmunity. *Nature* 2014; 509(7499):235–9.
3. Zheng W, Umitsu M, Jagan I, Tran CW, Ishiyama N, BeGora M, Araki K, Ohashi PS, Ikura M, Muthuswamy SK. An interaction between Scribble and the NADPH oxidase complex controls M1 macrophage polarization and function. *Nat Cell Biol* 2016; 18(11):1244–52.
4. Lambeth JD. NOX enzymes and the biology of reactive oxygen. *Nat Rev Immunol* 2004; 4(3):181–9.
5. Lambeth JD, Neish AS. Nox enzymes and new thinking on reactive oxygen: a double-edged sword revisited. *Annu Rev Pathol* 2014; 9:119–45.
6. Sirokmany G, Donko A, Geiszt M. Nox/Duox family of nadph oxidases: lessons from knockout mouse models. *Trends Pharmacol Sci* 2016; 37(4):318–27.
7. Faraci FM. Hydrogen peroxide: watery fuel for change in vascular biology. *Arterioscler Thromb Vasc Biol* 2006; 26(9):1931–3.
8. Takac I, Schroder K, Zhang L, Lardy B, Anilkumar N, Lambeth JD, Shah AM, Morel F, Brandes RP. The E-loop is involved in hydrogen peroxide formation by the NADPH oxidase Nox4. *J Biol Chem* 2011; 286(15):13304–13.
9. Bedard K, Krause KH. The NOX family of ROS-generating NADPH oxidases: physiology and pathophysiology. *Physiol Rev* 2007; 87(1):245–313.
10. Serrander L, Cartier L, Bedard K, Banfi B, Lardy B, Plastre O, Sienkiewicz A, Forro L, Schlegel W, Krause KH. NOX4 activity is determined by mRNA levels and reveals a unique pattern of ROS generation. *Biochem J* 2007; 406(1):105–14.
11. Lin MT, Beal MF. Mitochondrial dysfunction and oxidative stress in neurodegenerative diseases. *Nature* 2006; 443(7113):787–95.
12. Chouchani ET, Pell VR, Gaude E, Aksentijevic D, Sundier SY, Robb EL, Logan A, Nadtochiy SM, Ord EN, Smith AC, Eyassu F, Shirley R, et al. Ischaemic accumulation of succinate controls reperfusion injury through mitochondrial ROS. *Nature* 2014; 515(7527):431–5.
13. Li Y, Zhu H, Trush MA. Detection of mitochondria-derived reactive oxygen species production by the chemilumigenic probes lucigenin and luminol. *Biochim Biophys Acta* 1999; 1428(1):1–12.
14. Ambrosio G, Zweier JL, Duilio C, Kuppusamy P, Santoro G, Elia PP, Tritto I, Cirillo P, Condorelli M, Chiariello M, et al. Evidence that mitochondrial respiration is a source of potentially toxic oxygen free radicals in intact rabbit hearts subjected to ischemia and reflow. *J Biol Chem* 1993; 268(25):18532–41.
15. Chouchani ET, Pell VR, James AM, Work LM, Saeb-Parsy K, Frezza C, Krieg T, Murphy MP. A Unifying Mechanism for mitochondrial superoxide production during ischemia-reperfusion injury. *Cell Metab* 2016; 23(2):254–63.

16. Mills EL, Kelly B, Logan A, Costa AS, Varma M, Bryant CE, Tourlomousis P, Dabritz JH, Gottlieb E, Latorre I, Corr SC, McManus G, et al. Succinate dehydrogenase supports metabolic repurposing of mitochondria to drive inflammatory macrophages. *Cell* 2016; 167(2):457–70 e13.

17. Davies KJ, Doroshow JH. Redox cycling of anthracyclines by cardiac mitochondria. I. Anthracycline radical formation by NADH dehydrogenase. *J Biol Chem* 1986; 261(7):3060–7.

18. Block K, Gorin Y, Abboud HE. Subcellular localization of Nox4 and regulation in diabetes. *Proc Natl Acad Sci USA* 2009; 106(34):14385–90.

19. Elfering SL, Sarkela TM, Giulivi C. Biochemistry of mitochondrial nitric-oxide synthase. *J Biol Chem* 2002; 277(41):38079–86.

20. Migliaccio E, Giorgio M, Mele S, Pelicci G, Reboldi P, Pandolfi PP, Lanfrancone L, Pelicci PG. The p66^{shc} adaptor protein controls oxidative stress response and life span in mammals. *Nature* 1999; 402(6759):309–13.

21. Giorgio M, Migliaccio E, Orsini F, Paolucci D, Moroni M, Contursi C, Pelliccia G, Luzi L, Minucci S, Marcaccio M, Pinton P, Rizzuto R, et al. Electron transfer between cytochrome c and p66^{Shc} generates reactive oxygen species that trigger mitochondrial apoptosis. *Cell* 2005; 122(2):221–33.

22. Seitz HK, Stickel F. Acetaldehyde as an underestimated risk factor for cancer development: role of genetics in ethanol metabolism. *Genes Nutr* 2010; 5(2):121–8.

23. Lu Y, Cederbaum AI. Alcohol upregulation of CYP2A5: role of reactive oxygen species. *Reactive Oxygen Species* 2016; 1(2):117–30.

24. De Henau S, Tilleman L, Vangheel M, Luyckx E, Trashin S, Pauwels M, Germani F, Vlaeminck C, Vanfleteren JR, Bert W, Pesce A, Nardini M, et al. A redox signalling globin is essential for reproduction in Caenorhabditis elegans. *Nat Commun* 2015; 6:8782.

25. McCord JM. Oxygen-derived free radicals in postischemic tissue injury. *N Engl J Med* 1985; 312(3):159–63.

26. Dvash E, Har-Tal M, Barak S, Meir O, Rubinstein M. Leukotriene C4 is the major trigger of stress-induced oxidative DNA damage. *Nat Commun* 2015; 6:10112.

27. Matsushima S, Kuroda J, Ago T, Zhai P, Park JY, Xie LH, Tian B, Sadoshima J. Increased oxidative stress in the nucleus caused by Nox4 mediates oxidation of HDAC4 and cardiac hypertrophy. *Circ Res* 2013; 112(4):651–63.

28. Spencer NY, Yan Z, Boudreau RL, Zhang Y, Luo M, Li Q, Tian X, Shah AM, Davisson RL, Davidson B, Banfi B, Engelhardt JF. Control of hepatic nuclear superoxide production by glucose 6-phosphate dehydrogenase and NADPH oxidase-4. *J Biol Chem* 2011; 286(11):8977–87.

29. Tsang CK, Liu Y, Thomas J, Zhang Y, Zheng XF. Superoxide dismutase 1 acts as a nuclear transcription factor to regulate oxidative stress resistance. *Nat Commun* 2014; 5:3446.

30. Xia T, Li N, Nel AE. Potential health impact of nanoparticles. *Annu Rev Public Health* 2009; 30:137–50.

31. Liu J, Finkel T. Stem cells and oxidants: too little of a bad thing. *Cell Metab* 2013; 18(1):1–2.

32. Bitner BR, Marcano DC, Berlin JM, Fabian RH, Cherian L, Culver JC, Dickinson ME, Robertson CS, Pautler RG, Kent TA, Tour JM. Antioxidant carbon particles improve cerebrovascular dysfunction following traumatic brain injury. *ACS Nano* 2012; 6(9):8007–14.

33. Kumar A, Wu H, Collier-Hyams LS, Hansen JM, Li T, Yamoah K, Pan ZQ, Jones DP, Neish AS. Commensal bacteria modulate cullin-dependent signaling via generation of reactive oxygen species. *EMBO J* 2007; 26(21):4457–66.

34. Rai P, Parrish M, Tay IJ, Li N, Ackerman S, He F, Kwang J, Chow VT, Engelward BP. Streptococcus pneumoniae secretes hydrogen peroxide leading to DNA damage and apoptosis in lung cells. *Proc Natl Acad Sci USA* 2015; 112(26):E3421–30.

35. Mardinoglu A, Shoaie S, Bergentall M, Ghaffari P, Zhang C, Larsson E, Backhed F, Nielsen J. The gut microbiota modulates host amino acid and glutathione metabolism in mice. *Mol Syst Biol* 2015; 11(10):834.

36. Berger MM, Jia XY, Legay V, Aymard M, Tilles JG, Lina B. Nutrition- and virus-induced stress represses the expression of manganese superoxide dismutase in vitro. *Exp Biol Med (Maywood)* 2004; 229(8):843–9.

37. Abdalla MY, Britigan BE, Wen F, Icardi M, McCormick ML, LaBrecque DR, Voigt M, Brown KE, Schmidt WN. Down-regulation of heme oxygenase-1 by hepatitis C virus infection in vivo and by the in vitro expression of hepatitis C core protein. *J Infect Dis* 2004; 190(6):1109–18.

38. Hosakote YM, Jantzi PD, Esham DL, Spratt H, Kurosky A, Casola A, Garofalo RP. Viral-mediated inhibition of antioxidant enzymes contributes to the pathogenesis of severe respiratory syncytial virus bronchiolitis. *Am J Respir Crit Care Med* 2011; 183(11):1550–60.

39. Jones RM, Luo L, Ardita CS, Richardson AN, Kwon YM, Mercante JW, Alam A, Gates CL, Wu H, Swanson PA, Lambeth JD, Denning PW, et al. Symbiotic lactobacilli stimulate gut epithelial proliferation via Nox-mediated generation of reactive oxygen species. *EMBO J* 2013; 32(23):3017–28.

40. Patel PH, Maldera JA, Edgar BA. Stimulating cROSstalk between commensal bacteria and intestinal stem cells. *EMBO J* 2013; 32(23):3009–10.

41. Shaked Y, Rose A. Microbiology. Seas of superoxide. *Science* 2013; 340(6137):1176–7.

42. Diaz JM, Hansel CM, Voelker BM, Mendes CM, Andeer PF, Zhang T. Widespread production of extracellular superoxide by heterotrophic bacteria. *Science* 2013; 340(6137):1223–6.

43. Georgiou CD, Sun HJ, McKay CP, Grintzalis K, Papapostolou I, Zisimopoulos D, Panagiotidis K, Zhang G, Koutsopoulou E, Christidis GE, Margiolaki I. Evidence for photochemical production of reactive oxygen species in desert soils. *Nat Commun* 2015; 6:7100.

44. Yen AS, Kim SS, Hecht MH, Frant MS, Murray B. Evidence that the reactivity of the martian soil is due to superoxide ions. *Science* 2000; 289(5486):1909–12.

45. Prinn R, Huang J, Weiss R, Cunnold D, Fraser P, Simmonds P, McCulloch A, Harth C, Reimann S, Salameh P. Evidence for variability of atmospheric hydroxyl radicals over the past quarter century. *Geophys Res Lett* 2005; 32(7):LO7809

46. Jackson A, Hewitt C. Atmosphere hydrogen peroxide and organic hydroperoxides: a review. *Crit Rev Environ Sci Tech* 1999; 29(2):175–228.

47. Li S, Matthews J, Sinha A. Atmospheric hydroxyl radical production from electronically excited NO_2 and H_2O. *Science* 2008; 319(5870):1657–60.

48. Bergman P, Parise B, Liseau R, Larsson B, Olofsson H, Menten K, Güsten R. Detection of interstellar hydrogen peroxide. *Astronomy Astrophysics* 2011; 531:L8.

49. Gligorovski S, Strekowski R, Barbati S, Vione D. Environmental implications of hydroxyl radicals (·OH). *Chem Rev* 2015; 115(24):13051–92.

Biological Effects of Free Radicals and Related Reactive Species

ABSTRACT | The biological effects of free radicals and related reactive species (FRRS) are determined by various factors, including the types of FRRS, the sites, levels and duration of FRRS exposure, and the intrinsic susceptibility of the molecular targets as well as the availability of the antioxidant defenses. FRRS have the potential to damage a spectrum of cellular biomolecules, including lipids, proteins, and nucleic acids. At the molecular levels, FRRS can cause lipid peroxidation, protein oxidation, and oxidative DNA damage. At the cellular levels, exposure to FRRS may result in cell death, cell dysfunction, cell senescence, cell transformation, as well as cell proinflammatory responses, depending on the factors noted above. These cellular events and responses dictate the development of tissue injury and disease process associated with FRRS. While FRRS are involved in tissue injury and disease development, it should be borne in mind that these reactive species may also play important physiological roles under specific conditions.

KEYWORDS | Adaptive immunity; Cell senescence; Cell transformation; Free radicals and related reactive species; 8-Hydroxy-2′-deoxyguanosine; Lifespan; Lipid peroxidation; microRNAs; 3-Nitrotyrosine; Proinflammatory response; Protein carbonyl; Protein oxidation; Reactive oxygen species; Redox signaling; Tumorigenesis

CITATION | *Hopkins RZ and Li YR. Essentials of Free radical Biology and Medicine. Cell Med Press, Raleigh, NC, USA. 2017. http://dx.doi.org/10.20455/efrbm.2017.07*

ABBREVIATIONS | GPx, glutathione peroxidase; GST, glutathione S-transferase; NF-κB, nuclear factor kappaB; Nrf2, nuclear factor E2-related factor 2; NRROS, negative regulator of ROS; 8-OH-dG, 8-hydroxy-2′-deoxyguanosine; FRRS, free radicals and related reactive species; ROS, reactive oxygen species

CHAPTER AT A GLANCE

1. OVERVIEW

Free radicals and related reactive species (FRRS), in particular, reactive oxygen species (ROS) can exert both detrimental and beneficial effects in biological systems. The nature of the biological effects depends on various factors, including the types of the FRRS, the concentrations and duration of the FRRS exposure, the types of cells and tissues that the FRRS act on, and the levels of the endogenous antioxidant defenses. In general, large increases in the levels of FRRS for a sustained period of time cause severe damage to cellular constituents, leading to cell injury or death. In contrast, small increases in the levels of FRRS, especially ROS can be employed as a signaling mechanism to mediate cell signal transduction. On the one hand, such a signaling role of FRRS contributes to the maintenance of normal functions of cells and tissues. On the other hand, modulation of cell signaling by FRRS can also lead to pathophysiological processes, such as tumorigenesis and tissue fibrosis. Another scenario regarding the biological effects of FRRS is the production of large amounts of these reactive species by professional phagocytes for destroying invading microorganisms. When this response is under control, it plays an important role in innate immunity. However, the uncontrolled prolonged stimulation of respiratory burst causes sustained production of large amounts of FRRS, which may cause tissue injury. To provide an overview of the biological effects of FRRS, this chapter first considers the molecular targets of FRRS. It then discusses FRRS-mediated detrimental cellular responses. For the purpose of completion, the chapter ends with a brief description of the physiological effects of FRRS, a topic also covered to various degrees in preceding chapters.

2. MOLECULAR TARGETS

As illustrated in **Figure 7.1**, the molecular targets of FRRS include such cellular constituents as lipids, proteins, and nucleic acids, as well as nucleotide pools and carbohydrates. The range of biomolecules damaged by FRRS is dependent on the types of FRRS and their levels and duration of exposure. For example, due to its extremely high oxidizing capacity (Table 5.1 of Chapter 5), hydroxyl radical is able to oxidize any biomolecule that it first bumps into. On the other hand, due to its limited reactivity, superoxide only directly reacts with a limited number of biomolecules, such as the proteins containing iron-sulfur clusters (see Chapter 8).

2.1. Oxidative Damage to Lipids

Lipid molecules are important components of biomembranes including plasma membranes and the membranes of cellular organelles. They are also components of lipoproteins. FRRS, especially ROS attack lipid molecules, causing lipid peroxidation. Lipid peroxidation refers to the oxidative deterioration of lipid molecules containing two or more carbon-carbon double bonds, i.e., polyunsaturated fatty acids. The propensity of polyunsaturated fatty acids to undergo lipid peroxidation is due to the bis-allylic methylene hydrogens which are more susceptible to hydrogen abstraction by FRRS than fully saturated lipids. The FRRS that can cause lipid peroxidation include free radicals, such as hydroxyl, alkyoxyl, peroxyl, perhydroxyl, and nitrogen dioxide radicals. The non-free radical ROS such as peroxynitrite, ozone, and singlet oxygen are also able to cause lipid peroxidation. In contrast, neither superoxide nor nitric oxide directly causes lipid peroxidation due to limited reactivity. This section focuses on free radical-mediated lipid peroxidation. Free radical-triggered lipid peroxidation proceeds through the following three steps: initiation, propagation, and termination. A diverse array of reactive products is generated by lipid peroxidation in biological systems (**Figure 7.2**).

2.1.1. Initiation

The initiation step is caused by hydrogen atom abstraction from a polyunsaturated fatty acid side-chain of a lipid (LH) by a free radical, such as a hydroxyl radical, alkyoxyl radical, or peroxyl radical. This converts the polyunsaturated fatty acid to a carbon-centered radical (L˙) (Reaction 1).

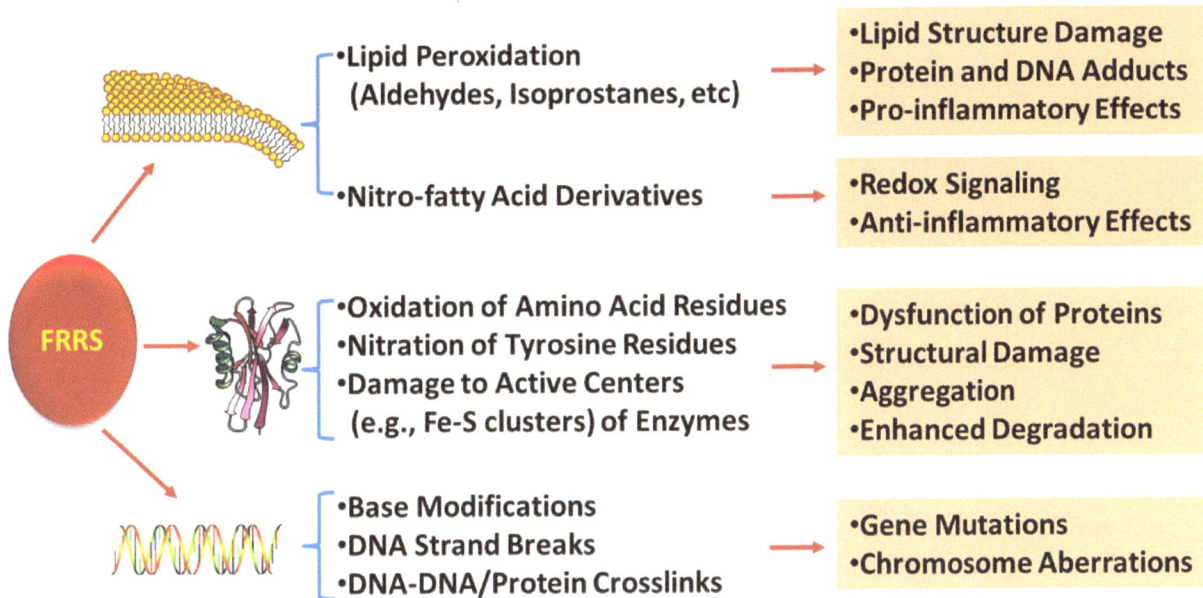

FIGURE 7.1. Molecular targets of free radicals and related reactive species (FRRS). The major molecular targets of FRRS include lipids, proteins, and nucleic acids. Reaction of FRRS with these cellular constituents causes oxidative modifications or damage, resulting in the formation of various secondary products. Some of the secondary products, such as reactive aldehydes can cause further adverse effects.

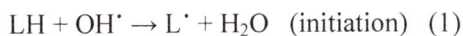

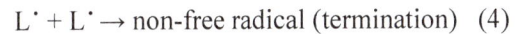

$$LH + OH^{\cdot} \rightarrow L^{\cdot} + H_2O \quad \text{(initiation)} \quad (1)$$

2.1.2. Propagation

In the presence of molecular oxygen, the above carbon-centered radical ($L^{\cdot}$) is converted to a peroxyl radical ($LOO^{\cdot}$). The peroxyl radical is able to cause hydrogen atom abstraction from an adjacent polyunsaturated fatty acid side-chain of lipid, yielding another carbon-centered radical ($L^{\cdot}$). This thus triggers a chain reaction that leads to the propagation of lipid peroxidation, and the peroxyl radical acts as a chain-carrying free radical. The peroxyl radical after combining with a hydrogen atom is converted to a lipid hydroperoxide ($LOOH$) (Reactions 2 and 3).

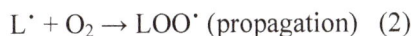

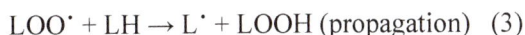

$$L^{\cdot} + O_2 \rightarrow LOO^{\cdot} \quad \text{(propagation)} \quad (2)$$

$$LOO^{\cdot} + LH \rightarrow L^{\cdot} + LOOH \quad \text{(propagation)} \quad (3)$$

2.1.3. Termination

The free radicals produced in the above propagation step can react with each other to form non-free radical products, thus causing termination of the chain reactions (Reactions 4 and 5).

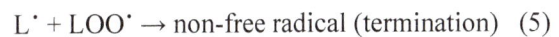

$$L^{\cdot} + L^{\cdot} \rightarrow \text{non-free radical (termination)} \quad (4)$$

$$L^{\cdot} + LOO^{\cdot} \rightarrow \text{non-free radical (termination)} \quad (5)$$

In addition, other free radicals can react with the free radicals produced during the propagation step to cause termination. For example, nitric oxide ($NO^{\cdot}$) may act as a chain-terminating antioxidant by reacting with chain-carrying peroxyl radical ($LOO^{\cdot}$) to form lipid peroxynitrite ($LOONO$) (Reaction 6).

$$LOO^{\cdot} + NO^{\cdot} \rightarrow LOONO \quad (6)$$

2.1.4. Reactive Products and Biological Effects

A number of diverse peroxidation products are formed during lipid peroxidation of biomembranes and lipoproteins in cells and tissues. In the presence of transition metal ions, lipid hydroperoxides can be converted to peroxyl and alkoxyl radicals. The decomposition of lipid hydroperoxides also gives rise to many other reactive species, including electrophilic aldehydes (e.g., acrolein, 4-hydroxy-2-nonenal, and malondialdehyde). Another class of peroxidation products formed in abundance is the isoprostanes. Isoprostanes are a series of prostaglandin-like com-

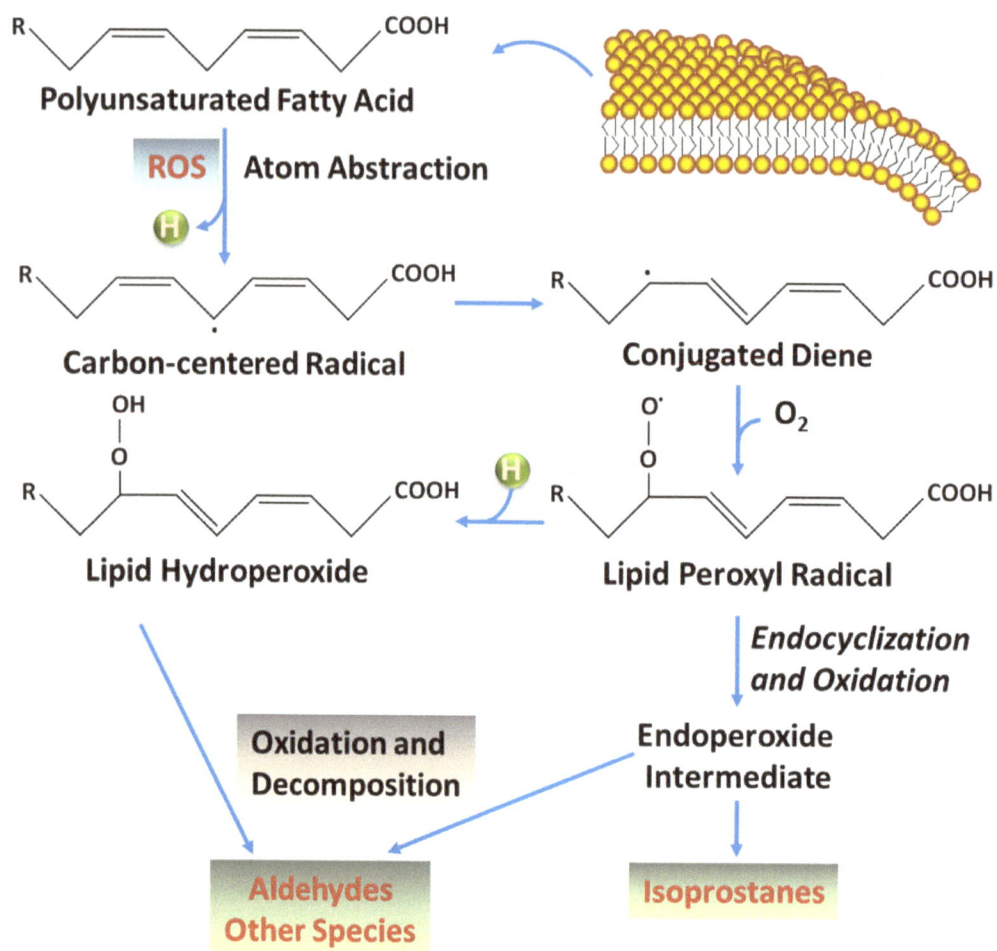

FIGURE 7.2. **Lipid peroxidation caused by reactive oxygen species (ROS).** ROS cause lipid peroxidation that proceeds through initiation, propagation, and termination, resulting in the formation of diverse reactive products. Some of the products, such as isoprostanes are measured in the body fluids to serve as molecular biomarkers of oxidative stress.

pounds produced by the free radical-mediated perox-idation of arachidonic acid independent of the cy-clooxygenase. Levels of isoprostanes are increased in a number of human diseases, and measurement of these molecules is considered the most reliable way to assess oxidative injury in vivo [1]. In addition, both native and oxidized fatty acids react with nitro-gen dioxide radicals, leading to the formation of ni-tro-fatty acid derivatives.

Lipid peroxidation causes damage to cell mem-branes and associated proteins. Lipid peroxidation products, such as reactive aldehydes also cause dam-age to other cellular molecules, including non-membrane-associated proteins and DNA. The prod-ucts of lipid peroxidation are able to also modulate cell signaling. In this regard, the reactive aldehydes (e.g., 4-hydroxy-2-nonenal and acrolein), isopros-tanes, and nitro-fatty acid derivatives are all able to cause redox modulation of cell signal transduction [2, 3]. In contrast to reactive aldehydes and isoprostanes, which are generally pro-inflammatory, the nitro-fatty acid derivatives are anti-inflammatory [4].

2.1.5. Cell and Tissue Defenses

A number of cellular defenses are involved in pro-tecting against the adverse effects of lipid peroxida-tion. These include (1) the enzymes that remove and detoxify lipid hydroperoxides, and (2) the enzymes and non-enzyme factors that detoxify the reactive products of lipid peroxidation. For example, lipid hydroperoxides in membranes can be converted to lipid alcohols by phospholipid hydroperoxide glutathione peroxidase (GPx4). Lipid hydroperoxides can also be cleaved from the membranes by phospholipases, and the released lipid hydroperoxides can be further converted to lipid alcohols by either cytosolic GPx (also known as GPx2) or glutathione S-transferase (GST). The reactive aldehydes are detoxified by glutathione conjugation. This reaction is catalyzed by GST. Thus, GST detoxifies both lipid hydroperoxides and the reactive aldehydes derived from lipid peroxidation. Detailed discussion of these antioxidants is provided in Appendix B.

2.2. Oxidative Damage to Proteins

2.2.1. Targeting Sites

Proteins are another class of important targets of FRRS [5]. The attack by FRRS on proteins can lead to (1) oxidation of the amino acid residues of proteins, such as oxidation of cysteine and methionine residues to form disulfides and methionine sulfoxide, respectively; (2) nitration of tyrosine residues to 3-nitrotyrosines; (3) oxidation of other amino acid residues (e.g., lysine, arginine, proline, threonine) to form protein carbonyls [6, 7]; and (4) damage of the active centers of certain enzymes, such as oxidation of the iron-sulfur clusters in some hydratases (e.g., aconitase) to lead to the release of iron from the enzyme and consequent enzyme inactivation [8–10] (**Figure 7.3**).

2.2.2. Molecular Consequences

The consequences of protein damage by FRRS include: (1) altered structures and functions of the proteins; (2) aggregation of the proteins; and (3) increased degradation of the proteins by the proteasome pathway. Oxidative modifications of proteins usually lead to inhibition of the protein functions, such as inhibition of enzyme activity. Under certain circumstances, modifications of proteins by FRRS also cause activation of the enzymes.

2.2.3. Molecular Biomarkers

As noted earlier, oxidation of proteins by FRRS leads to the formation of protein carbonyl derivatives. In addition, carbonyl groups may be introduced into proteins by reactions with aldehydes (4-hydroxy-2-nonenal, malondialdehyde) produced during lipid

peroxidation or with reactive carbonyl derivatives (ketoamines, ketoaldehydes, deoxyosones) generated as a consequence of the reaction of reducing sugars or their oxidation products with lysine residues of proteins (glycation and glycoxidation reactions) [7]. The carbonyl content of proteins has become the most commonly used indicator for the estimation of protein oxidation by ROS and under oxidative stress conditions in biological systems. Likewise, formation of 3-nitrotyrosine is used as a molecular biomarker for protein damage by reactive nitrogen species (RNS), such as peroxynitrite [11].

2.2.4. Cell and Tissue Defenses

Various cellular defenses exist to protect against protein damage by FRRS. For example, the reduced form of glutathione (GSH) and thioredoxin can reduce the disulfide bridges formed by aberrant oxidative cross-linking of thiol groups of cysteine residues of proteins. Another example is the repair of oxidized methionine residues by methionine sulfoxide reductase. FRRS oxidize methionine residues in proteins yielding methionine sulfoxide. The enzyme methionine sulfoxide reductase reduces the methionine sulfoxide in proteins back to the normal methionine. The reduced form of thioredoxin provides the reducing equivalent to this enzyme. Methionine sulfoxide reductase protects against oxidative injury in vivo [12] (see Appendix B).

2.3. Oxidative Damage to Nucleic Acids

2.3.1. Molecular Targets

Both the backbone and bases of nucleic acids can be targeting sites of FRRS, especially ROS. FRRS not only damage nuclear DNA, but also mitochondrial DNA [13]. Damage of mitochondrial DNA by FRRS is implicated in degenerative disorders, including aging, neurodegeneration, and cancer [14, 15]. In addition to nuclear and mitochondrial DNA, RNA molecules are also targets of FRRS. Because they are less protected, RNA molecules are in fact more susceptible to FRRS-induced damage. The oxidation of rRNA, tRNA, and mRNA may have serious effects on cellular homeostasis, because oxidation of these RNA molecules could impair the overall integrity of translational processes [16]. Oxidation of RNA molecules is implicated in several degenerative diseases, such as neurodegeneration [17]. A recent study shows that microRNAs can be oxidatively modified by ROS and oxidized miR-184 becomes associated

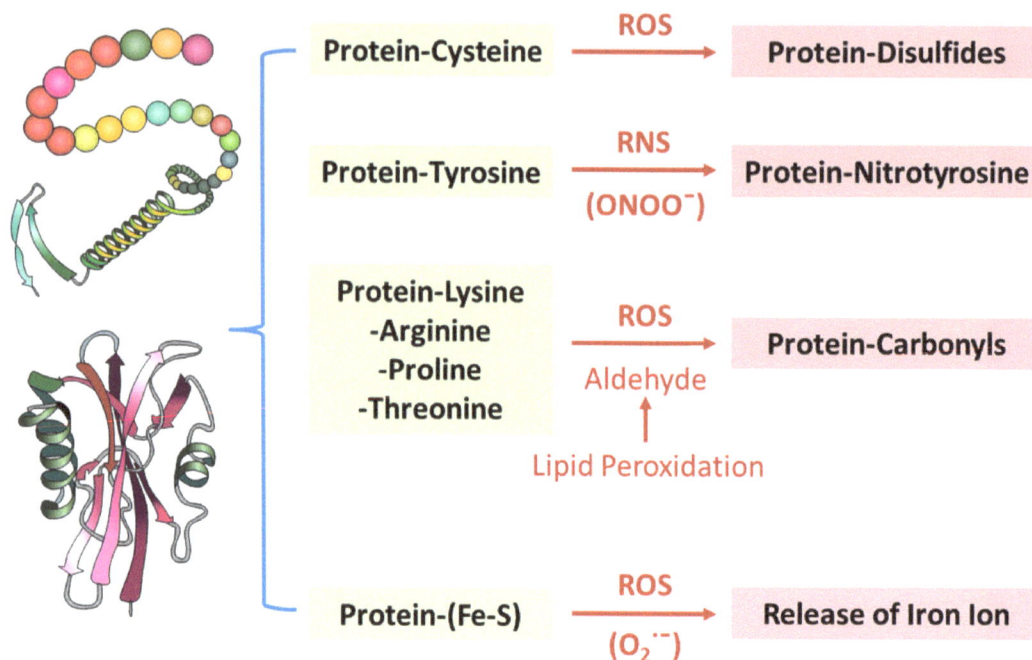

FIGURE 7.3. Protein oxidation by free radicals and related reactive species (FRRS). The attack by FRRS, including reactive oxygen and nitrogen species (ROS, RNS) on proteins can lead to oxidation of the amino acid residues of proteins (such as oxidation of cysteine to form disulfides, nitration of tyrosine residues to form 3-nitrotyrosines, and oxidation of lysine, arginine, proline, and threonine to form protein carbonyls) as well as damage of the active centers of certain enzymes (such as oxidation of the iron-sulfur clusters in mitochondrial aconitase to lead to the release of iron ion from the enzyme and consequent enzyme inactivation).

with Bcl-xL and Bcl-w, resulting in apoptosis in cardiac cells [18].

2.3.2. Molecular Consequences

Direct DNA damage by FRRS can be manifested as (1) DNA base modifications, such as formation of 8-hydroxy-2′-deoxyguanosine (8-OH-dG) (**Figure 7.4**), (2) DNA strand breaks, including both single- and double-stranded breakage, and (3) DNA-DNA or DNA-protein crosslinks. Notably, measurement of 8-OH-dG in tissue and body fluid samples is a widely used biomarker for assessing oxidative DNA damage in both experimental animals and humans (also see Section 2.2.1 of Chapter 5). In this context, ROS, including hydroxyl radicals, peroxyl radicals, peroxynitrite, and singlet oxygen are known to cause the increased formation of 8-OH-dG in biological systems. In addition, as discussed above, oxidation of other cellular constituents, such as lipids by FRRS leads to the formation of reactive aldehydes that can form DNA adducts [19].

The consequences of DNA damage by FRRS are essentially two-fold: (1) after mispair or replication of the damaged template, surviving cells may be subject to permanent changes in the genetic code in the form of gene mutations or chromosomal aberrations, both of which increase the risk of cancer development; and (2) alternatively, damage may interfere with the vital process of transcription or induce cell cycle arrest, which may trigger cell death or cell senescence, contributing to aging or other degenerative disorders.

2.3.3. Cell and Tissue Defenses

Mammalian cells are equipped with a variety of repair pathways that control DNA damage to ensure faithful transmission of genetic information to progeny cells. These pathways include the base-excision repair, nucleotide-excision repair, transcription-coupled repair, non-homologous end joining, and homologous recombination repair [20]. These various repairing mechanisms, especially base-excision

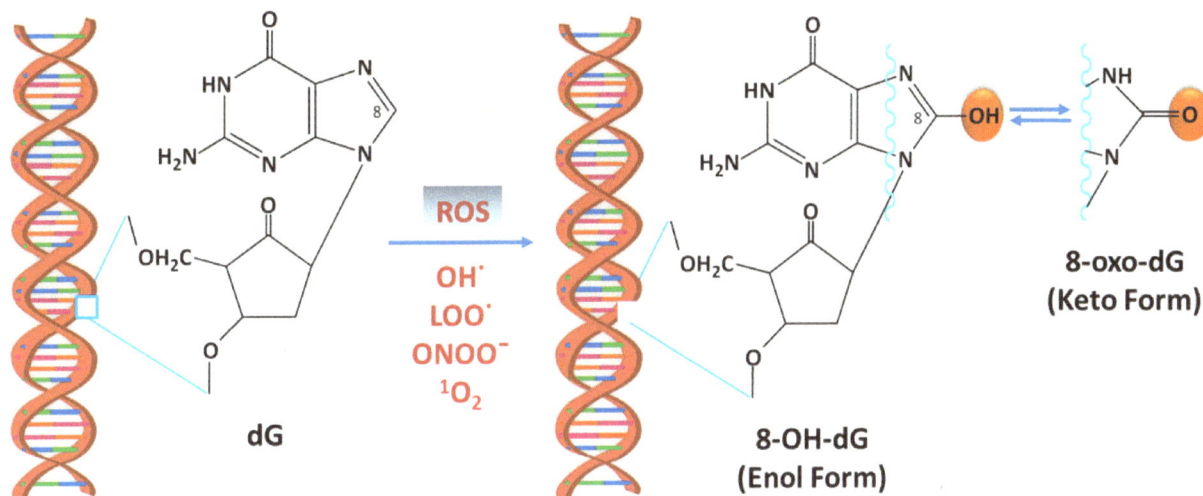

FIGURE 7.4. Formation of 8-hydroxy-2′-deoxyguanosine (8-OH-dG) induced by free radicals and related reactive species (FRRS). FRRS, including hydroxyl radicals (OH·), lipid peroxyl radicals (LOO·), peroxynitrite (ONOO⁻), and singlet oxygen ($^1O_2$) cause oxidation of deoxyguanosine in DNA, resulting in the formation of 8-OH-dG. 8-OH-dG is in equilibrium with its keto form, also known as 8-oxo-2′-deoxyguanosine (8-oxo-dG). Measurement of the levels of 8-OH-dG or 8-oxo-dG in tissue samples and body fluids (e.g., serum and urine) has been widely used as a molecular biomarker for assessing oxidative DNA damage by reactive oxygen species (ROS) in both experimental animals and human subjects.

and nucleotide-excision repair systems, play an important role in controlling DNA damage induced by FRRS in biological systems [21].

2.4. Oxidative Damage to Other Biomolecules

In addition to such vital cellular constituents as proteins, lipids, and nucleic acids, FRRS also cause damage to other biomolecules, including free amino acids, carbohydrates, nicotinamide adenine dinucleotide (NADH), nicotinamide adenine dinucleotide phosphate (NADPH), and the nucleotide pool [22]. Reactions of FRRS with these biomolecules may lead to the formation of various products, including secondary free radicals and related reactive species.

3. DETRIMENTAL EFFECTS AT THE CELLULAR LEVEL

The detrimental effects mediated by FRRS at the cellular level include cell death, cell dysfunction, cell senescence, cell transformation, and cell proinflammatory responses. The above detrimental effects constitute the cellular basis for FRRS-induced disease process (**Figure 7.5**).

3.1. Cell Death

As stated before, FRRS are able to cause damage to biomolecules, including lipids, proteins, and nucleic acids. When cells are exposed to large amounts of FRRS for prolonged periods of time, the FRRS overwhelm the normal cellular antioxidant defenses. This induces severe oxidative stress, leading to irreversible cell injury and eventually the death of the cells. The most widely used classification of mammalian cell death recognizes two types: (1) apoptosis and (2) oncosis. The term oncosis (derived from ónkos, meaning swelling) was proposed in 1910 by Friedrich Daniel von Reckling-hausen (1833–1910), a German pathologist to mean cell death with swelling. Oncosis leads to necrosis with karyolysis and stands in contrast to apoptosis, which leads to necrosis with karyorrhexis and cell shrinkage [23].

Autophagy, which has been recognized as a third mode of cell death, is a process in which cells generate energy and metabolites by digesting their own organelles and macromolecules [24, 25]. FRRS-induced cell death can occur through any of the above three modes. Upon attack by FRRS, occurrence of cell death depends on the types of FRRS, the concentrations and duration of FRRS exposure,

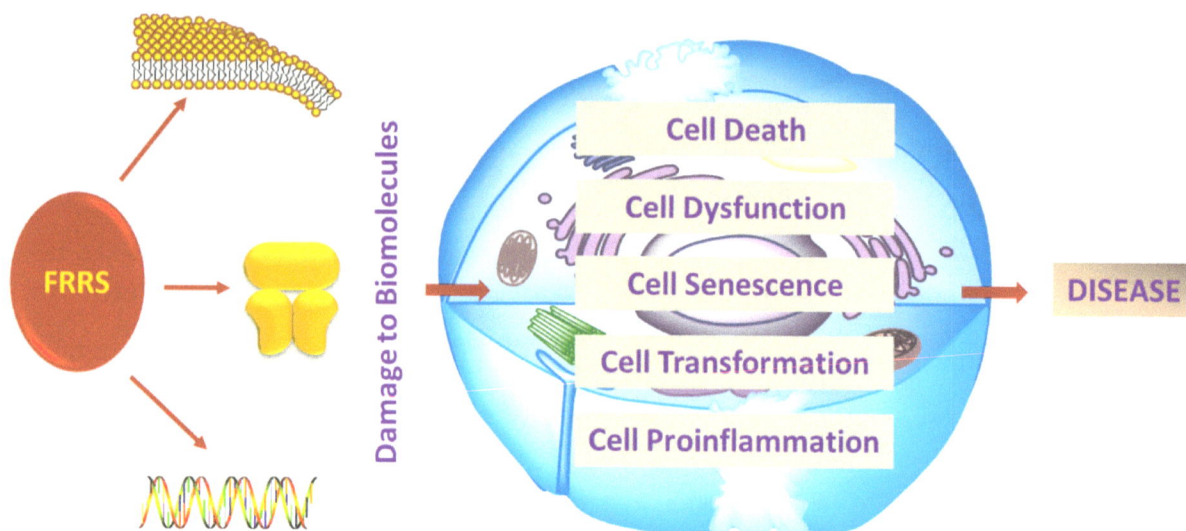

FIGURE 7.5. Cellular consequences of free radicals and related reactive species (FRRS)-mediated molecular damage in biological systems. Via oxidatively damaging or modifying cellular constituents, especially lipids, proteins, and nucleic acids, FRRS can cause a number of detrimental responses at the cellular level. These include cell death, cell dysfunction, cell senescence, cell transformation, and cell proinflammatory responses.

and the types of cells that the FRRS act on, as well as the status of cellular antioxidant defenses.

3.2. Cell Dysfunction

When cells are exposed to moderate amounts of FRRS, damage to cellular constituents may significantly compromise normal cell function though it is not severe enough to cause cell death. Cell dysfunction can result from FRRS-mediated inhibition of enzymes, dysregulation of ion transport, and altered signal transduction and gene expression. Dysregulated cell signal transduction and gene expression may also lead to uncontrolled cell proliferation, contributing to tumorigenesis and tissue fibrosis [26, 27].

3.3. Cell Senescence

Cell senescence refers to the phenomenon by which normal diploid cells lose the ability to divide, normally after certain numbers of cell divisions in vitro. Exposure of cells to FRRS, such as hydrogen peroxide can cause senescence. Inhibition of telomerase is one important mechanism by which FRRS induce cell senescence. Cell senescence is a hallmark of aging. FRRS-induced cell senescence may contribute to aging and other degenerative disorders [28, 29].

3.4. Cell Transformation

Cell transformation refers to the change that a normal cell undergoes as it becomes malignant. Exposure of cells to exogenous FRRS causes cell transformation. Production of ROS by overexpression of NADPH oxidase (NOX) enzymes also results in cell mitogenesis and transformation [30]. As discussed above in Section 2.3, FRRS are able to cause DNA damage, including base modifications, leading to gene mutations. FRRS also modify cell signaling molecules, including protein kinase cascades and transcription factors, resulting in dysregulated cell proliferation and death. Both DNA damage and dysregulated cell signal transduction contribute to FRRS-induced cell transformation and tumorigenesis [31, 32].

3.5. Cell Proinflammatory Responses

It is known that inflammatory responses result in the formation of large amounts of ROS from phagocytic cell respiratory burst. In addition, certain inflammatory cytokines, such as tumor necrosis factor-alpha (TNF-α) can induce ROS formation from cellular sources, including mitochondria [33, 34]. On the other hand, ROS stimulate expression of inflammatory cytokines and adhesion molecules via activation of nuclear factor kappaB (NF-κB, a central regulator of inflammatory cytokine genes), thereby promoting inflammatory responses [35]. Notably, NF-κB regulates phagocytic NADPH oxidase by inducing the expression of gp91^{phox}. This may provide a positive feedback loop in which NF-κB activation by oxidative stress leads to further radical production via NADPH oxidase [36].

A recent study also shows that release of glutathionylated peroxiredoxin-2 acts as a danger signal to link oxidative stress and inflammation, thereby revealing a novel molecular mechanism linking ROS and inflammation [37]. Hence, oxidative stress and inflammation are closely intertwined. As such, the compound term "oxidative/inflammatory stress" is often used in the literature to describe the pathophysiological processes involving ROS and inflammation (see Section 4.3 of Chapter 2).

4. PHYSIOLOGICAL EFFECTS

To understand the biological effects of FRRS, the physiological functions of these species (especially ROS) cannot be ignored. In fact, this represents a rapidly evolving area of free radical biology and medicine. For the purpose of completion, this section outlines the major physiological roles played by ROS, including immunity, redox signaling (also see Section 3 of Chapter 3 and Section 2.4 of Chapter 4), suppression of cancer development, and prolongation of lifespan.

4.1. Immunity

4.1.1. Phagocytic NADPH Oxidases and Immunity

Although FRRS contribute to tissue injury and disease pathophysiology, under certain circumstances, they are also useful species playing important physiological roles. One typical scenario where FRRS play a physiological role is the ROS formed during respiratory burst of phagocytic cells. The ROS formed are involved in the killing of invading microorganisms. Thus, formation of ROS by phagocytic cells is an important component of innate immunity. Deficiency of phagocytic NADPH oxidase, as seen in chronic granulomatous disease, is associated with increased susceptibility to infections [38].

Phagocytic NADPH oxidase-derived ROS are essential for killing invading microorganisms; however, overstimulation of the ROS production also causes tissue injury, contributing to various disease processes associated with inflammation. Hence, tight regulation of phagocytic ROS formation is essential to maintaining physiological homeostasis. In this context, a regulatory protein, known as negative regulator of ROS (NRROS), has been recently identified to limit ROS generation by phagocytes during inflammatory responses [39].

NRROS expression in phagocytes can be repressed by inflammatory signals. NRROS-deficient phagocytes produce increased ROS upon inflammatory challenges, and mice lacking NRROS in their phagocytes show enhanced bactericidal activity against *Escherichia coli* and *Listeria monocytogenes* [39]. Conversely, these mice develop severe experimental autoimmune encephalomyelitis owing to oxidative tissue damage in the central nervous system. NRROS is localized to the endoplasmic reticulum, where it directly interacts with nascent NOX2 monomer, one of the membrane-bound subunits of the NADPH oxidase complex, and facilitates the degradation of NOX2 through the endoplasmic reticulum-associated degradation pathway. Thus, NRROS provides a novel mechanism for regulating ROS production. This regulatory mechanism enables phagocytes to produce higher amounts of ROS, if required to control invading pathogens, while minimizing unwanted collateral tissue damage [39].

4.1.2. Mitochondrial ROS and Immunity

Mitochondria-derived ROS also play a role in immunity [40]. The engagement of a subset of Toll-like receptors (TLR1, TLR2, and TLR4) results in the recruitment of mitochondria to macrophage phagosomes and augments mitochondrial ROS production. The increased production of mitochondrial ROS is required for the bactericidal activity of macrophages, implicating mitochondrial ROS as an important component of antibacterial responses [41]. More recently, mitochondrial ROS are found to mediate the lymphocyte expansion molecule (LEM)-promoted, antigen-dependent expansion of proliferative CD8^{+} T cells and memory cell generation [42].

4.2. Redox Signaling and Redox Modulation

The term cell signaling or signal transduction refers to part of a complex system of communication that governs basic cellular activities and coordinates cell actions. The role of the free radical nitric oxide in cell signal transduction in mammals, including humans is well-established. Under certain conditions,

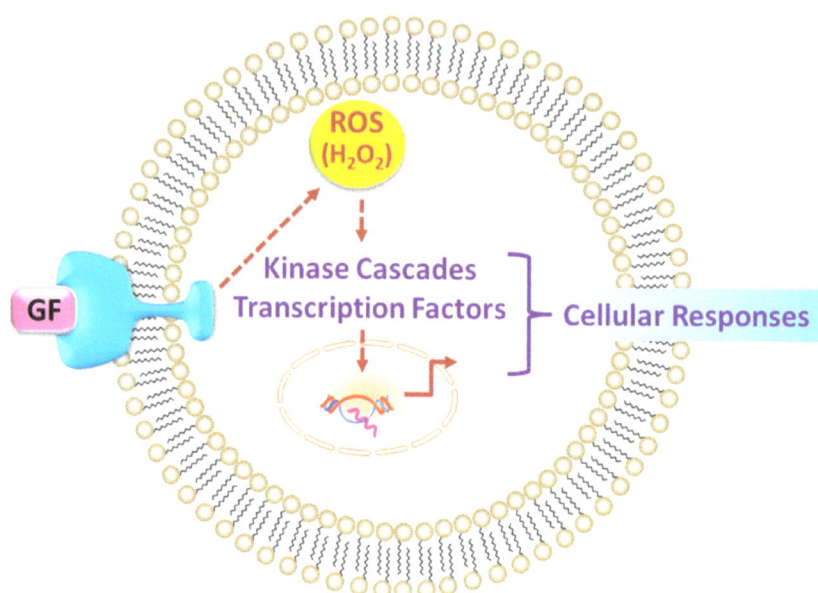

FIGURE 7.6. Reactive oxygen species (ROS) act as second messengers in cell signal transduction. As illustrated, a growth factor (GF) (e.g., platelet-derived growth factor) binds to its receptor, leading to the formation of ROS, especially hydrogen peroxide (H_2O_2). The H_2O_2 formed then acts as a second messenger to cause activation of signaling proteins (e.g., protein kinases and transcription factors), resulting in physiological cellular responses (e.g., cell proliferation). The dashed arrows indicate multiple steps.

besides nitric oxide, other ROS are also able to act as second messengers to participate in cell signal transduction, leading to physiological cellular responses (also see Chapter 2). For example, interaction of certain growth factors with specific receptors in cells results in increased formation of ROS, and the ROS formed then mediate the growth factor-induced cellular responses [43] (**Figure 7.6**).

Another scenario is the ability of ROS to mediate activation of cellular antioxidant enzyme genes via, at least partly, a nuclear factor E2-related factor 2 (Nrf2)-dependent mechanism [44, 45]. Indeed, many of the antioxidant enzyme genes are subject to redox regulation. This adaptive mechanism plays an important role in protecting cells and tissues from overt oxidative stress. The biochemical basis for ROS-mediated redox regulation lies primarily in their ability to modulate the activities of protein kinase cascades as well as transcription factors. The concept of ROS as redox modulators has implications not only in physiological processes, but also in pathophysiological conditions [46–48]. As noted earlier, through interfering with cell signal transduction, ROS may cause dysregulated cell growth, differentiation, and death, thereby contributing to pathophysiological

processes, including tumorigenesis and tissue fibrosis (see Section 3.2).

4.3. Suppression of Cancer Development

While oxidative stress is an important mechanism of carcinogenesis, ROS may also play a beneficial role in controlling tumor development. This notion is supported by the finding that oncogene-induced Nrf2 transcription promotes ROS detoxification and tumorigenesis in animal models [49]. The antioxidant gene regulator Nrf2 is also necessary to maintain pancreatic cancer proliferation by regulating mRNA translation. Specifically, loss of Nrf2 leads to defects in autocrine epidermal growth factor receptor (EGFR) signaling and oxidation of specific translational regulatory proteins, resulting in impaired cap-dependent and cap-independent mRNA translation in pancreatic cancer cells [50]. These findings suggest that constitutive production of ROS might serve as a protective mechanism against tumor development.

The above findings also highlight the potential of antioxidants to adversely impact cancer via stimulating cancer cell growth and metastasis. Indeed, it shows that in a mouse model, successfully metastasizing melanomas undergo reversible metabolic changes during metastasis that increase their capacity to withstand oxidative stress, and treatment with antioxidants promotes distal metastasis [51]. The potential of endogenous ROS in protecting against cancer development is also in line with the emerging concept of using ROS-enhancing agents to treat cancer [52]. The seemingly paradoxical roles of ROS in cancer development point to the complex nature of ROS homeostasis and a reason for maintaining their physiological levels to achieve optimal health.

4.4. Prolongation of Lifespan

As noted earlier (Section 3.3), ROS can cause cell senescence contributing to aging. Indeed, oxidative stress is a widely accepted theory of aging. Since ROS may act physiologically as signaling molecules regulating cell signal transduction, it is possible that well-controlled production of ROS may contribute to the maintenance of normal cell function and cell longevity. Studies in *Caenorhabditis elegans* suggest that elevation of ROS generated from mitochondria may trigger a unique pattern of gene expression that modulates stress sensitivity and promotes the survival of the organisms [53, 54]. Substantial evidence supports that mitochondria may act as a signaling organelle via releasing ROS to epigenetically regulate the expression of nuclear pro-lifespan genes so as to achieve optimal lifespan [55, 56].

5. SUMMARY OF CHAPTER KEY POINTS

- FRRS, in particular, ROS can exert both detrimental and beneficial effects in biological systems.
- The biological effects of FRRS are affected by a number of factors, including the levels and time of exposure to FRRS, the availability of antioxidant defenses, and the types of molecular targets that FRRS act on.
- The molecular targets of FRRS include such cellular constituents as lipids, proteins, and nucleic acids, as well as nucleotide pools and carbohydrates. Lipids, nucleic acids, and proteins are generally considered the three major types of molecular targets of FRRS.
- FRRS cause oxidation of lipids, resulting in lipid peroxidation. Lipid peroxidation proceeds through three steps: initiation, propagation, and termination. Lipid peroxidation also generates secondary free radicals and other reactive species, such as electrophilic aldehydes.

- The attack by FRRS on proteins can lead to oxidation of the amino acid residues of proteins as well as disruption of the active centers of certain enzymes (such as the iron-sulfur cluster in mitochondrial aconitase).
- Oxidative damage of proteins by FRRS may lead to altered structures and functions of the proteins, protein aggregations, and increased degradation of the oxidatively modified proteins.
- Both the backbone and bases of nucleic acids can be targeting sites of FRRS. Attack of DNA by FRRS may cause DNA base modifications, resulting in gene mutations. In addition to DNA, RNA and the nucleotide pools, as well as microRNAs can be oxidatively damaged by FRRS, which may contribute to disease pathogenesis.
- The detrimental effects mediated by FRRS at the cellular level include cell death, cell dysfunction, cell senescence, cell transformation, and cell proinflammatory responses. The above detrimental effects constitute the cellular basis of FRRS-induced disease pathogenesis and progression.
- An important aspect of FRRS-mediated biological effects is the physiological roles played by these reactive species under certain specific conditions. These emerging physiological functions of FRRS range from adaptive immunity and redox signaling to suppression of cancer development and prolongation of lifespan.

6. SELF-ASSESSMENT QUESTIONS

6.1. Free radical-triggered lipid peroxidation proceeds through initiation, propagation, and termination. Initiation is typically caused by which of the following reactions?

A. Dismutation
B. Electron transfer
C. Free radical addition
D. Hydrogen atom abstraction
E. Reduction

6.2. A number of diverse peroxidation products are formed during lipid peroxidation of biomembranes and lipoproteins in cells and tissues. Which of the following chemical species may be formed during lipid peroxidation?

A. 4-Hydroxy-2-nonenal
B. Ascorbic acid
C. Glutathione (GSH)

D. Nitric dioxide

E. α-Tocopherol

6.3. Attack of which of the following molecular targets by FRRS can lead to the release of iron from the target?

A. Aconitase

B. Glutathione reductase

C. NADPH oxidase

D. Superoxide dismutase

E. Xanthine oxidoreductase

6.4. FRRS can cause oxidative damage to DNA, resulting in DNA base modifications, strand breaks, as well as DNA-DNA and DNA-protein crosslinks. Detection of which of the following chemical species is widely used to assess oxidative DNA damage in biological systems?

A. Acrolein

B. 8-Hydroxy-2'-deoxyguanosine

C. 4-Hydroxy-2-nonenal

D. Malondialdehyde

E. 3-Nitrotyrosine

6.5. It is well established that oxidative stress and inflammation are two closely intertwined processes. In this context, which of the following transcription factors is known to be activated by ROS, thereby leading to the increased expression of pro-inflammatory cytokines?

A. AP-1

B. NF-κB

C. Nrf2

D. TFIIA

E. TFIIF

ANSWERS AND EXPLANATIONS

6.1. The answer is D. The initiation step of lipid peroxidation occurs as a result of hydrogen atom abstraction from a polyunsaturated fatty acid side-chain of a lipid (LH) by a free radical, such as a hydroxyl radical, alkyoxyl radical, or peroxyl radical. This converts the polyunsaturated fatty acid to a carbon-centered radical (L$^•$): LH + OH$^•$ → L$^•$ + H$_2$O.

6.2. The answer is A. Various peroxidation products are formed during lipid peroxidation. For instance, in the presence of transition metal ions, lipid hydroper-oxides can be converted to peroxyl and alkoxyl radicals. The decomposition of lipid hydroperoxides also gives rise to many other reactive species, including electrophilic aldehydes (e.g., acrolein, 4-hydroxy-2-nonenal, and malondialdehyde).

6.3. The answer is A. Oxidation of the iron-sulfur cluster in mitochondrial aconitase by superoxide can lead to the release of iron ion from the enzyme and the consequent enzyme inactivation.

6.4. The answer is B. Measurement of the levels of 8-OH-dG in tissue and body fluid samples is a widely used biomarker for assessing oxidative DNA damage in both experimental animals and humans.

6.5. The answer is B. ROS stimulate the expression of inflammatory cytokines and adhesion molecules via activation of NF-κB, a central regulator of inflammatory cytokine genes, thereby promoting inflammatory responses.

REFERENCES

1. Milne GL, Yin H, Morrow JD. Human biochemistry of the isoprostane pathway. *J Biol Chem* 2008; 283(23):15533–7.
2. Milne GL, Dai Q, Roberts LJ, 2nd. The isoprostanes: 25 years later. *Biochim Biophys Acta* 2015; 1851(4):433–45.
3. Charles RL, Rudyk O, Prysyazhna O, Kamynina A, Yang J, Morisseau C, Hammock BD, Freeman BA, Eaton P. Protection from hypertension in mice by the Mediterranean diet is mediated by nitro fatty acid inhibition of soluble epoxide hydrolase. *Proc Natl Acad Sci USA* 2014; 111(22):8167–72.
4. Rudolph V, Freeman BA. Cardiovascular consequences when nitric oxide and lipid signaling converge. *Circ Res* 2009; 105(6):511–22.
5. Stadtman ER. Protein oxidation and aging. *Science* 1992; 257(5074):1220–4.
6. Davies MJ. Protein oxidation and peroxidation. *Biochem J* 2016; 473(7):805–25.
7. Berlett BS, Stadtman ER. Protein oxidation in aging, disease, and oxidative stress. *J Biol Chem* 1997; 272(33):20313–6.
8. Gardner PR, Nguyen DD, White CW. Aconitase is a sensitive and critical target of oxygen poisoning in cultured mammalian cells and in rat lungs. *Proc Natl Acad Sci USA* 1994;

91(25):12248–52.

9. Gardner PR, Raineri I, Epstein LB, White CW. Superoxide radical and iron modulate aconitase activity in mammalian cells. *J Biol Chem* 1995; 270(22):13399–405.

10. Vasquez-Vivar J, Kalyanaraman B, Kennedy MC. Mitochondrial aconitase is a source of hydroxyl radical: an electron spin resonance investigation. *J Biol Chem* 2000; 275(19):14064–9.

11. Radi R. Nitric oxide, oxidants, and protein tyrosine nitration. *Proc Natl Acad Sci USA* 2004; 101(12):4003–8.

12. Moskovitz J, Bar-Noy S, Williams WM, Requena J, Berlett BS, Stadtman ER. Methionine sulfoxide reductase (MsrA) is a regulator of antioxidant defense and lifespan in mammals. *Proc Natl Acad Sci USA* 2001; 98(23):12920–5.

13. Yakes FM, Van Houten B. Mitochondrial DNA damage is more extensive and persists longer than nuclear DNA damage in human cells following oxidative stress. *Proc Natl Acad Sci USA* 1997; 94(2):514–9.

14. Wallace DC. Mitochondrial diseases in man and mouse. *Science* 1999; 283(5407):1482–8.

15. Henchcliffe C, Beal MF. Mitochondrial biology and oxidative stress in Parkinson disease pathogenesis. *Nat Clin Pract Neurol* 2008; 4(11):600–9.

16. Tanaka M, Chock PB, Stadtman ER. Oxidized messenger RNA induces translation errors. *Proc Natl Acad Sci USA* 2007; 104(1):66–71.

17. Chang Y, Kong Q, Shan X, Tian G, Ilieva H, Cleveland DW, Rothstein JD, Borchelt DR, Wong PC, Lin CL. Messenger RNA oxidation occurs early in disease pathogenesis and promotes motor neuron degeneration in ALS. *PLoS One* 2008; 3(8):e2849.

18. Wang JX, Gao J, Ding SL, Wang K, Jiao JQ, Wang Y, Sun T, Zhou LY, Long B, Zhang XJ, Li Q, Liu JP, et al. Oxidative modification of miR-184 enables it to target Bcl-xL and Bcl-w. *Mol Cell* 2015; 59(1):50–61.

19. Chaudhary AK, Nokubo M, Reddy GR, Yeola SN, Morrow JD, Blair IA, Marnett LJ. Detection of endogenous malondialdehyde-deoxyguanosine adducts in human liver. *Science* 1994; 265(5178):1580–2.

20. Hoeijmakers JH. DNA damage, aging, and cancer. *N Engl J Med* 2009; 361(15):1475–85.

21. David SS, O'Shea VL, Kundu S. Base-excision repair of oxidative DNA damage. *Nature* 2007; 447(7147):941–50.

22. Rai P, Onder TT, Young JJ, McFaline JL, Pang B, Dedon PC, Weinberg RA. Continuous elimination of oxidized nucleotides is necessary to prevent rapid onset of cellular senescence. *Proc Natl Acad Sci USA* 2009; 106(1):169–74.

23. Majno G, Joris I. Apoptosis, oncosis, and necrosis. An overview of cell death. *Am J Pathol* 1995; 146(1):3–15.

24. Hotchkiss RS, Strasser A, McDunn JE, Swanson PE. Cell death. *N Engl J Med* 2009; 361(16):1570–83.

25. Galluzzi L, Pietrocola F, Levine B, Kroemer G. Metabolic control of autophagy. *Cell* 2014; 159(6):1263–76.

26. Burgoyne JR, Mongue-Din H, Eaton P, Shah AM. Redox signaling in cardiac physiology and pathology. *Circ Res* 2012; 111(8):1091–106.

27. Holmstrom KM, Finkel T. Cellular mechanisms and physiological consequences of redox-dependent signalling. *Nat Rev Mol Cell Biol* 2014; 15(6):411–21.

28. Lu T, Finkel T. Free radicals and senescence. *Exp Cell Res* 2008; 314(9):1918–22.

29. Jurk D, Wilson C, Passos JF, Oakley F, Correia-Melo C, Greaves L, Saretzki G, Fox C, Lawless C, Anderson R, Hewitt G, Pender SL, et al. Chronic inflammation induces telomere dysfunction and accelerates ageing in mice. *Nat Commun* 2014; 2:4172.

30. Arnold RS, Shi J, Murad E, Whalen AM, Sun CQ, Polavarapu R, Parthasarathy S, Petros JA, Lambeth JD. Hydrogen peroxide mediates the cell growth and transformation caused by the mitogenic oxidase Nox1. *Proc Natl Acad Sci USA* 2001; 98(10):5550–5.

31. Sabharwal SS, Schumacker PT. Mitochondrial ROS in cancer: initiators, amplifiers or an Achilles' heel? *Nat Rev Cancer* 2014; 14(11):709–21.

32. Ma C, Kesarwala AH, Eggert T, Medina-Echeverz J, Kleiner DE, Jin P, Stroncek DF, Terabe M, Kapoor V, ElGindi M, Han M, Thornton AM, et al. NAFLD causes selective CD4$^+$ T lymphocyte loss and promotes hepatocarcinogenesis. *Nature* 2016; 531(7593):253–7.

33. Goossens V, Grooten J, De Vos K, Fiers W. Direct evidence for tumor necrosis factor-induced mitochondrial reactive oxygen intermediates and their involvement in cytotoxicity. *Proc Natl Acad Sci USA* 1995; 92(18):8115–9.

34. Roca FJ, Ramakrishnan L. TNF dually mediates resistance and susceptibility to mycobacteria via mitochondrial reactive oxygen species. *Cell* 2013; 153(3):521–34.

35. Schreck R, Rieber P, Baeuerle PA. Reactive oxygen intermediates as apparently widely used messengers in the activation of the NF-kappa B transcription factor and HIV-1. *EMBO J* 1991; 10(8):2247–58.

36. Anrather J, Racchumi G, Iadecola C. NF-kappaB regulates phagocytic NADPH oxidase by inducing the expression of gp91phox. *J Biol Chem* 2006; 281(9):5657–67.

37. Salzano S, Checconi P, Hanschmann EM, Lillig CH, Bowler LD, Chan P, Vaudry D, Mengozzi M, Coppo L, Sacre S, Atkuri KR, Sahaf B, et al. Linkage of inflammation and oxidative stress via release of glutathionylated peroxiredoxin-2, which acts as a danger signal. *Proc Natl Acad Sci USA* 2014; 111(33):12157–62.

38. Kuhns DB, Alvord WG, Heller T, Feld JJ, Pike KM, Marciano BE, Uzel G, DeRavin SS, Priel DA, Soule BP, Zarember KA, Malech HL, et al. Residual NADPH oxidase and survival in chronic granulomatous disease. *N Engl J Med* 2010; 363(27):2600–10.

39. Noubade R, Wong K, Ota N, Rutz S, Eidenschenk C, Valdez PA, Ding J, Peng I, Sebrell A, Caplazi P, DeVoss J, Soriano RH, et al. NRROS negatively regulates reactive oxygen species during host defence and autoimmunity. *Nature* 2014; 509(7499):235–9.

40. Sena LA, Chandel NS. Physiological roles of mitochondrial reactive oxygen species. *Mol Cell* 2012; 48(2):158–67.

41. West AP, Brodsky IE, Rahner C, Woo DK, Erdjument-Bromage H, Tempst P, Walsh MC, Choi Y, Shadel GS, Ghosh S. TLR signalling augments macrophage bactericidal activity through mitochondrial ROS. *Nature* 2011; 472(7344):476–80.

42. Okoye I, Wang L, Pallmer K, Richter K, Ichimura T, Haas R, Crouse J, Choi O, Heathcote D, Lovo E, Mauro C, Abdi R, et al. The protein LEM promotes CD8$^+$ T cell immunity through effects on mitochondrial respiration. *Science* 2015.

43. Sundaresan M, Yu ZX, Ferrans VJ, Irani K, Finkel T. Requirement for generation of H_2O_2 for platelet-derived growth factor signal transduction. *Science* 1995; 270(5234):296–9.

44. Nguyen T, Sherratt PJ, Nioi P, Yang CS, Pickett CB. Nrf2 controls constitutive and inducible expression of ARE-driven genes through a dynamic pathway involving nucleocytoplasmic shuttling by Keap1. *J Biol Chem* 2005; 280(37):32485–92.

45. Nguyen T, Nioi P, Pickett CB. The Nrf2-antioxidant response element signaling pathway and its activation by oxidative stress. *J Biol Chem* 2009; 284(20):13291–5.

46. Dickinson BC, Peltier J, Stone D, Schaffer DV, Chang CJ. Nox2 redox signaling maintains essential cell populations in the brain. *Nat Chem Biol* 2011; 7(2):106–12.

47. Hamalainen RH, Ahlqvist KJ, Ellonen P, Lepisto M, Logan A, Otonkoski T, Murphy MP, Suomalainen A. mtDNA mutagenesis disrupts pluripotent stem cell function by altering redox signaling. *Cell Rep* 2015; 11(10):1614–24.

48. Gouge J, Satia K, Guthertz N, Widya M, Thompson AJ, Cousin P, Dergai O, Hernandez N, Vannini A. Redox signaling by the RNA polymerase III TFIIB-related factor Brf2. *Cell* 2015; 163(6):1375–87.

49. DeNicola GM, Karreth FA, Humpton TJ, Gopinathan A, Wei C, Frese K, Mangal D, Yu KH, Yeo CJ, Calhoun ES, Scrimieri F, Winter JM, et al. Oncogene-induced Nrf2 transcription promotes ROS detoxification and tumorigenesis. *Nature* 2011; 475(7354):106–9.

50. Chio, II, Jafarnejad SM, Ponz-Sarvise M, Park Y, Rivera K, Palm W, Wilson J, Sangar V, Hao Y, Ohlund D, Wright K, Filippini D, et al. NRF2 promotes tumor maintenance by modulating mRNA translation in pancreatic cancer. *Cell* 2016; 166(4):963–76.

51. Piskounova E, Agathocleous M, Murphy MM, Hu Z, Huddlestun SE, Zhao Z, Leitch AM, Johnson TM, DeBerardinis RJ, Morrison SJ. Oxidative stress inhibits distant metastasis by human melanoma cells. *Nature* 2015; 527(7577):186–91.

52. Kasiappan R, Safe SH. ROS-inducing agents for cancer chemotherapy. *Reactive Oxygen Species* 2016; 1(1):22–37.

53. Yee C, Yang W, Hekimi S. The intrinsic apoptosis pathway mediates the pro-longevity response to mitochondrial ROS in *C. elegans*. *Cell* 2014; 157(4):897–909.

54. Wang Y, Hekimi S. Mitochondrial dysfunction and longevity in animals: untangling the knot. *Science* 2015; 350(6265):1204–7.

55. Schroeder EA, Raimundo N, Shadel GS. Epigenetic silencing mediates mitochondria stress-induced longevity. *Cell Metab* 2013;

17(6):954–64.

56. Zarse K, Schmeisser S, Groth M, Priebe S, Beuster G, Kuhlow D, Guthke R, Platzer M, Kahn CR, Ristow M. Impaired insulin/IGF1 signaling extends life span by promoting mitochondrial L-proline catabolism to induce a transient ROS signal. *Cell Metab* 2012; 15(4):451–65.

UNIT III

COMMON FREE RADICALS AND RELATED REACTIVE SPECIES

Chapter 8

Superoxide in Biology and Medicine

ABSTRACT | Since 1933 when Linus Pauling, a twice-honored Nobel laureate, proposed its existence based on the theory of quantum mechanics, superoxide has gradually taken central stage in the research field of free radical biology and medicine. Indeed, superoxide is considered the primary reactive oxygen species (ROS) that gives rise to secondary ROS in biological systems. Superoxide is produced from one electron reduction of molecular oxygen during various metabolic processes and by diverse enzymes, including the mitochondrial electron transport chain, NADPH oxidase, cytochrome P450 enzyme system, xanthine oxidoreductase, and uncoupled nitric oxide synthase, among others. Because of its low reduction potential, superoxide often acts as a reducing agent rather than an oxidizing species. However, superoxide is able to oxidize the iron-sulfur clusters in certain enzymes, such as mitochondrial aconitase and electron transport chain enzyme complexes. Superoxide reacts with nitric oxide to form the potent oxidant, peroxynitrite. Superoxide is also a reactant in iron-catalyzed Haber–Weiss reaction, leading to the production of hydroxyl radical, the most potent ROS. These chemical and biochemical properties of superoxide dictate the biological effects of this oxygen radical. In fact, superoxide is now recognized as an important molecule that is formed via defined mechanisms and metabolized by specific enzymes, and involved in diverse physiological and pathophysiological processes.

KEYWORDS | Cytochrome P450 system; Disease process; Fenton reaction; Haber–Weiss reaction; Innate immunity; Mitochondria; NADPH oxidase; Reactive oxygen species; Redox signaling; Superoxide; Superoxide dismutase; Uncoupled endothelial nitric oxide synthase; Xanthine oxidoreductase

CITATION | Hopkins RZ and Li YR. *Essentials of Free Radical Biology and Medicine. Cell Med Press, Raleigh, NC, USA. 2017. http://dx.doi.org/10.20455/efrbm.2017.08*

ABBREVIATIONS | CuZnSOD, Cu,Zn superoxide dismutase; ECSOD, extracellular superoxide dismutase; METC, mitochondrial electron transport chain; MnSOD, manganese superoxide dismutase; NOS, nitric oxide synthase; ROS, reactive oxygen species; SOD, superoxide dismutase

CHAPTER AT A GLANCE

1. OVERVIEW

Superoxide, also known as superoxide anion or superoxide anion radical, is designated as $O_2^{\cdot-}$, where the dot denotes the unpaired electron and the minus sign denotes that the species is negatively charged. The above three names for $O_2^{\cdot-}$ are used interchangeably in the literature, and for simplicity, superoxide is used throughout this chapter. Superoxide can exist in a protonated form, known as perhydroxyl or hydroperoxyl radical ($HO_2^{\cdot}$) with a pKa of 4.8. Because of this pKa, superoxide exists predominantly in the non-protonated form ($O_2^{\cdot-}$) under a physiological pH.

Linus Pauling, a twice-honored Nobel laureate (Chemistry in 1954; Peace in 1962) proposed the existence of superoxide based on the theory of quantum mechanics in 1933 (see in ref. [1]). Two decades after Linus Pauling's proposal, in 1954, Rebecca Gershman and associates suggested that superoxide might be responsible for both oxygen toxicity and the deleterious effects of x-irradiation [2]. Subsequently, xanthine oxidase was proposed to produce superoxide in 1962 [3], and this was proved by electron paramagnetic resonance (EPR) studies in 1969 [4]. Meanwhile, methods involving electrolytic univalent reduction of molecular oxygen were used to produce superoxide.

With superoxide generated via the above approaches, Joe McCord and Irvine Fridovich discovered Cu,Zn superoxide dismutase (CuZnSOD) in 1969 [5]. Subsequently, Bernard Babior and coworkers reported superoxide generation by respiratory burst (activation of NADPH oxidase) of leukocytes as a potential mechanism of bactericidal activity [6]. Now superoxide is considered one of the most important reactive oxygen species (ROS) that plays significant roles in a variety of biological processes and disease conditions. This chapter provides an overview on the sources of superoxide and discusses the basic chemistry and biochemistry of this ubiquitous oxygen free radical. The chapter then considers its roles in biology and medicine.

2. SOURCES

Superoxide is produced from one electron reduction of molecular dioxygen (oxygen for simplicity): $O_2 + e^- \rightarrow O_2^{\cdot-}$ [7] (**Figure 8.1**). In biological systems, superoxide is generated from various metabolic processes. These include the mitochondrial electron transport chain (METC) complexes, NADPH oxidases (also known as NOXs), cytochrome P450 en-

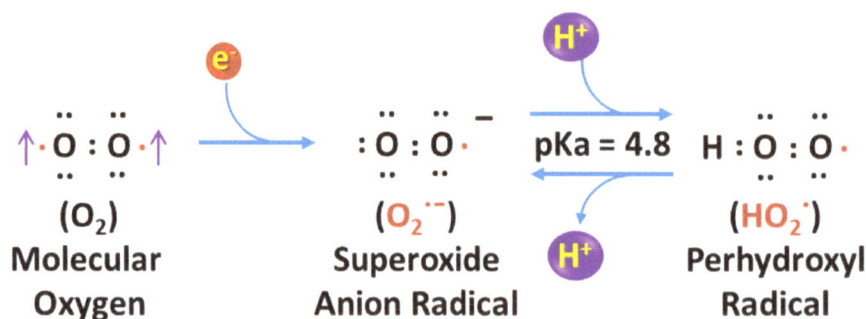

FIGURE 8.1. Electron configuration illustration of one-electron reduction of molecular oxygen to form superoxide. Molecular oxygen (O_2) is in fact a di-radical because it contains two unpaired electrons. The same spin direction of the two unpaired electrons in O_2 causes spin restriction, making O_2 less reactive. On the other hand, superoxide ($O_2^{\cdot-}$) contains one unpaired electron and has one more electron than O_2, and as such, superoxide is negatively charged. Superoxide can become protonated to form perhydroxyl radical ($HO_2^{\cdot}$), which is believed to be more reactive than $O_2^{\cdot-}$.

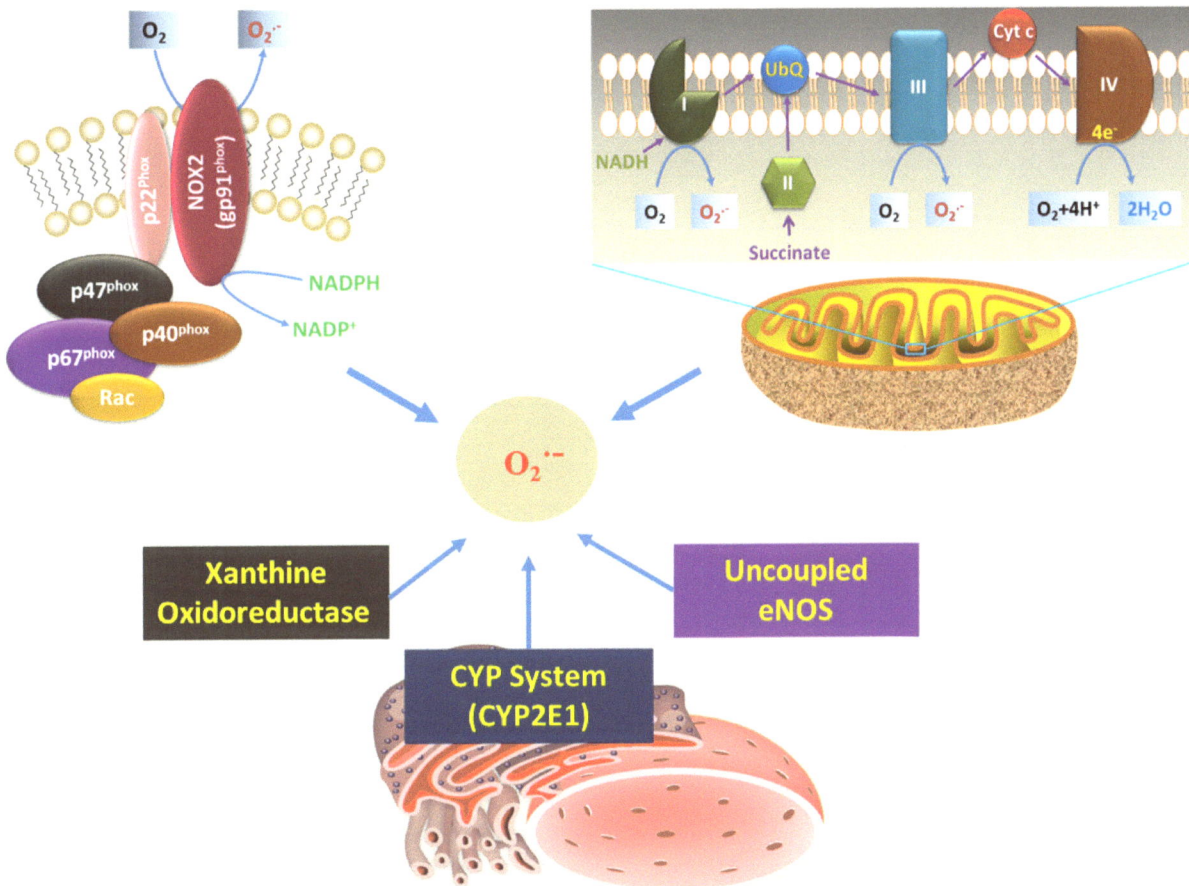

FIGURE 8.2. Major sources of cellular superoxide. NADPH oxidases (NOXs) and mitochondria are considered the major cellular sources of superoxide. Many other enzymes and cellular processes also contribute to cellular superoxide production, such as xanthine oxidoreductase, cytochrome P450 (CYP) enzyme system (especially CYP2E1), and uncoupled endothelial nitric oxide synthase (eNOS).

zyme system, xanthine oxidoreductase, uncoupled endothelial nitric oxide synthase (eNOS), among others (e.g., Rac) (**Figure 8.2**). In addition to the above cellular processes and enzymes, superoxide is also generated from various exogenous sources, including environmental toxicants and drugs. The various sources of superoxide as well as other free radicals and related reactive species are covered in Chapter 6.

3. CHEMISTRY AND BIOCHEMISTRY

Although it is called "super-oxide", superoxide is in fact not a strong oxidizing species. Because of its lower reduction potential (–330 mV for the $O_2/O_2^{\cdot-}$ redox couple), superoxide often acts as a reducing agent rather than an oxidizing species. Indeed, the ferricytochrome c reduction assay, a method for detecting superoxide, is based on the ability of superoxide to reduce this small heme-containing protein [8]. The ability of superoxide to directly oxidize biomolecules, including lipids, proteins, and nucleic acids is much limited. However, superoxide is an important ROS that can result in cell and tissue injury [9]. As outlined below, the biologically damaging potential of superoxide is attributed to its several unique chemical and biochemical properties (**Figure 8.3**).

3.1. Oxidation of Iron-Sulfur Clusters

Although it generally acts as a reducing agent, superoxide does oxidize the iron-sulfur clusters in several enzymes, including aconitase, an enzyme of the

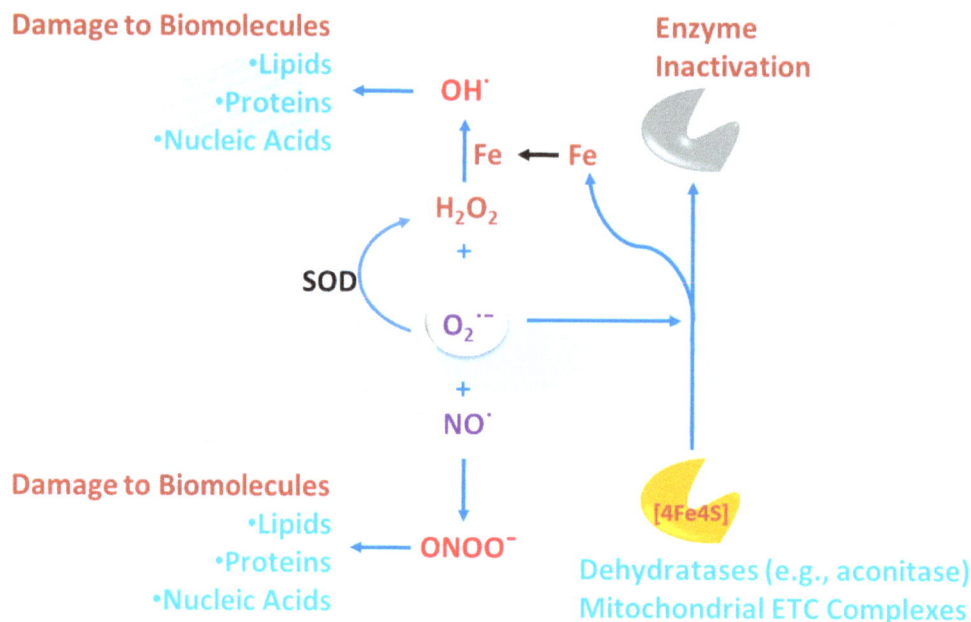

FIGURE 8.3. Chemical reactivity of superoxide. As illustrated, superoxide ($O_2^{\cdot-}$) reacts with iron-sulfur [4Fe4S] clusters in enzymes, leading to enzyme inactivation. It reacts with nitric oxide (NO$^{\cdot}$) at a diffusion-limited rate to form peroxynitrite (ONOO$^-$), a potent oxidant. Superoxide is also a reactant of the iron-catalyzed Haber-Weiss reaction, giving rise to hydroxyl radical (OH$^{\cdot}$), the most potent ROS formed in biological systems. Spontaneous or superoxide dismutase (SOD)-catalyzed dismutation of superoxide produces hydrogen peroxide, another important ROS.

tricarboxylic acid cycle [10, 11], and the mitochondrial electron transport chain enzyme complexes [12]. Oxidation of the iron-sulfur clusters by superoxide in these enzymes leads to the release of iron from the enzymes and the enzyme inactivation. The released iron ions may participate in the Fenton reaction, resulting in the formation of hydroxyl radicals (see Section 3.3). In contrast, reversible oxidation of the iron-sulfur cluster in prokaryotic transcription factors SoxR/SoxS leads to their activation (see Section 4.2).

3.2. Reaction with Nitric Oxide

Superoxide reacts with nitric oxide (NO$^{\cdot}$) at an almost diffusion-limited rate to form peroxynitrite ani-

on (ONOO$^-$), which is frequently called peroxynitrite for simplicity. The reaction is as following: $O_2^{\cdot-}$ + NO$^{\cdot}$ → ONOO$^-$. Peroxynitrite is a potent oxidant that causes damage to various biomolecules [13]. The fast reaction between superoxide and nitric oxide also contributes to the decreased bioavailability of nitric oxide under diverse pathophysiological conditions. Nitric oxide is generally regarded as a cardiovascular protective molecule, whose deficiency might contribute, at least partly, to such diseases as atherosclerosis, hypertension, coronary artery disease, and erectile dysfunction [14]. Hence, the consequence of the reaction between superoxide and nitric oxide is two-fold: production of a much more potent oxidant and depletion of a beneficial molecule.

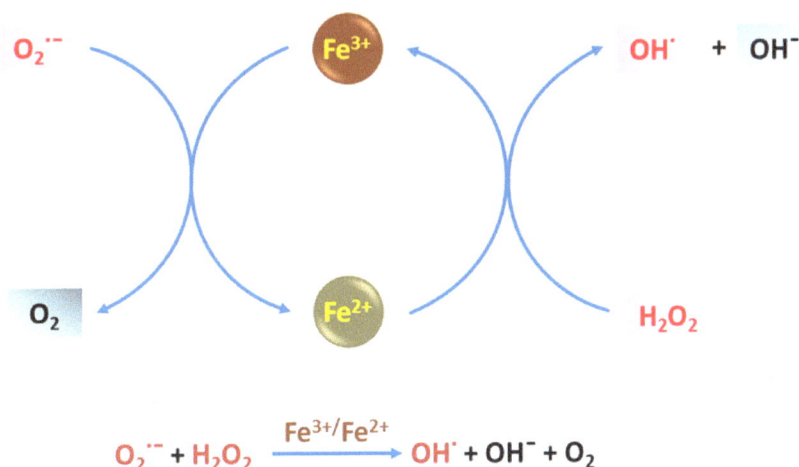

FIGURE 8.4. Iron-catalyzed Haber-Weiss reaction. The reaction between superoxide ($O_2^{\bullet-}$) and hydrogen peroxide (H_2O_2) to form hydroxyl radical ($OH^{\bullet}$) is commonly referred to as the Haber–Weiss reaction. This reaction proceeds slowly, but can be dramatically accelerated by the presence of iron (Fe) ions. The reaction on the right side of the scheme is also called the Fenton reaction.

3.3. Haber–Weiss Reaction and Fenton Reaction

In the presence of transition metal ions, such as iron ions, superoxide and hydrogen peroxide together can give rise to hydroxyl radical ($OH^{\bullet}$), the most potent ROS capable of damaging the entire spectrum of biomolecules. The reaction of superoxide and hydrogen peroxide in the presence of iron ions to produce hydroxyl radical is known as iron-catalyzed Haber–Weiss reaction, which was first proposed by Fritz Haber and Joseph Weiss in 1934 [15] (**Figure 8.4**). In addition to his contributions to the field of free radical biology, Fritz Haber received the Nobel Prize in Chemistry in 1918 for the synthesis of ammonia from its elements.

In the absence of iron ions, the above reaction proceeds slowly. The presence of iron ions markedly accelerates the reaction to produce hydroxyl radical. The iron ion-catalyzed Haber–Weiss reaction can be written in two sequential sub-reactions: (1) $O_2^{\bullet-}$ + Fe^{3+} → O_2 + Fe^{2+}, and (2) Fe^{2+} + H_2O_2 → Fe^{3+} + $OH^{\bullet}$ + OH^-. The second reaction is commonly referred to as the Fenton reaction, which is also frequently called the Fenton chemistry.

By definition, Fenton chemistry refers to the oxidation of organic substrates by Fe^{2+} and H_2O_2. In 1894, Henry J.H. Fenton first observed the oxidation of tartaric acid by H_2O_2 in the presence of Fe^{2+} [16], indicating that a potent oxidant(s) is formed by the reaction between H_2O_2 and Fe^{2+}, which are also known as the Fenton reagent. The Fenton reagent is commonly used to oxidize (destroy) organic chemicals, such as wastes in water. Later in the 1930s, Fritz Haber and Joseph Weiss proposed the formation of hydroxyl radical from the Fenton reagent, which is known today to be a major ultimate free radical species responsible for oxidative damage of a wide range of biomolecules. Indeed, hydroxyl radical is considered the most potent oxidant formed in biological systems.

In addition to Fe^{2+}, other transition metal ions, such as cuprous ion (Cu^{1+}), also react with H_2O_2, forming hydroxyl radical or its equivalent: $M^{(n-1)+}$ + H_2O_2 → M^{n+} + $OH^{\bullet}$ + OH^-, where M denotes the transition metal ion. For example: Cu^{1+} + H_2O_2 → Cu^{2+} + $OH^{\bullet}$ + OH^-. Such reactions are commonly referred to as Fenton-type reactions.

3.4. Half-Life, Diffusion, Membrane Permeability, and Protonation

In general, free radicals are short-lived, especially in biological milieu. The half-life of free radicals, including superoxide is an important factor in determining the biological activity of the radical species. In biological systems, the half-life of superoxide is estimated to be in the range of 10^{-6}–10^{-5} s depending on the components of the biological milieu (such as

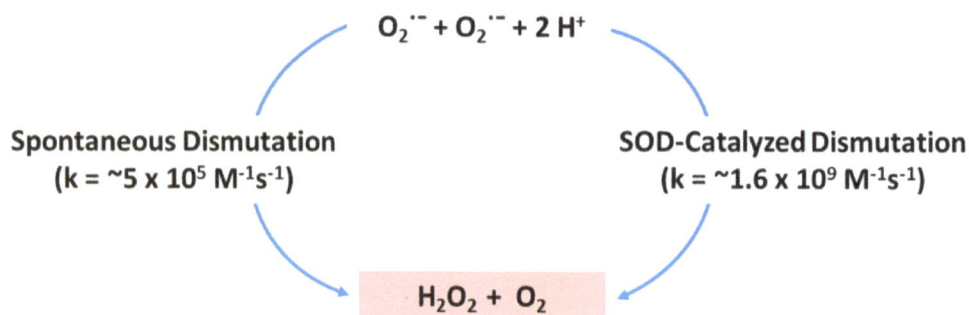

FIGURE 8.5. Spontaneous and superoxide dismutase (SOD)-catalyzed dismutation of superoxide. As illustrated, the dismutation reaction of superoxide ($O_2^{\cdot-}$) is greatly accelerated by SOD with a reaction rate constant being over three orders of magnitude greater than that of spontaneous dismutation.

superoxide dismutase which catalyzes the dismutation of superoxide at a nearly diffusion-limited rate).

Another factor influencing the biological activities of superoxide is its limited ability to cross biomembranes due to the negative charge as well as short half-life of this free radical species. However, superoxide may cross cell membranes through anion channels, such as the 4-diisothiocyano-2,2-disulfonic acid stilbene (DIDS)-sensitive chloride channel [17]. In contrast, perhydroxyl radical, the protonated form of superoxide, is highly membrane permeable, and is also a potent oxidizing species [18].

Perhydroxy radical has a pKa of 4.8, and as such, may reach high levels in cellular compartments with high concentrations of protons, including the mitochondrial intermembrane space. A recent study by Li et al. provides direct evidence for the METC-derived superoxide to exit mitochondria and cross cell membranes to enter the extracellular milieu [19]. Exit of superoxide from mitochondria and its subsequent crossing of cell membranes to enter extracellular milieu provide a basis for superoxide to participate in diverse intracellular and intercellular processes under physiological and pathophysiological conditions.

4. CELL AND TISSUE DEFENSES

Superoxide undergoes spontaneous dismutation to form hydrogen peroxide and molecular oxygen with a reaction rate constant of $\sim 5 \times 10^5$ $M^{-1}s^{-1}$ at pH 7.0 (**Figure 8.5**). The term dismutation reaction refers to a chemical reaction in which the same reactant is both oxidized and reduced. In superoxide dismutation reaction, one molecule of superoxide is oxidized

to molecular oxygen, and another is reduced to hydrogen peroxide. The dismutation reaction of superoxide is catalyzed by superoxide dismutase (SOD) with a reaction rate constant of $\sim 1.6 \times 10^9$ $M^{-1}s^{-1}$ which is over three orders of magnitude greater than that of spontaneous dismutation (**Figure 8.5**).

In mammalian species, including humans, there are three types of SOD: (1) CuZnSOD, (2) manganese (MnSOD), and (3) extracellular SOD (ECSOD). All three forms of SOD catalyze dismutation of superoxide to hydrogen peroxide and molecular oxygen at a similar reaction rate constant (see Appendix B).

Recently, NAD(P)H oxidoreductase 1 (NQO1), an enzyme that catalyzes 2-electron reduction of quinone compounds, has been suggested to scavenge biological superoxide possibly by catalyzing its conversion to hydrogen peroxide [29, 30]. NQO1 appears to play a role in scavenging superoxide in tissues, such as vascular endothelium and myocardium, where SOD is relatively deficient and NQO1 is, on the other hand, highly expressed [30].

The fate of cellular superoxide (derived from the chief source—METC) is illustrated in **Figure 8.6**. The presence of the multiple layers of SOD defenses suggests that tight control of superoxide levels is essential for cell physiological homeostasis.

5. BIOLOGY AND MEDICINE

Superoxide is one of the most extensively investigated ROS in biology and medicine. A PubMed search on December 14, 2016 revealed 86.436 entries containing the term "superoxide" in title/abstract. The number of entries for "hydrogen peroxide" and "hy-

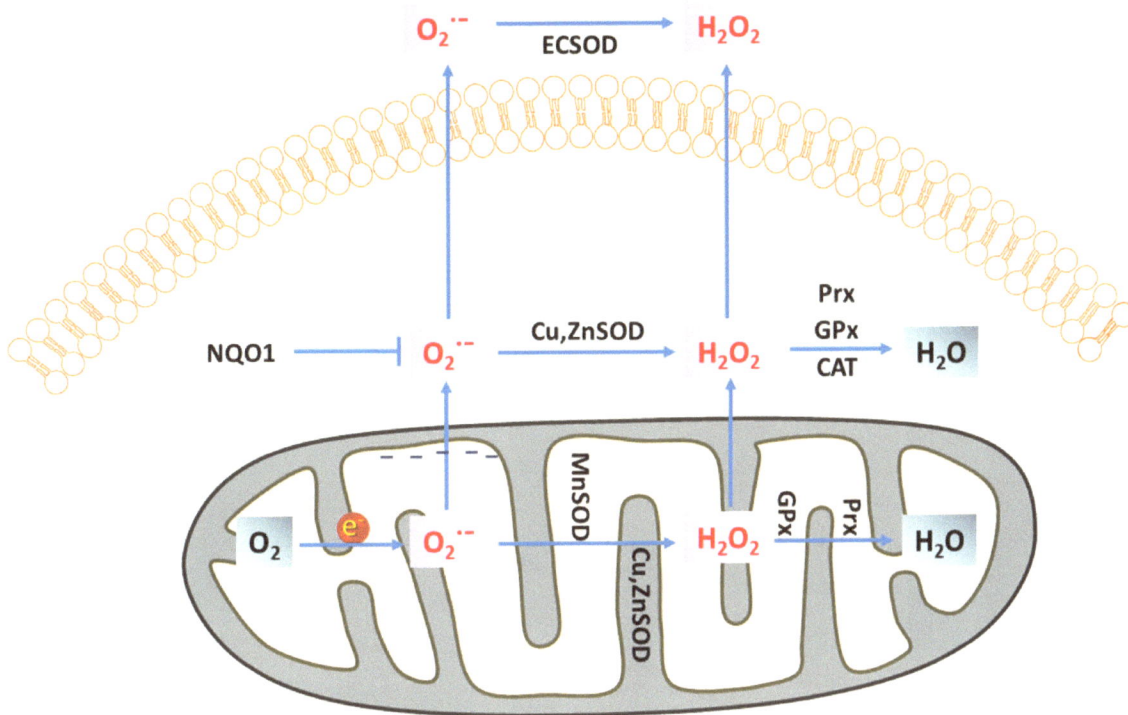

FIGURE 8.6. The cellular fate of mitochondria-derived superoxide. Mitochondrial electron transport chain (METC) is the major source of cellular superoxide ($O_2{}^{\cdot-}$) formation. The METC-derived superoxide undergoes MnSOD-catalyzed dismutation to form hydrogen peroxide (H_2O_2), which is then converted to water by glutathione peroxidase (GPx) or peroxiredoxin (Prx) in mitochondrial matrix. Superoxide is able to cross the mitochondrial inner membrane and enter the cytosol, where CuZnSOD catalyzes its dismutation to H_2O_2, and the H_2O_2 formed in the cytosol or escaped from mitochondria is converted to water by enzymes, including GPx, Prx, and catalase (CAT), in the cytoplasm. CuZnSOD present in the mitochondrial intermembrane space also catalyzes the dismutation of superoxide present in the intermembrane space. ECSOD acts on extracellular superoxide. In addition to SOD, NAD(P)H:quinone oxidoreductase 1 (NQO1) may also scavenge superoxide.

droxyl radical" was 80,594 and 10,438, respectively. As outlined below, biological superoxide plays important roles in both physiological and pathophysiological processes.

5.1. Phagocyte-Mediated Immunity

Superoxide produced from phagocytic NADPH oxidase during respiratory burst is an important precursor molecule leading to the formation of more potent ROS, especially hypochlorous acid (HOCl), peroxynitrite, and hydroxyl radical that kill the invading microorganisms (**Figure 8.7**). Dismutation of superoxide generates hydrogen peroxide, which in turn reacts with chloride ion in the presence of the phagocyte-derived myeloperoxidase (MPO), forming hypochlorous acid. Likewise, superoxide released from

the NADPH oxidase reacts with nitric oxide generated by inducible nitric oxide synthase (iNOS), resulting in the formation of peroxynitrite. In the presence of iron ions, reaction of superoxide with hydrogen peroxide generates hydroxyl radical via the iron-catalyzed Haber–Weiss reaction (see Section 3.3). Failure to generate phagocyte-derived superoxide and related ROS is the major defect in chronic granulomatous disease, causing recurrent infections and granulomatous complications [20].

5.2. Redox Modulation and Signaling

The role of superoxide in redox regulation in prokaryotes is well established. In bacteria, SoxR and SoxS are activated by superoxide via reversible one-electron oxidation of the [2Fe-2S] cluster and then

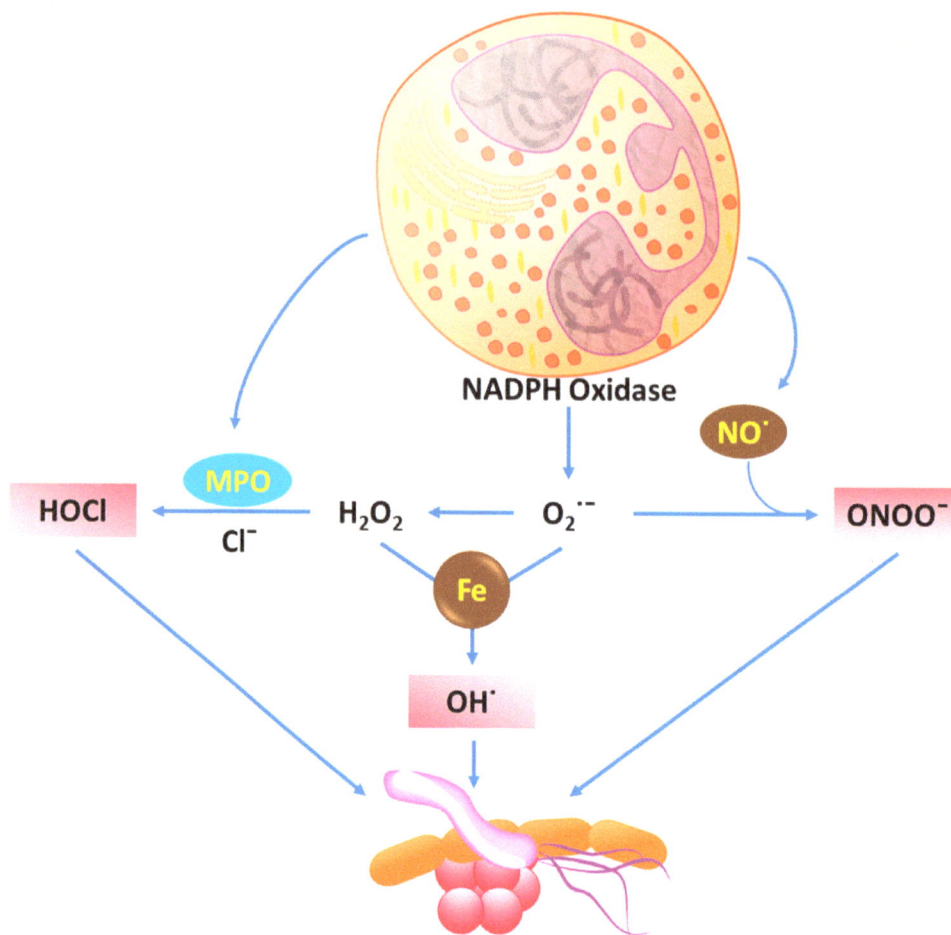

FIGURE 8.7. Phagocytic NADPH oxidase-derived superoxide as a precursor of secondary reactive species for killing invading pathogens. As illustrated, phagocytic respiratory burst results in the formation of superoxide ($O_2^{\cdot-}$) via activation of the membrane-associated NADPH oxidase. Superoxide undergoes dismutation to give rise to hydrogen peroxide (H_2O_2), which, in the presence of phagocytic myeloperoxidase (MPO), reacts with chloride ion to form hypochlorous acid (HOCl), a potent oxidant and pathogen-killing compound. Superoxide also reacts with nitric oxide (NO$^\cdot$) derived from phagocytic inducible nitric oxide synthase to form peroxynitrite ($ONOO^-$), another potent oxidant capable of killing pathogens. Lastly, iron-catalyzed Haber–Weiss reaction gives rise to hydroxyl radical, the most potent oxidizing species formed in biological systems. The above potent oxidants collectively contribute to phagocytic cell-mediated innate immunity against invading microorganisms.

enhance the production of various antioxidant proteins through the soxRS regulon [21, 22].

Superoxide stimulates mitogenesis and promotes cell proliferation. Overexpression of superoxide-producing NADPH oxidase induces cell transformation [23] although the responsible ROS seems to be hydrogen peroxide derived from the dismutation of superoxide [24]. Superoxide may also relay Ras protein's oncogenic message, resulting in uncon-

trolled cell proliferation and malignant cell transformation [25].

5.3. Autoregulation

Superoxide may regulate its own production. On the one hand, superoxide activates mitochondrial uncoupling proteins, leading to decreased formation of superoxide from the mitochondrial electron transport chain [26, 27]. On the other hand, superoxide flux across the endothelial cell plasma membrane occurs through chloride ion channels and induces intracellular calcium ion release, which in turn increases mitochondrial superoxide generation [28]. However, the significance of superoxide-regulated superoxide production in physiology and pathophysiology remains to be elucidated.

5.4. Disease Process

Although superoxide possesses physiological functions, dysregulated formation of this oxygen radical leads to tissue injury. In fact, formation of superoxide is an important mechanism of oxygen toxicity. The tissue damage may occur as a result of direct effects of superoxide on molecular targets but more likely due to the secondary formation of hydrogen peroxide from superoxide dismutation or the formation of peroxynitrite from the reaction of superoxide with nitric oxide (**Figure 8.3**).

The causal involvement of superoxide in disease pathogenesis is supported by numerous studies showing that genetic deletion of SOD causes diverse disease processes and transgenic overexpression of SOD renders resistance to disease pathogenesis in animal models [31–33]. The diseases or conditions whose pathogenesis is impacted by the alterations of SOD expression or activity involve diverse organs and systems, and include aging [34, 35], cancer [36–38], cardiovascular diseases [39, 40], diabetes [32, 41], neurodegeneration [42, 43], immunological disorders [44, 45], pulmonary disorders [46, 47], hepatic disorders [48, 49], gastrointestinal diseases [50, 51], and kidney diseases [41, 52, 53], among many others.

Although substantial evidence supports a causal involvement of superoxide in diverse disease processes in animal models, the exact role of superoxide and SOD in disease pathogenesis in humans remains to be established. The only human disease that is, thus far, known to be affected by mutations in the SOD (CuZnSOD) gene is familial amyotrophic lateral sclerosis (ALS) [54]. Large-scale, well-designed, randomized controlled trials on using SOD (either native protein or biomimetic) in human disease intervention are currently lacking. Clinical research on the role of superoxide in disease process is hampered by the limited bioavailability of native SOD. In this context, recent development in selective SOD biomimetics with favorable pharmacokinetic properties [55] would facilitate research on the role of superoxide in human diseases.

6. SUMMARY OF CHAPTER KEY POINTS

- Superoxide, also known as superoxide anion or superoxide anion radical, is designated as $O_2^{\cdot-}$. Since 1933 when Linus Pauling, a twice-honored Nobel laureate, proposed its existence based on the theory of quantum mechanics, superoxide has gradually taken central stage in the research field of free radical biology and medicine.
- In biological systems, superoxide is generated from various metabolic processes. These include METC complexes, NADPH oxidases, cytochrome P450 enzyme system, xanthine oxidoreductase, uncoupled eNOS, among others (e.g., Rac).
- Although it is called "super-oxide", superoxide is in fact not a strong oxidizing species. Because of its lower reduction potential (-330 mV for the $O_2/O_2^{\cdot-}$ redox couple), superoxide often acts as a reducing agent rather than an oxidizing species.
- Several biochemical properties determine the biological effects of superoxide. These include: (1) oxidation of iron-sulfur cluster (this is a particular case where superoxide acts as an oxidant); (2) reaction with nitric oxide to form peroxynitrite (a potent oxidant); and (3) acting as a reactant in the Haber–Weiss reaction, giving rise to hydroxyl radical, the most potent ROS formed in biological systems.
- The biological effects of superoxide are also affected by the antioxidant enzymes, especially superoxide dismutase.
- Superoxide plays important physiological roles. For example, it is the primary radical species produced during phagocytic respiratory burst, leading to the formation of secondary reactive species that kill invading pathogens.
- Uncontrolled production of superoxide may be responsible, at least partially, for the pathogenesis of various disease processes and related conditions in animal models. These include aging, cancer, cardiovascular diseases, diabetes, neurodegeneration, immunological disorders, pulmonary disorders, hepatic disorders, gastrointestinal diseases, and kidney diseases, among others.

7. SELF-ASSESSMENT QUESTIONS

7.1. It is now well known that superoxide is constitutively formed in diverse biological systems, including animals, plants, as well as microorganisms. This oxygen free radical has become a topic of intensive research in biology and medicine. Which of the following scientists first proposed the existence of superoxide based on the theory of quantum mechanics in the early 1930s?

A. Babior, Bernard
B. Fridovich, Irvine
C. Gershman, Rebecca
D. Murad, Ferid
E. Pauling, Linus

7.2. The biologically damaging potential of superoxide is attributed to its several unique chemical and biochemical properties. Which of the following best describes the chemical property of superoxide in biology and medicine?

A. Superoxide does not react with nitric oxide
B. Superoxide frequently acts as a reducing agent
C. Superoxide is a di-radical
D. Superoxide is a potent oxidant
E. Superoxide oxidizes ferric iron

7.3. The iron-catalyzed Haber–Weiss reaction was first proposed by Fritz Haber and Joseph Weiss in 1934. Which of the following reactive species is largely responsible for the oxidative damaging potential of the above reaction?

A. Hydroxyl radical
B. Hypochlorous acid
C. Nitric oxide
D. Peroxynitrite
E. Singlet oxygen

7.4. The biological effects of superoxide are affected by the presence of its cell and tissue defense system. Which of the following is the best characterized cellular defense against superoxide toxicity in mammals?

A. Glutathione S-transferase
B. NADPH:quinone oxidoreductase 1
C. Superoxide dismutase
D. Vitamin C
E. Vitamin E

7.5. Superoxide produced from phagocytic NADPH oxidase during respiratory burst is an important precursor molecule leading to the formation of more potent oxidizing species, especially hypochlorous acid, that kill the invading pathogenic microorganisms. Which of the following proteins is directly involved in catalyzing the formation of the above hypochlorous acid?

A. Catalase
B. Glutathione S-transferase
C. Myeloperoxidase
D. NADPH:quinone oxidoreductase 1
E. Superoxide dismutase

ANSWERS AND EXPLANATIONS

7.1. The answer is E. Linus Pauling, a twice-honored Nobel laureate (Chemistry in 1954; Peace in 1962) proposed the existence of superoxide based on the theory of quantum mechanics in 1933. He is also known for his proposal of using high doses of vitamin C to treat cancer.

7.2. The answer is B. Although it is called "superoxide", superoxide is in fact not a strong oxidizing species. Because of its lower reduction potential (-330 mV for the $O_2/O_2^{\cdot-}$ redox couple), this free radical often acts as a reducing agent rather than an oxidizing species.

7.3. The answer is A. Iron-catalyzed Haber–Weiss reaction produces hydroxyl radical, which is one of the most potent ROS that causes oxidation of all types of biomolecules, resulting in tissue injury.

7.4. The answer is C. The dismutation reaction of superoxide is catalyzed by SOD with a reaction rate constant of ~1.6×10^9 $M^{-1}s^{-1}$ which is over three orders of magnitude greater than that of spontaneous dismutation. In mammalian species, there are three types of SOD: CuZnSOD, MnSOD, and ECSOD, all of which catalyze dismutation of superoxide at a similar reaction rate constant, and represent the best known cellular defense system against superoxide toxicity.

7.5. The answer is C. Dismutation of phagocytic NADPH oxidase-derived superoxide generates hydrogen peroxide, which in turn reacts with chloride ion in the presence of the phagocyte-derived myeloperoxidase, forming hypochlorous acid.

REFERENCES

1. Pauling L. The discovery of the superoxide radical. *Trends Biochem Sci* 1979; 4(11):N270–N1.
2. Gerschman R, Gilbert DL, Nye SW, Dwyer P, Fenn WO. Oxygen poisoning and x-irradiation: a

mechanism in common. *Science* 1954; 119(3097):623–6.

3. Fridovich I, Handler P. Xanthine oxidase. V. Differential inhibition of the reduction of various electron acceptors. *J Biol Chem* 1962; 237:916–21.

4. Knowles PF, Gibson JF, Pick FM, Bray RC. Electron-spin-resonance evidence for enzymic reduction of oxygen to a free radical, the superoxide ion. *Biochem J* 1969; 111(1):53–8.

5. McCord JM, Fridovich I. Superoxide dismutase: an enzymic function for erythrocuprein (hemocuprein). *J Biol Chem* 1969; 244(22):6049–55.

6. Babior BM, Kipnes RS, Curnutte JT. Biological defense mechanisms. The production by leukocytes of superoxide, a potential bactericidal agent. *J Clin Invest* 1973; 52(3):741–4.

7. Li YR, Trush MA. Defining ROS in biology and medicine. *Reactive Oxygen Species* 2016; 1(1):9–21.

8. Zhu H. Assays for detecting biological superoxide. *Reactive Oxygen Species* 2016; 1(1):65–80.

9. Fridovich I. Superoxide anion radical ($O_2^{\cdot-}$), superoxide dismutases, and related matters. *J Biol Chem* 1997; 272(30):18515–7.

10. Gardner PR, Fridovich I. Superoxide sensitivity of the Escherichia coli aconitase. *J Biol Chem* 1991; 266(29):19328–33.

11. Gardner PR, Nguyen DD, White CW. Aconitase is a sensitive and critical target of oxygen poisoning in cultured mammalian cells and in rat lungs. *Proc Natl Acad Sci USA* 1994; 91(25):12248–52.

12. Diaz F, Enriquez JA, Moraes CT. Cells lacking Rieske iron-sulfur protein have a reactive oxygen species-associated decrease in respiratory complexes I and IV. *Mol Cell Biol* 2012; 32(2):415–29.

13. Radi R. Peroxynitrite, a stealthy biological oxidant. *J Biol Chem* 2013; 288(37):26464–72.

14. Murad F. Shattuck Lecture. Nitric oxide and cyclic GMP in cell signaling and drug development. *N Engl J Med* 2006; 355(19):2003–11.

15. Haber F, Weiss J. The catalytic decomposition of hydrogen peroxide by iron salts. *Proc R Soc A* 1934. p. 332–51.

16. Fenton HJ. Oxidation of tartaric acid in presence of iron. *J Chem Soc Trans* 1894; 65:899–910.

17. Mumbengegwi DR, Li Q, Li C, Bear CE, Engelhardt JF. Evidence for a superoxide permeability pathway in endosomal membranes. *Mol Cell Biol* 2008; 28(11):3700–12.

18. De Grey AD. $HO_2^{\cdot}$: the forgotten radical. *DNA Cell Biol* 2002; 21(4):251–7.

19. Li Y, Zhu H, Kuppusamy P, Zweier JL, Trush MA. Mitochondrial electron transport chain-derived superoxide exits macrophages: implications for mononuclear cell-mediated pathophysiological processes. *Reactive Oxygen Species* 2016; 1(1):81–98.

20. Kuhns DB, Alvord WG, Heller T, Feld JJ, Pike KM, Marciano BE, Uzel G, DeRavin SS, Priel DA, Soule BP, Zarember KA, Malech HL, et al. Residual NADPH oxidase and survival in chronic granulomatous disease. *N Engl J Med* 2010; 363(27):2600–10.

21. Watanabe S, Kita A, Kobayashi K, Miki K. Crystal structure of the [2Fe-2S] oxidative-stress sensor SoxR bound to DNA. *Proc Natl Acad Sci USA* 2008; 105(11):4121–6.

22. Demple B, Amabile-Cuevas CF. Redox redux: the control of oxidative stress responses. *Cell* 1991; 67(5):837–9.

23. Suh YA, Arnold RS, Lassegue B, Shi J, Xu X, Sorescu D, Chung AB, Griendling KK, Lambeth JD. Cell transformation by the superoxide-generating oxidase Mox1. *Nature* 1999; 401(6748):79–82.

24. Arnold RS, Shi J, Murad E, Whalen AM, Sun CQ, Polavarapu R, Parthasarathy S, Petros JA, Lambeth JD. Hydrogen peroxide mediates the cell growth and transformation caused by the mitogenic oxidase Nox1. *Proc Natl Acad Sci USA* 2001; 98(10):5550–5.

25. Pennisi E. Superoxides relay Ras protein's oncogenic message. *Science* 1997; 275(5306):1567–8.

26. Echtay KS, Roussel D, St-Pierre J, Jekabsons MB, Cadenas S, Stuart JA, Harper JA, Roebuck SJ, Morrison A, Pickering S, Clapham JC, Brand MD. Superoxide activates mitochondrial uncoupling proteins. *Nature* 2002; 415(6867):96–9.

27. Echtay KS, Murphy MP, Smith RA, Talbot DA, Brand MD. Superoxide activates mitochondrial uncoupling protein 2 from the matrix side: studies using targeted antioxidants. *J Biol Chem* 2002; 277(49):47129–35.

28. Hawkins BJ, Madesh M, Kirkpatrick CJ, Fisher AB. Superoxide flux in endothelial cells via the chloride channel-3 mediates intracellular signaling. *Mol Biol Cell* 2007; 18(6):2002–12.

29. Siegel D, Gustafson DL, Dehn DL, Han JY,

Boonchoong P, Berliner LJ, Ross D. NAD(P)H:quinone oxidoreductase 1: role as a superoxide scavenger. *Mol Pharmacol* 2004; 65(5):1238–47.

30. Zhu H, Jia Z, Mahaney JE, Ross D, Misra HP, Trush MA, Li Y. The highly expressed and inducible endogenous NAD(P)H:quinone oxidoreductase 1 in cardiovascular cells acts as a potential superoxide scavenger. *Cardiovasc Toxicol* 2007; 7(3):202–11.

31. Melov S, Schneider JA, Day BJ, Hinerfeld D, Coskun P, Mirra SS, Crapo JD, Wallace DC. A novel neurological phenotype in mice lacking mitochondrial manganese superoxide dismutase. *Nat Genet* 1998; 18(2):159–63.

32. Shen X, Zheng S, Metreveli NS, Epstein PN. Protection of cardiac mitochondria by overexpression of MnSOD reduces diabetic cardiomyopathy. *Diabetes* 2006; 55(3):798–805.

33. Li Y, Huang TT, Carlson EJ, Melov S, Ursell PC, Olson JL, Noble LJ, Yoshimura MP, Berger C, Chan PH, Wallace DC, Epstein CJ. Dilated cardiomyopathy and neonatal lethality in mutant mice lacking manganese superoxide dismutase. *Nat Genet* 1995; 11(4):376–81.

34. Orr WC, Sohal RS. Extension of life-span by overexpression of superoxide dismutase and catalase in *Drosophila melanogaster*. *Science* 1994; 263(5150):1128–30.

35. Melov S, Ravenscroft J, Malik S, Gill MS, Walker DW, Clayton PE, Wallace DC, Malfroy B, Doctrow SR, Lithgow GJ. Extension of life-span with superoxide dismutase/catalase mimetics. *Science* 2000; 289(5484):1567–9.

36. Kim SH, Kim MO, Gao P, Youm CA, Park HR, Lee TS, Kim KS, Suh JG, Lee HT, Park BJ, Ryoo ZY, Lee TH. Overexpression of extracellular superoxide dismutase (EC-SOD) in mouse skin plays a protective role in DMBA/TPA-induced tumor formation. *Oncol Res* 2005; 15(7–8):333–41.

37. Kensler TW, Bush DM, Kozumbo WJ. Inhibition of tumor promotion by a biomimetic superoxide dismutase. *Science* 1983; 221(4605):75–7.

38. Van Remmen H, Ikeno Y, Hamilton M, Pahlavani M, Wolf N, Thorpe SR, Alderson NL, Baynes JW, Epstein CJ, Huang TT, Nelson J, Strong R, et al. Life-long reduction in MnSOD activity results in increased DNA damage and higher incidence of cancer but does not accelerate aging. *Physiol Genomics* 2003; 16(1):29–37.

39. Yen HC, Oberley TD, Vichitbandha S, Ho YS, St Clair DK. The protective role of manganese superoxide dismutase against adriamycin-induced acute cardiac toxicity in transgenic mice. *J Clin Invest* 1996; 98(5):1253–60.

40. Lebovitz RM, Zhang H, Vogel H, Cartwright J, Jr., Dionne L, Lu N, Huang S, Matzuk MM. Neurodegeneration, myocardial injury, and perinatal death in mitochondrial superoxide dismutase-deficient mice. *Proc Natl Acad Sci USA* 1996; 93(18):9782–7.

41. Kubisch HM, Wang J, Luche R, Carlson E, Bray TM, Epstein CJ, Phillips JP. Transgenic copper/zinc superoxide dismutase modulates susceptibility to type I diabetes. *Proc Natl Acad Sci USA* 1994; 91(21):9956–9.

42. Murakami K, Murata N, Noda Y, Tahara S, Kaneko T, Kinoshita N, Hatsuta H, Murayama S, Barnham KJ, Irie K, Shirasawa T, Shimizu T. SOD1 (copper/zinc superoxide dismutase) deficiency drives amyloid beta protein oligomerization and memory loss in mouse model of Alzheimer disease. *J Biol Chem* 2011; 286(52):44557–68.

43. Massaad CA, Washington TM, Pautler RG, Klann E. Overexpression of SOD-2 reduces hippocampal superoxide and prevents memory deficits in a mouse model of Alzheimer's disease. *Proc Natl Acad Sci USA* 2009; 106(32):13576–81.

44. Marikovsky M, Ziv V, Nevo N, Harris-Cerruti C, Mahler O. Cu/Zn superoxide dismutase plays important role in immune response. *J Immunol* 2003; 170(6):2993–3001.

45. Iuchi Y, Okada F, Takamiya R, Kibe N, Tsunoda S, Nakajima O, Toyoda K, Nagae R, Suematsu M, Soga T, Uchida K, Fujii J. Rescue of anaemia and autoimmune responses in SOD1-deficient mice by transgenic expression of human SOD1 in erythrocytes. *Biochem J* 2009; 422(2):313–20.

46. Folz RJ, Abushamaa AM, Suliman HB. Extracellular superoxide dismutase in the airways of transgenic mice reduces inflammation and attenuates lung toxicity following hyperoxia. *J Clin Invest* 1999; 103(7):1055–66.

47. Yao H, Arunachalam G, Hwang JW, Chung S, Sundar IK, Kinnula VL, Crapo JD, Rahman I. Extracellular superoxide dismutase protects against pulmonary emphysema by attenuating oxidative fragmentation of ECM. *Proc Natl Acad Sci USA* 2010; 107(35):15571–6.

48. Wheeler MD, Nakagami M, Bradford BU,

Uesugi T, Mason RP, Connor HD, Dikalova A, Kadiiska M, Thurman RG. Overexpression of manganese superoxide dismutase prevents alcohol-induced liver injury in the rat. *J Biol Chem* 2001; 276(39):36664–72.

49. Laukkanen MO, Leppanen P, Turunen P, Tuomisto T, Naarala J, Yla-Herttuala S. EC-SOD gene therapy reduces paracetamol-induced liver damage in mice. *J Gene Med* 2001; 3(4):321–5.

50. Carroll IM, Andrus JM, Bruno-Barcena JM, Klaenhammer TR, Hassan HM, Threadgill DS. Anti-inflammatory properties of Lactobacillus gasseri expressing manganese superoxide dismutase using the interleukin 10-deficient mouse model of colitis. *Am J Physiol Gastrointest Liver Physiol* 2007; 293(4):G729–38.

51. Horie Y, Wolf R, Flores SC, McCord JM, Epstein CJ, Granger DN. Transgenic mice with increased copper/zinc-superoxide dismutase activity are resistant to hepatic leukostasis and capillary no-reflow after gut ischemia/reperfusion. *Circ Res* 1998; 83(7):691–6.

52. DeRubertis FR, Craven PA, Melhem MF, Salah EM. Attenuation of renal injury in db/db mice overexpressing superoxide dismutase: evidence for reduced superoxide- nitric oxide interaction. *Diabetes* 2004; 53(3):762–8.

53. Yin M, Wheeler MD, Connor HD, Zhong Z, Bunzendahl H, Dikalova A, Samulski RJ, Schoonhoven R, Mason RP, Swenberg JA, Thurman RG. Cu/Zn-superoxide dismutase gene attenuates ischemia-reperfusion injury in the rat kidney. *J Am Soc Nephrol* 2001; 12(12):2691–700.

54. Rosen DR, Siddique T, Patterson D, Figlewicz DA, Sapp P, Hentati A, Donaldson D, Goto J, O'Regan JP, Deng HX, et al. Mutations in Cu/Zn superoxide dismutase gene are associated with familial amyotrophic lateral sclerosis. *Nature* 1993; 362(6415):59–62.

55. Bird HZ, Hopkins RZ. Nanomaterials for selective superoxide dismutation. *Reactive Oxygen Species* 2016; 1(1):59–64.

Chapter 9

Hydrogen Peroxide in Biology and Medicine

ABSTRACT | Hydrogen peroxide (H_2O_2) is one of the most extensively investigated reactive oxygen species (ROS) in biology and medicine. It is generated constitutively from various cellular processes either directly through two-electron reduction of molecular oxygen or indirectly via dismutation of superoxide. The notable direct cellular sources for H_2O_2 include xanthine oxidoreductase, monoamine oxidase, endoplasmic reticulum oxidoreductin 1, oxidases in peroxisomes, and possibly certain members of the NOX/DUOX family. Because of the high activation energy, H_2O_2 reacts poorly with most cellular constituents. However, it may oxidize the cysteine thiol groups in certain proteins and enzymes, including those involved in cell signaling transduction. The potential of H_2O_2 to cause oxidative stress and tissue injury primarily results from its reactions with other molecules to form secondary more potent reactive species, including hydroxyl radical and hypochlorous acid. While the tightly controlled production of H_2O_2 plays important roles in various physiological responses, overproduction of this ROS contributes to the pathophysiology of a variety of disease processes and related conditions, including cardiovascular diseases, diabetes, neurodegeneration, cancer, and aging, among many others.

KEYWORDS | Catalase; Circadian rhythm; Disease pathophysiology; Endoplasmic reticulum oxidoreductin 1; Fenton reaction; Hydrogen peroxide; Hypochlorous acid; Immunity; Reactive oxygen species; Redox signaling; Stem cells; Superoxide; Wound healing; Xanthine oxidoreductase

CITATION | Hopkins RZ and Li YR. *Essentials of Free Radical Biology and Medicine. Cell Med Press, Raleigh, NC, USA. 2017. http://dx.doi.org/10.20455/efrbm.2017.09*

ABBREVIATIONS | CYP, cytochrome P450; ERO1, endoplasmic reticulum oxidoreductin 1; MAO, monoamine oxidase; MPO, myeloperoxidase; METC, mitochondrial electron transport chain; NOX, NADPH oxidase; ROS, reactive oxygen species; SOD, superoxide dismutase; XOR, xanthine oxidoreductase

CHAPTER AT A GLANCE

1. OVERVIEW

Hydrogen peroxide (H_2O_2) was discovered in 1818 by Louis Jacques Thénard (1777-1857), a French chemist [1], and the biological catalyst of H_2O_2 was identified and named as catalase in 1900 by Oscar Loew (1844-1941), a German chemist [2]. In the early 1970s, H_2O_2 was shown to be produced by animal cells and tissues [3-5]. It is now known that formation of H_2O_2 occurs ubiquitously in both animal and plant cells, as well as microorganisms. The past two decades have witnessed the explosion of knowledge on H_2O_2 in biology and medicine, ranging from its well established ability to cause oxidative stress and tissue injury to its emerging roles in cell signaling and normal physiology. Indeed, like superoxide (see Chapter 8), H_2O_2 is also among the most extensively investigated reactive oxygen species (ROS) in biology and medicine. A PubMed search using hydrogen peroxide or H_2O_2 as the key word in title/abstract resulted in 80,594 entries on December 14, 2016.

In biological systems, H_2O_2 is the primary product of superoxide dismutation, which occurs either spontaneously or catalyzed by superoxide dismutase (SOD). Hence, the sources of production as well as the biological activities of these two ROS overlap significantly. Different from superoxide, H_2O_2 is a non-radical species with a relatively long half-life in biological milieu and is able to readily cross cell membranes and diffuse into different cellular compartments. As such, H_2O_2 may act as a novel second messenger in cell signal transduction. This chapter considers the source, chemistry and biochemistry, as well as biology and medicine of this simple, but biologically unique molecule.

2. SOURCES

H_2O_2 is a major ROS formed in animal cells from various intracellular sources, which are discussed next. It is noteworthy that H_2O_2 is also formed in plant cells, with mitochondria and chloroplasts being the major sources [6]. In addition to the animal and plant kingdoms, H_2O_2 is found in Earth's atmosphere as well as interstellar space [7]. Regarding the cellular production of H_2O_2 in animals including humans, both direct and indirect mechanisms have been identified (**Figure 9.1**).

2.1. Indirect Formation via Superoxide Dismutation

H_2O_2 is formed through either the spontaneous or SOD-catalyzed dismutation of superoxide (see Figure 8.5 of Chapter 8). Therefore, the chief sources for superoxide formation are also the main ones for H_2O_2. In this context, NADPH oxidases (also known as NOXs) and mitochondrial electron transport chain (METC) are the primary sources of superoxide-derived H_2O_2 in mammalian cells. Other sources of superoxide-derived H_2O_2 include xanthine oxidoreductase, cytochrome P450 enzyme system, and uncoupled endothelial nitric oxide synthase (eNOS), among others (see Chapter 8).

2.2. Direct Formation via Two-Electron Reduction

Some enzymes in mammals including humans may directly catalyze the two-electron reduction of molecular oxygen to form H_2O_2 or predominately produce H_2O_2 via an unclear mechanism. These include xanthine oxidoreductase, monoamine oxidase, some members of the NOX/DUOX family (e.g., NOX4, DUOX1, DUOX2), and multiple oxidases in peroxisomes, among others.

2.2.1. Xanthine Oxidoreductase

As noted above, xanthine oxidoreductase catalyzes the one-electron reduction of molecular oxygen to form superoxide. This enzyme also directly catalyzes the two electron-reduction of molecular oxygen to form H_2O_2. Hence, xanthine oxidoreductase is capa-

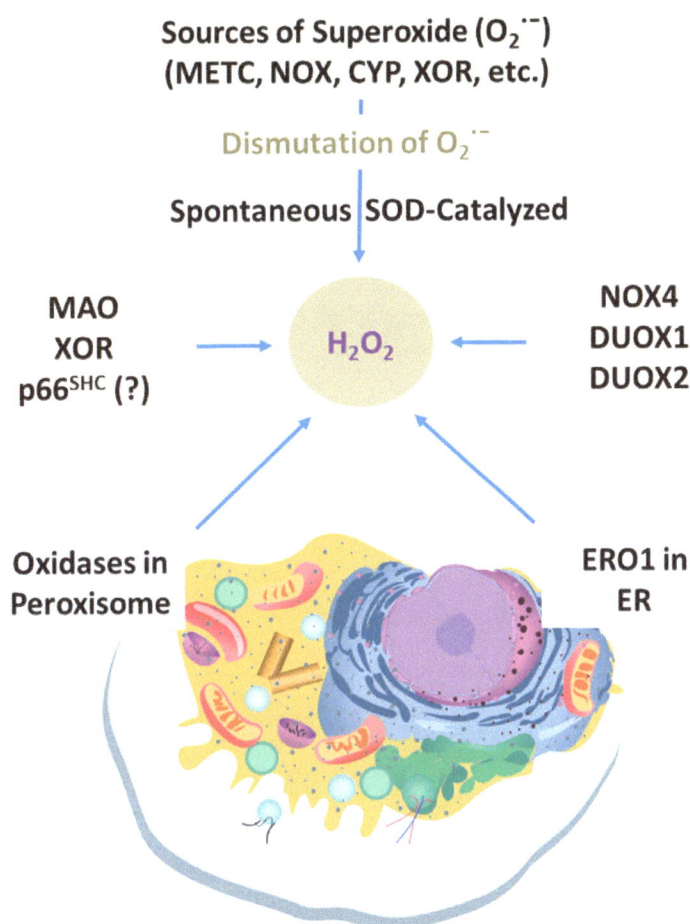

FIGURE 9.1. Cellular sources of hydrogen peroxide (H_2O_2). Cellular H_2O_2 production may result from either dismutation of superoxide or directly via two-electron reduction of molecular oxygen. Enzymes that directly catalyze two-electron reduction of molecular oxygen to form H_2O_2 include xanthine oxidoreductase (XOR), monoamine oxidase (MAO), endoplasmic reticulum (ER) oxidoreductin 1 (ERO1), and oxidases in the peroxisome, as well as possibly p66[SHC] and some members of the NADPH oxidase (NOX)/DUOX family (e.g., NOX4, DUOX1, DUOX2). XOR is also capable of catalyzing one-electron reduction of molecular oxygen to superoxide. METC, mitochondrial electron transport chain; CYP, cytochrome P450 system.

ble of causing both one- and two-electron reduction of molecular oxygen to form superoxide and H_2O_2, respectively [8].

2.2.2. Monoamine Oxidase

Another enzyme directly producing H_2O_2 is the flavin-dependent monoamine oxidase (MAO), which catalyzes deamination of dopamine via two-electron reduction of molecular oxygen to H_2O_2 [9]. There are two types of MAO: MAOA and MAOB, and both are located in mitochondrial outer membrane.

2.2.3. NOX/DUOX Family

While superoxide is the primary product of most NOX enzymes, NOX4 may predominantly produce H_2O_2 rather than superoxide [10, 11]. Dual oxidases 1 and 2 (DUOX1 and DUOX 2), members of the NOX/DUOX family, may also primarily generate H_2O_2 [12]. However, it remains unclear whether these enzymes can directly catalyze the two-electron reduction of oxygen to H_2O_2 or they produce H_2O_2 via a possible superoxide intermediate that may not be detected by current techniques due to rapid intramolecular dismutation or inaccessibility to the superoxide-detecting probes [12, 13].

2.2.4. Endoplasmic Reticulum

Endoplasmic reticulum (ER) is a significant source of cellular H_2O_2 due to the presence of various oxidoreductases in this organelle. While the cytochrome P450 enzyme (CYP) system associated with ER is a major indirect source of H_2O_2 (from dismutation of CYP-derived superoxide), oxidoreductases present in the ER lumen can directly reduce oxygen to form H_2O_2. For instance, the endoplasmic reticulum oxidoreductin 1 (ERO1), also known as endoplasmic reticulum oxidase 1, is a major source of H_2O_2 formed in the ER lumen [14]. The H_2O_2 produced by ERO1 plays an important role in oxidative protein folding in the ER. However, in cells lacking ERO1, H_2O_2 is also formed in the ER lumen and fuels peroxiredoxin 4-mediated oxidative protein folding, suggesting the existence of an unrecognized luminal source of H_2O_2 [15].

2.2.5. Oxidases in Peroxisomes

Peroxisomes contain various enzymes that produce H_2O_2 as part of their normal catalytic cycle. These enzymes include acyl-CoA oxidases, urate oxidase, D-amino acid oxidase, D-aspartate oxidase, L-pipecolic acid oxidase, L-α-hydroxyacid oxidase, polyamine oxidase, and xanthine oxidase [16]. The primary localization of catalase in peroxisomes is also in line with the notion that peroxisome is a H_2O_2-generating organelle.

2.2.6. Others

The mitochondria-associated redox protein p66^{SHC} is a genetic determinant of lifespan in mammals [17]. This redox protein may reduce oxygen to H_2O_2 by utilizing the reducing equivalents of the mitochondrial electron transport chain via oxidation of cytochrome c [18].

Although not naturally occurring in mammalian tissues, glucose oxidase, an enzyme expressed in certain fungal species, is among the best known enzymes for producing H_2O_2. Glucose oxidase catalyzes the oxidation of beta-D-glucose to gluconic acid, by utilizing molecular oxygen as an electron acceptor with simultaneous production of H_2O_2 [19, 20]. This enzyme has a number of industrial and biotechnological applications, with its use in measurement of blood glucose being most notable [19, 20].

3. CHEMISTRY AND BIOCHEMISTRY

3.1. General Aspects

H_2O_2 is a strong two-electron oxidant, with a standard reduction potential (H_2O_2/H_2O) of 1.32 V at pH 7.0. It is therefore more oxidizing than hypochlorous acid (OCl^-/Cl^-) and peroxynitrite ($ONOO^-/NO_2^-$), for which the standard reduction potentials are 1.28 and 1.20 V, respectively. However, in contrast to the above two oxidants, H_2O_2 reacts poorly or not at all with most biological molecules, including proteins, nucleic acids, and lipids, as well as low-molecular-weight antioxidants. This is because a high activation energy barrier must be overcome to release its oxidizing power, or in other words, the reactions of H_2O_2 are kinetically rather than thermodynamically driven [21].

Nevertheless, as discussed below, via two-electron oxidation, H_2O_2 reacts readily with certain biological molecules especially protein thiols to account for much of its signaling function. On the other hand, H_2O_2 is a weak one-electron oxidant with the standard reduction potential of 0.32 V ($H_2O_2/OH^•$). But, its reaction with transition metals (e.g., iron and copper) generates the highly reactive hydroxyl radical which may account for much of the detrimental effects of H_2O_2 in biological systems.

3.2. Oxidation of Protein Thiol Groups

Although in general the reaction between H_2O_2 and proteins is much limited, the cysteine thiol groups (also known as sulfhydryl groups) in certain proteins are readily oxidized by H_2O_2. These proteins include antioxidant enzymes (e.g., peroxiredoxins) and cell signaling molecules (e.g., certain transcription factors) [22–24]. Protein thiol oxidation is now recognized as a major chemical basis behind H_2O_2 sensing and signaling [25, 26] (see section below). However, extensive oxidation of protein thiols by large amounts of H_2O_2 causes irreversible oxidative protein damage, resulting in cell injury. **Figure 9.2** depicts the redox modifications of protein thiols by H_2O_2.

As illustrated in the above figure as well as **Figure 9.3**, mild oxidation of protein thiols by H_2O_2 results in the formation of protein sulfenic acid, which is unstable and readily reacts with an adjacent protein thiol group (either on the same protein or another protein) to form protein disulfides or with reduced form of glutathione (GSH) to become glutathionylated. The above redox modifications of proteins are

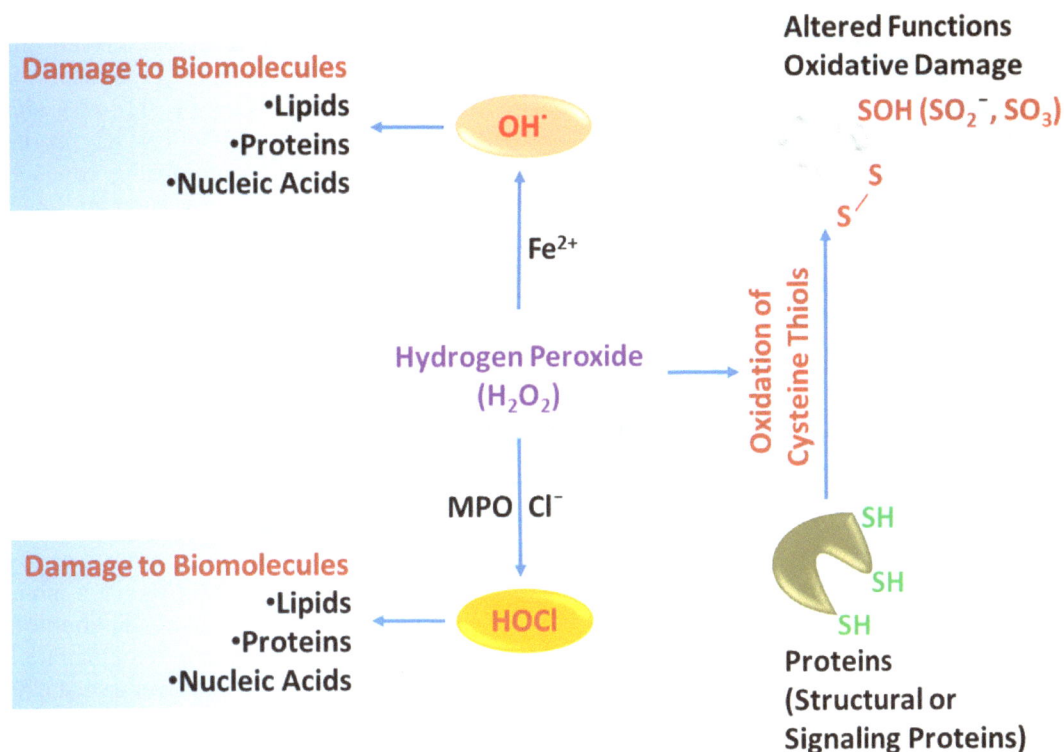

FIGURE 9.2. Chemical and biochemical reactivity of hydrogen peroxide (H_2O_2). As illustrated, H_2O_2 may directly react with the thiol groups of the cysteine residues in certain proteins, resulting in the formation of protein sulfenic acid (protein–SOH), sulfinic acid (protein–SO_2H), and sulfonic acid (protein–SO_3H). These modifications may cause altered protein function and oxidative protein damage depending on the levels and duration of H_2O_2 exposure (also see the legend of **Figure 9.3**). H_2O_2 reacts with transition metal ions, such as ferrous iron ion (Fe^{2+}), producing the highly reactive hydroxyl radical (OH·). Likewise, reaction between H_2O_2 and chloride ion (Cl^-) in the presence of myeloperoxidase (MPO) results in the formation of hypochlorous acid (HOCl), another potent oxidant. Production of these secondary reactive species is largely responsible for H_2O_2-induced oxidative damage in biological systems. Although hydrogen peroxide at high levels causes damage to cells and tissues, under certain circumstances, at lower levels it can act as a signaling molecule to participate in cell signal transduction

reversible via the actions of antioxidant enzymes, including thioredoxin and glutaredoxin systems (see Chapters 18 and 19). Such a reversible nature is instrumental in H_2O_2-mediated redox signaling.

On the other hand, prolonged exposure to large amounts of H_2O_2 can cause further oxidation of the protein sulfenic acid to form sulfinic acid and oxidation of sulfinic acid to form sulfonic acid. Such hyperoxidative modifications of protein thiols typically cause irreversible damage to the protein (**Figure 9.3**).

Hence, H_2O_2 serves as a signaling molecule only when its formation is tightly regulated. In this context, multiple families of enzymes are involved in the decomposition of H_2O_2 (see Section 4).

3.3. Fenton Reaction to Form Hydroxyl Radical

Reaction of H_2O_2 with transition metal ions gives rise to the formation of hydroxyl radical (OH·), an extremely potent oxidant. The Fenton reaction (Fe^{2+}

$+ H_2O_2 \rightarrow Fe^{3+} + OH^{\bullet} + OH^-$) is an important mechanism for H_2O_2-mediated oxidative damage (also see Section 3.3 of Chapter 8). Other metal ions such as cuprous ion (Cu^{1+}) can also catalyze the formation of hydroxyl radical from H_2O_2 via a similar reaction called Fenton-type reaction: $Cu^{1+} + H_2O_2 \rightarrow Cu^{2+} + OH^{\bullet} + OH^-$.

3.4. Reaction with Chloride Ion Forming Hypochlorous Acid

Reaction of H_2O_2 with chloride (Cl^-) generates hypochlorous acid (HOCl), a potent oxidant ($H_2O_2 + Cl^- \rightarrow HOCl + OH^-$). This reaction is catalyzed by myeloperoxidase (MPO) found in phagocytic cells. The HOCl formed is involved in the killing of invading microorganisms by phagocytic cells (also see Figure 8.7 of Chapter 8). On the other hand, abnormal formation of HOCl also contributes to tissue injury, such as atherosclerosis [27].

3.5. Reaction with Other Molecules

H_2O_2 oxidizes pyruvate to form acetate and CO_2 with a reaction rate constant of 2.2 $M^{-1}s^{-1}$ and as such, pyruvate may act as an efficient biological scavenger of H_2O_2 [28]. Indeed, pyruvate present in cell culture media or inside the cells has been shown to inhibit the biological activity of H_2O_2 [29–31].

H_2O_2 reacts with CO_2 to form peroxymonocarbonate ($H_2O_2 + CO_2 \rightarrow HCO_4^- + H^+$), which is much more reactive to thiols and methionine [21]. The biological significance of this reaction remains to be elucidated though peroxymonocarbonate may give rise to carbonate radical ($CO_3^{\bullet-}$), a potent oxidizing species. Reaction of H_2O_2 with CuZnSOD has also been shown to produce secondary oxidants and inactivation of the enzyme [32, 33].

3.6. Half-Life, Diffusion, and Membrane Permeability

In biological systems, H_2O_2 has a relatively long half-life in the range of minutes depending on the levels of surrounding H_2O_2-decomposing enzymes (e.g., catalase, glutathione peroxidase, peroxiredoxin). It has been long known that H_2O_2 readily crosses mammalian cell membranes. Recently, several specific aquaporin (water channel) isoforms (e.g., AQP3, AQP8, AQP9) are found to facilitate the passive diffusion of H_2O_2 across cell membranes and influence the cellular effects (e.g., cytotoxicity) of this ROS [34–36]. This is not surprising as water and H_2O_2

share similar physicochemical properties. Notably, aquaporin-facilitated H_2O_2 transport regulates H_2O_2 signaling [35, 37]. For example, a recent study shows that aquaporin-3-mediated H_2O_2 transport is required for nuclear factor kappaB (NF-κB) signaling in keratinocytes and development of psoriasis in an animal model [37]. Additionally, aquaporin-3 controls breast cancer cell migration and metastasis by regulating hydrogen peroxide transport and its downstream cell signaling (e.g., the Akt pathway) [38].

4. CELL AND TISSUE DEFENSES

H_2O_2 is decomposed to water by several enzymes in mammals including humans. These include catalase, glutathione peroxidase, and peroxiredoxin (see Appendix B). As noted earlier in Section 3.5, pyruvate (or pyruvic acid) present in biological systems can spontaneously detoxify H_2O_2 via a nonenzymatic decarboxylation reaction. In addition to pyruvate, other α-keto acids, such as α-ketoglutarate, oxaloacetate, glyoxylate may also scavenge H_2O_2 via a similar mechanism [39, 40].

5. BIOLOGY AND MEDICINE

As mentioned above, H_2O_2 is among the most extensively investigated ROS in biology and medicine. Substantial evidence points to that the important roles played by this ROS, ranging from both innate and adaptive immunity to cell signaling involved in stem cell proliferation and wound healing. On the other hand, abnormal production of H_2O_2 causes oxidative stress and tissue injury, thereby contributing to disease pathophysiology.

5.1. Innate Immunity

As a major product of phagocytic respiratory burst, H_2O_2 is involved in the killing of the invading pathogens via the formation of hypochlorous acid, a much more potent oxidant (see Section 3.4). H_2O_2 may also kill the microorganisms via the formation of hydroxyl radical through the Fenton reaction (see Section 3.3). In addition to its antiseptic role, a recent study using zebrafish shows that H_2O_2 formed by dual oxidase (DUOX) at the wound margin and the resulting H_2O_2 concentration gradient are required for the rapid recruitment of leukocytes to the wound [41]. This finding reveals a novel role for H_2O_2 in innate immunity.

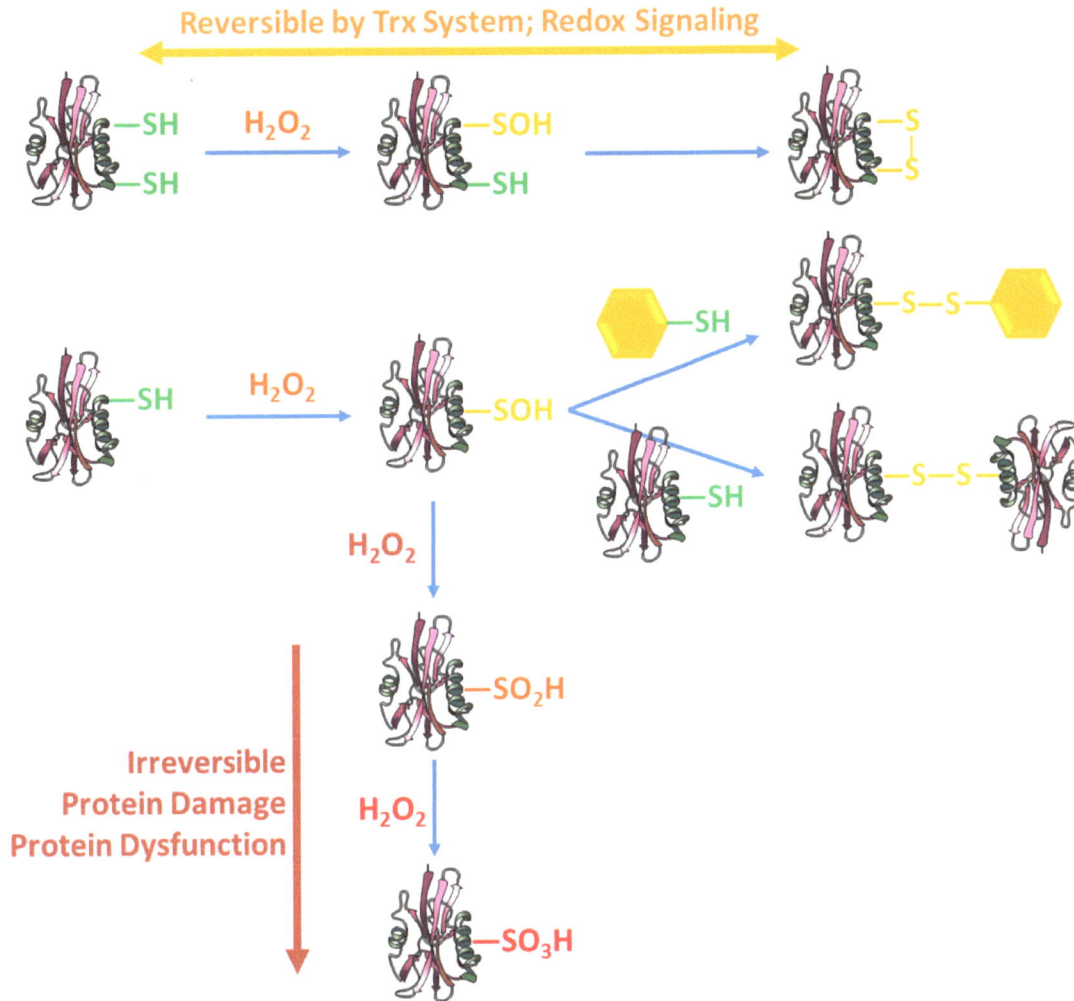

FIGURE 9.3. Thiol-dependent redox mechanisms of cell signaling mediated by hydrogen peroxide (H_2O_2). Oxidation of protein cysteine thiol groups by H_2O_2 is a major chemical basis for this ROS-mediated redox signaling. In this regard, a moderate and transient increase in the levels of H_2O_2 may cause oxidation of the cysteine thiols in certain signaling proteins, resulting in the formation of protein sulfenic acid (protein–SOH). Due to its high reactivity, the protein–SOH reacts with another cysteine thiol either on the same or another protein, forming protein disulfides (protein–S-S–protein). These reactions are reversible via the action of thioredoxin (Trx) system (see Appendix B). The reversibility of the above reactions makes it possible for H_2O_2 to transiently alter the functionality of the protein (e.g., a protein kinase or a transcription factor), ensuring redox signaling. On the other hand, high levels and prolonged duration of H_2O_2 exposure may cause further oxidation of protein sulfenic acid to form protein sulfinic acid (protein–SO_2H) and sulfonic acid (protein–SO_3H). These hyperoxidative reactions are generally irreversible and thereby cause significant protein dysfunction and oxidative damage.

5.2. Adaptive Immunity

Mitochondria-derived ROS have recently been demonstrated to play important roles in adaptive immunity, including regulation of T cell activation and CD8[+] memory T cell formation as well as B cell fate determination upon activation [42–44]. Although the exact ROS involved remain unclear, H_2O_2 appears to be the most likely ROS that acts as a signaling molecule to regulate adaptive immunity [45].

In this regard, H_2O_2 is among the best characterized ROS to be able to act as a second messenger in cell signal transduction.

5.3. Redox Signaling

It is well recognized that the regulated formation of H_2O_2 from various sources (including NOX and mitochondria) serves as an important mechanism of cell signaling. Oxidation of the cysteine thiol by H_2O_2 in signaling proteins (e.g., proteins kinases/phosphatase cascades, receptors, and transcription factors) appears to be a major molecular basis underlying H_2O_2-mediated cellular redox signal transduction [25, 26] (**Figure 9.3**).

Notably, a recent study shows that peroxiredoxin-2 (Prx2, a H_2O_2-decomposation enzyme) and STAT3 form a redox relay for H_2O_2 signaling. Specifically, H_2O_2 oxidizes Prx2, and the oxidized Prx2 forms a redox relay with the transcription factor STAT3 in which oxidative equivalents flow from Prx2 to STAT3. The redox relay generates disulfide-linked STAT3 oligomers with attenuated transcriptional activity. Cytokine-induced STAT3 signaling is accompanied by Prx2 and STAT3 oxidation and is modulated by Prx2 expression levels [46]. The redox signaling role of H_2O_2 explains its involvement in diverse conditions, such as stem cell proliferation and wound healing.

5.4. Stem Cell Biology

H_2O_2 is involved in stem cell biology. While high levels of H_2O_2 cause injury and shorten the lifespan of stem cells [47], regulated production of H_2O_2 may be essential for stem cell proliferation. In this regard, A study by Dickinson et al. shows that adult hippocampal stem/progenitor cells generate H_2O_2 through NOX2 to regulate intracellular growth signaling pathways, which in turn maintains their normal proliferation in vitro and in vivo [48].

5.5. Wound Healing

As noted above in Section 5.1, wounded epithelial cells release H_2O_2 and generate a tissue-scale gradient of H_2O_2, which guides leukocytes to the wound to kill invading pathogens, minimize infection, and promote healing [41]. In addition, low levels of H_2O_2 may also cause proliferation of keratinocytes and promote angiogenesis via augmenting epithelial growth factor and endothelial growth factor signaling, respectively [49, 50].

5.6. Circadian Rhythm

Light is the key entraining stimulus for the circadian clock, but several features of the signaling pathways that convert the photic signal to clock entrainment remain to be deciphered. Hirayama et al. show that light induces the production of H_2O_2 that acts as the second messenger coupling photoreception to the circadian clock in zebrafish [51]. Recent studies suggest that mitochondrial release of H_2O_2 is also likely a circadian event that conveys temporal information on steroidogenesis in the adrenal gland and on energy metabolism in the heart and brown adipose tissue to cytosolic signaling pathways [52, 53].

5.7. Disease Process

Due to its readily commercial availability, H_2O_2 is perhaps the most widely used chemical for studying oxidative stress in experimental models. Indeed, much of our current knowledge in oxidative stress results from studies using exogenous H_2O_2. Studies on the involvement of endogenously generated H_2O_2 in disease process have been frequently done with animal models of catalase gene knockout or overexpression. In this regard, like SOD for selectively metabolizing superoxide, catalase is a highly selective enzyme for the detoxification of H_2O_2. As such, the impact of manipulating cellular or tissue catalase on disease pathogenesis can be reasonably interpreted as a causal involvement of H_2O_2 in the disease process.

Using primarily catalase gene knockout or overexpression animal models, extensive studies over the past decades suggest an important role for H_2O_2-induced oxidative stress in a wide variety of disease processes and related conditions. These include various forms of cardiovascular disorders [54–58], diabetes and metabolic syndrome [59–61], multistage tumorigenesis [62–64], neurodegeneration [65, 66], pulmonary injury [67, 68], hepatic injury [69], and osteoporosis [70], as well as aging [71–74], among many others.

6. SUMMARY OF CHAPTER KEY POINTS

- H_2O_2 was discovered in 1818 by Louis Jacques Thénard (1777–1857), a French chemist, and it was first shown to be produced in animal tissues in the early 1970s.

- H_2O_2 production occurs as a result of either the spontaneous or the SOD-catalyzed dismutation of superoxide. Hence, the sources of superoxide formation in a biological system are typically also the sources for H_2O_2 production.

- Certain cellular enzymes may directly catalyze the two-electron reduction of molecular oxygen to form H_2O_2 or predominately produce H_2O_2 via an unclear mechanism. These include xanthine oxidoreductase, monoamine oxidase, some members of the NOX/DUOX family (e.g., NOX4, DUOX1, DUOX2), ERO1, and multiple oxidases in peroxisomes, among others.

- Owing to the high activation energy, H_2O_2 reacts poorly with most biomolecules. However, it may oxidize the thiol groups in certain proteins and enzymes, including those involved in cell signaling transduction.

- Reaction of H_2O_2 with transition metal ions gives rise to the formation of hydroxyl radical, an extremely potent oxidant. In the presence of MPO, H_2O_2 reacts with chloride ion to form hypochlorous acid, another potent oxidizing species. Formation of the above secondary reactive species is largely responsible for the damaging activity of H_2O_2 in biological systems.

- H_2O_2 has a relatively long half-life (~minutes) in most biological systems and readily crosses mammalian cell membranes via, at least partly, an aquaporin (water channel)-dependent mechanism.

- H_2O_2 is decomposed to water by several cellular antioxidant enzymes including catalase, glutathione peroxidase, and peroxiredoxin.

- Tightly controlled production of H_2O_2 plays important physiological roles, ranging from immunity and redox signaling to stem cell proliferation, wound healing, and circadian rhythm.

- Abnormal accumulation of H_2O_2 causes oxidative stress, contributing to the pathophysiology of diverse disease processes and related conditions, including cardiovascular disorders, diabetes, cancer, neurodegeneration, and aging, among many others.

7. SELF-ASSESSMENT QUESTIONS

7.1. In biological systems, H_2O_2 results from either dismutation of superoxide or via a direct two-electron reduction of molecular oxygen. Which of the following enzymes is known to be able to cause both one and two electron reduction of molecular oxygen to form superoxide and H_2O_2, respectively?

A. Catalase
B. Endothelial nitric oxide synthase
C. Monoamine oxidase
D. Superoxide dismutase
E. Xanthine oxidoreductase

7.2. Enzymes of the NOX/DUOX family are known as a major source of cellular ROS, including H_2O_2. In this context, which of the following NOX/DUOX members is also likely to produce H_2O_2 as the primary product?

A. NOX1
B. NOX2
C. NOX3
D. NOX4
E. NOX5

7.3. Endoplasmic reticulum (ER) is considered a significant source of cellular H_2O_2, and the H_2O_2 produced in the ER lumen is involved in the oxidative protein folding, a critical process leading to protein maturation. Which of the following enzymes contributes to the luminal production of H_2O_2?

A. DUOX1
B. ERO1
C. Myeloperoxidase
D. NOX3
E. Xanthine oxidase

7.4. H_2O_2 generally reacts poorly with most cellular macromolecules, including lipids, proteins, and nucleic acids. However, H_2O_2 reacts with chloride ions in the presence of phagocyte-derived myeloperoxidase to produce an extremely potent oxidizing species that may contribute to the killing of pathogens as well as oxidative tissue injury. Which of the following is this reactive species?

A. Hydroxyl radical
B. Hypochlorous acid
C. Nitric oxide
D. Peroxynitrite
E. Superoxide

7.5. It has long been known that H_2O_2 can readily cross cell membranes. Which of the following proteins may mediate the transport of this ROS across cell membranes?

A. Aquaporin 3
B. Ca^{2+}-ATPase
C. $CD4^+$ T cells
D. Interleukin-1 receptor
E. Sodium pump

ANSWERS AND EXPLANATIONS

7.1. The answer is C. Among the enzymes listed, only xanthine oxidoreductase is able to catalyze both one- and two-electron reduction of molecular oxygen to form superoxide and H_2O_2, respectively. Monoamine oxidase only catalyzes the two-electron reduction of oxygen to H_2O_2.

7.2. The answer is D. While superoxide is the primary product of most NOX enzymes, NOX4 may predominantly produce H_2O_2 rather than superoxide. However, it remains unclear whether NOX4 can directly catalyze the two-electron reduction of oxygen to H_2O_2 or it simply produces H_2O_2 via a possible superoxide intermediate that may not be detected by current techniques due to rapid intramolecular dismutation or inaccessibility to the superoxide-detecting probes.

7.3. The answer is B. The endoplasmic reticulum oxidoreductin 1 (ERO1), also known as endoplasmic reticulum oxidase 1, is a major source of H_2O_2 formed in the ER lumen.

7.4. The answer is B. Reaction of H_2O_2 with chloride (Cl^-) generates hypochlorous acid (HOCl), a highly potent oxidant ($H_2O_2 + Cl^- \rightarrow HOCl + OH^-$). This reaction is catalyzed by myeloperoxidase (MPO) found in phagocytic cells. The HOCl formed is a major reactive species for phagocyte-mediated killing of invading microorganisms.

7.5. The answer is A. Several specific aquaporin (water channel) isoforms (e.g., AQP3, AQP8, AQP9) are found to facilitate the passive diffusion of H_2O_2 across cell membranes as well as influence the cellular effects of H_2O_2.

REFERENCES

1. Thénard LJ. Observations sur des nouvelles combinaisons entre l'oxigène et divers acides. *Ann Chim Phys* 1818; 8:306–12.
2. Loew O. A new enzyme of general occurrence in organisms. *Science* 1900; 11:701–2.
3. Chance B, Oshino N. Kinetics and mechanisms of catalase in peroxisomes of the mitochondrial fraction. *Biochem J* 1971; 122(2):225–33.
4. Boveris A, Oshino N, Chance B. The cellular production of hydrogen peroxide. *Biochem J* 1972; 128(3):617–30.
5. Boveris A, Chance B. The mitochondrial generation of hydrogen peroxide: general properties and effect of hyperbaric oxygen. *Biochem J* 1973; 134(3):707–16.
6. Apel K, Hirt H. Reactive oxygen species: metabolism, oxidative stress, and signal transduction. *Annu Rev Plant Biol* 2004; 55:373–99.
7. Bergman P, Parise B, Liseau R, Larsson B, Olofsson H, Menten K, Güsten R. Detection of interstellar hydrogen peroxide. *Astronomy Astrophysics* 2011; 531:L8.
8. Porras AG, Olson JS, Palmer G. The reaction of reduced xanthine oxidase with oxygen: kinetics of peroxide and superoxide formation. *J Biol Chem* 1981; 256(17):9006–103.
9. Maker HS, Weiss C, Silides DJ, Cohen G. Coupling of dopamine oxidation (monoamine oxidase activity) to glutathione oxidation via the generation of hydrogen peroxide in rat brain homogenates. *J Neurochem* 1981; 36(2):589–93.
10. Faraci FM. Hydrogen peroxide: watery fuel for change in vascular biology. *Arterioscler Thromb Vasc Biol* 2006; 26(9):1931–3.
11. Takac I, Schroder K, Zhang L, Lardy B, Anilkumar N, Lambeth JD, Shah AM, Morel F, Brandes RP. The E-loop is involved in hydrogen peroxide formation by the NADPH oxidase Nox4. *J Biol Chem* 2011; 286(15):13304–13.
12. Bedard K, Krause KH. The NOX family of ROS-generating NADPH oxidases: physiology and pathophysiology. *Physiol Rev* 2007; 87(1):245–313.
13. Serrander L, Cartier L, Bedard K, Banfi B, Lardy B, Plastre O, Sienkiewicz A, Forro L, Schlegel W, Krause KH. NOX4 activity is determined by mRNA levels and reveals a unique pattern of ROS generation. *Biochem J* 2007; 406(1):105–14.
14. Gross E, Sevier CS, Heldman N, Vitu E, Bentzur M, Kaiser CA, Thorpe C, Fass D. Generating disulfides enzymatically: reaction products and electron acceptors of the endoplasmic reticulum thiol oxidase Ero1p. *Proc Natl Acad Sci USA* 2006; 103(2):299–304.
15. Konno T, Pinho Melo E, Lopes C, Mehmeti I, Lenzen S, Ron D, Avezov E. ERO1-independent production of H_2O_2 within the endoplasmic reticulum fuels Prdx4-mediated oxidative protein folding. *J Cell Biol* 2015; 211(2):253–9.
16. Fransen M, Nordgren M, Wang B, Apanasets O. Role of peroxisomes in ROS/RNS-metabolism: implications for human disease. *Biochim*

Biophys Acta 2012; 1822(9):1363–73.

17. Migliaccio E, Giorgio M, Mele S, Pelicci G, Reboldi P, Pandolfi PP, Lanfrancone L, Pelicci PG. The p66^{shc} adaptor protein controls oxidative stress response and life span in mammals. *Nature* 1999; 402(6759):309–13.

18. Giorgio M, Migliaccio E, Orsini F, Paolucci D, Moroni M, Contursi C, Pelliccia G, Luzi L, Minucci S, Marcaccio M, Pinton P, Rizzuto R, et al. Electron transfer between cytochrome c and p66^{Shc} generates reactive oxygen species that trigger mitochondrial apoptosis. *Cell* 2005; 122(2):221–33.

19. Bankar SB, Bule MV, Singhal RS, Ananthanarayan L. Glucose oxidase: an overview. *Biotechnol Adv* 2009; 27(4):489–501.

20. Wong CM, Wong KH, Chen XD. Glucose oxidase: natural occurrence, function, properties and industrial applications. *Appl Microbiol Biotechnol* 2008; 78(6):927–38.

21. Winterbourn CC. The biological chemistry of hydrogen peroxide. *Methods Enzymol* 2013; 528:3–25.

22. Calvo IA, Boronat S, Domenech A, Garcia-Santamarina S, Ayte J, Hidalgo E. Dissection of a redox relay: H$_2$O$_2$-dependent activation of the transcription factor Pap1 through the peroxidatic Tpx1-thioredoxin cycle. *Cell Rep* 2013; 5(5):1413–24.

23. Toledano MB, Delaunay-Moisan A. Keeping oxidative metabolism on time: mitochondria as an autonomous redox pacemaker animated by H$_2$O$_2$ and peroxiredoxin. *Mol Cell* 2015; 59(4):517–9.

24. Garcia-Santamarina S, Boronat S, Hidalgo E. Reversible cysteine oxidation in hydrogen peroxide sensing and signal transduction. *Biochemistry* 2014; 53(16):2560–80.

25. Veal EA, Day AM, Morgan BA. Hydrogen peroxide sensing and signaling. *Mol Cell* 2007; 26(1):1–14.

26. Rhee SG. Cell signaling. H$_2$O$_2$, a necessary evil for cell signaling. *Science* 2006; 312(5782):1882–3.

27. Binder V, Ljubojevic S, Haybaeck J, Holzer M, El-Gamal D, Schicho R, Pieske B, Heinemann A, Marsche G. The myeloperoxidase product hypochlorous acid generates irreversible high-density lipoprotein receptor inhibitors. *Arterioscler Thromb Vasc Biol* 2013; 33(5):1020–7.

28. Lopalco A, Dalwadi G, Niu S, Schowen RL, Douglas J, Stella VJ. Mechanism of decarboxylation of pyruvic acid in the presence of hydrogen peroxide. *J Pharm Sci* 2016; 105(2):705–13.

29. Desagher S, Glowinski J, Premont J. Pyruvate protects neurons against hydrogen peroxide-induced toxicity. *J Neurosci* 1997; 17(23):9060–7.

30. Salahudeen AK, Clark EC, Nath KA. Hydrogen peroxide-induced renal injury: a protective role for pyruvate in vitro and in vivo. *J Clin Invest* 1991; 88(6):1886–93.

31. Troxell B, Zhang JJ, Bourret TJ, Zeng MY, Blum J, Gherardini F, Hassan HM, Yang XF. Pyruvate protects pathogenic spirochetes from H$_2$O$_2$ killing. *PLoS One* 2014; 9(1):e84625.

32. Bonini MG, Gabel SA, Ranguelova K, Stadler K, Derose EF, London RE, Mason RP. Direct magnetic resonance evidence for peroxymonocarbonate involvement in the Cu,Zn-superoxide dismutase peroxidase catalytic cycle. *J Biol Chem* 2009; 284(21):14618–27.

33. Liochev SI, Fridovich I. Copper, zinc superoxide dismutase and H$_2$O$_2$: effects of bicarbonate on inactivation and oxidations of NADPH and urate, and on consumption of H$_2$O$_2$. *J Biol Chem* 2002; 277(38):34674–8.

34. Bienert GP, Moller AL, Kristiansen KA, Schulz A, Moller IM, Schjoerring JK, Jahn TP. Specific aquaporins facilitate the diffusion of hydrogen peroxide across membranes. *J Biol Chem* 2007; 282(2):1183–92.

35. Miller EW, Dickinson BC, Chang CJ. Aquaporin-3 mediates hydrogen peroxide uptake to regulate downstream intracellular signaling. *Proc Natl Acad Sci USA* 2010; 107(36):15681–6.

36. Watanabe S, Moniaga CS, Nielsen S, Hara-Chikuma M. Aquaporin-9 facilitates membrane transport of hydrogen peroxide in mammalian cells. *Biochem Biophys Res Commun* 2016; 471(1):191–7.

37. Hara-Chikuma M, Satooka H, Watanabe S, Honda T, Miyachi Y, Watanabe T, Verkman AS. Aquaporin-3-mediated hydrogen peroxide transport is required for NF-kappaB signalling in keratinocytes and development of psoriasis. *Nat Commun* 2015; 6:7454.

38. Satooka H, Hara-Chikuma M. Aquaporin-3 controls breast cancer cell migration by regulating hydrogen peroxide transport and its downstream cell signaling. *Mol Cell Biol* 2016; 36(7):1206–18.

39. Nath KA, Ngo EO, Hebbel RP, Croatt AJ, Zhou

B, Nutter LM. alpha-Ketoacids scavenge H_2O_2 in vitro and in vivo and reduce menadione-induced DNA injury and cytotoxicity. *Am J Physiol* 1995; 268(1 Pt 1):C227–36.

40. Kim JG, Park SJ, Sinninghe Damste JS, Schouten S, Rijpstra WI, Jung MY, Kim SJ, Gwak JH, Hong H, Si OJ, Lee S, Madsen EL, et al. Hydrogen peroxide detoxification is a key mechanism for growth of ammonia-oxidizing archaea. *Proc Natl Acad Sci USA* 2016; 113(28):7888–93.

41. Niethammer P, Grabher C, Look AT, Mitchison TJ. A tissue-scale gradient of hydrogen peroxide mediates rapid wound detection in zebrafish. *Nature* 2009; 459(7249):996–9.

42. Sena LA, Li S, Jairaman A, Prakriya M, Ezponda T, Hildeman DA, Wang CR, Schumacker PT, Licht JD, Perlman H, Bryce PJ, Chandel NS. Mitochondria are required for antigen-specific T cell activation through reactive oxygen species signaling. *Immunity* 2013; 38(2):225–36.

43. Okoye I, Wang L, Pallmer K, Richter K, Ichimura T, Haas R, Crouse J, Choi O, Heathcote D, Lovo E, Mauro C, Abdi R, et al. T cell metabolism. The protein LEM promotes $CD8^+$ T cell immunity through effects on mitochondrial respiration. *Science* 2015; 348(6238):995–1001.

44. Jang KJ, Mano H, Aoki K, Hayashi T, Muto A, Nambu Y, Takahashi K, Itoh K, Taketani S, Nutt SL, Igarashi K, Shimizu A, et al. Mitochondrial function provides instructive signals for activation-induced B-cell fates. *Nat Commun* 2015; 6:6750.

45. Gill T, Levine AD. Mitochondria-derived hydrogen peroxide selectively enhances T cell receptor-initiated signal transduction. *J Biol Chem* 2013; 288(36):26246–55.

46. Sobotta MC, Liou W, Stocker S, Talwar D, Oehler M, Ruppert T, Scharf AN, Dick TP. Peroxiredoxin-2 and STAT3 form a redox relay for H_2O_2 signaling. *Nat Chem Biol* 2015; 11(1):64–70.

47. Ito K, Hirao A, Arai F, Takubo K, Matsuoka S, Miyamoto K, Ohmura M, Naka K, Hosokawa K, Ikeda Y, Suda T. Reactive oxygen species act through p38 MAPK to limit the lifespan of hematopoietic stem cells. *Nat Med* 2006; 12(4):446–51.

48. Dickinson BC, Peltier J, Stone D, Schaffer DV, Chang CJ. Nox2 redox signaling maintains essential cell populations in the brain. *Nat Chem Biol* 2011; 7(2):106–12.

49. Lisse TS, King BL, Rieger S. Comparative transcriptomic profiling of hydrogen peroxide signaling networks in zebrafish and human keratinocytes: implications toward conservation, migration and wound healing. *Sci Rep* 2016; 6:20328.

50. Brauchle M, Funk JO, Kind P, Werner S. Ultraviolet B and H_2O_2 are potent inducers of vascular endothelial growth factor expression in cultured keratinocytes. *J Biol Chem* 1996; 271(36):21793–7.

51. Hirayama J, Cho S, Sassone-Corsi P. Circadian control by the reduction/oxidation pathway: catalase represses light-dependent clock gene expression in the zebrafish. *Proc Natl Acad Sci USA* 2007; 104(40):15747–52.

52. Kil IS, Ryu KW, Lee SK, Kim JY, Chu SY, Kim JH, Park S, Rhee SG. Circadian oscillation of sulfiredoxin in the mitochondria. *Mol Cell* 2015; 59(4):651–63.

53. Kil IS, Lee SK, Ryu KW, Woo HA, Hu MC, Bae SH, Rhee SG. Feedback control of adrenal steroidogenesis via H_2O_2-dependent, reversible inactivation of peroxiredoxin III in mitochondria. *Mol Cell* 2012; 46(5):584–94.

54. Kang YJ, Chen Y, Epstein PN. Suppression of doxorubicin cardiotoxicity by overexpression of catalase in the heart of transgenic mice. *J Biol Chem* 1996; 271(21):12610–6.

55. Yang H, Shi M, VanRemmen H, Chen X, Vijg J, Richardson A, Guo Z. Reduction of pressor response to vasoconstrictor agents by overexpression of catalase in mice. *Am J Hypertens* 2003; 16(1):1–5.

56. Yang H, Roberts LJ, Shi MJ, Zhou LC, Ballard BR, Richardson A, Guo ZM. Retardation of atherosclerosis by overexpression of catalase or both Cu/Zn-superoxide dismutase and catalase in mice lacking apolipoprotein E. *Circ Res* 2004; 95(11):1075–81.

57. Qin F, Lennon-Edwards S, Lancel S, Biolo A, Siwik DA, Pimentel DR, Dorn GW, Kang YJ, Colucci WS. Cardiac-specific overexpression of catalase identifies hydrogen peroxide-dependent and -independent phases of myocardial remodeling and prevents the progression to overt heart failure in G(alpha)q-overexpressing transgenic mice. *Circ Heart Fail* 2010; 3(2):306–13.

58. Dai DF, Santana LF, Vermulst M, Tomazela DM, Emond MJ, MacCoss MJ, Gollahon K, Martin GM, Loeb LA, Ladiges WC, Rabinovitch

PS. Overexpression of catalase targeted to mitochondria attenuates murine cardiac aging. *Circulation* 2009; 119(21):2789–97.

59. Ye G, Metreveli NS, Donthi RV, Xia S, Xu M, Carlson EC, Epstein PN. Catalase protects cardiomyocyte function in models of type 1 and type 2 diabetes. *Diabetes* 2004; 53(5):1336–43.

60. Gurgul E, Lortz S, Tiedge M, Jorns A, Lenzen S. Mitochondrial catalase overexpression protects insulin-producing cells against toxicity of reactive oxygen species and proinflammatory cytokines. *Diabetes* 2004; 53(9):2271–80.

61. Anderson EJ, Lustig ME, Boyle KE, Woodlief TL, Kane DA, Lin CT, Price JW, 3rd, Kang L, Rabinovitch PS, Szeto HH, Houmard JA, Cortright RN, et al. Mitochondrial H_2O_2 emission and cellular redox state link excess fat intake to insulin resistance in both rodents and humans. *J Clin Invest* 2009; 119(3):573–81.

62. Arnold RS, Shi J, Murad E, Whalen AM, Sun CQ, Polavarapu R, Parthasarathy S, Petros JA, Lambeth JD. Hydrogen peroxide mediates the cell growth and transformation caused by the mitogenic oxidase Nox1. *Proc Natl Acad Sci USA* 2001; 98(10):5550–5.

63. Preston TJ, Muller WJ, Singh G. Scavenging of extracellular H_2O_2 by catalase inhibits the proliferation of HER-2/Neu-transformed rat-1 fibroblasts through the induction of a stress response. *J Biol Chem* 2001; 276(12):9558–64.

64. Hart PC, Mao M, de Abreu AL, Ansenberger-Fricano K, Ekoue DN, Ganini D, Kajdacsy-Balla A, Diamond AM, Minshall RD, Consolaro ME, Santos JH, Bonini MG. MnSOD upregulation sustains the Warburg effect via mitochondrial ROS and AMPK-dependent signalling in cancer. *Nat Commun* 2015; 6:6053.

65. Sheikh FG, Pahan K, Khan M, Barbosa E, Singh I. Abnormality in catalase import into peroxisomes leads to severe neurological disorder. *Proc Natl Acad Sci USA* 1998; 95(6):2961–6.

66. Anderson PR, Kirby K, Orr WC, Hilliker AJ, Phillips JP. Hydrogen peroxide scavenging rescues frataxin deficiency in a Drosophila model of Friedreich's ataxia. *Proc Natl Acad Sci USA* 2008; 105(2):611–6.

67. Kozower BD, Christofidou-Solomidou M, Sweitzer TD, Muro S, Buerk DG, Solomides CC, Albelda SM, Patterson GA, Muzykantov VR. Immunotargeting of catalase to the pulmonary endothelium alleviates oxidative stress and reduces acute lung transplantation injury. *Nat Biotechnol* 2003; 21(4):392–8.

68. Rai P, Parrish M, Tay IJ, Li N, Ackerman S, He F, Kwang J, Chow VT, Engelward BP. Streptococcus pneumoniae secretes hydrogen peroxide leading to DNA damage and apoptosis in lung cells. *Proc Natl Acad Sci USA* 2015; 112(26):E3421–30.

69. Koliaki C, Szendroedi J, Kaul K, Jelenik T, Nowotny P, Jankowiak F, Herder C, Carstensen M, Krausch M, Knoefel WT, Schlensak M, Roden M. Adaptation of hepatic mitochondrial function in humans with non-alcoholic fatty liver is lost in steatohepatitis. *Cell Metab* 2015; 21(5):739–46.

70. Bartell SM, Kim HN, Ambrogini E, Han L, Iyer S, Serra Ucer S, Rabinovitch P, Jilka RL, Weinstein RS, Zhao H, O'Brien CA, Manolagas SC, et al. FoxO proteins restrain osteoclastogenesis and bone resorption by attenuating H_2O_2 accumulation. *Nat Commun* 2014; 5:3773.

71. Orr WC, Sohal RS. Extension of life-span by overexpression of superoxide dismutase and catalase in Drosophila melanogaster. *Science* 1994; 263(5150):1128–30.

72. Sohal RS, Agarwal A, Agarwal S, Orr WC. Simultaneous overexpression of copper- and zinc-containing superoxide dismutase and catalase retards age-related oxidative damage and increases metabolic potential in *Drosophila melanogaster. J Biol Chem* 1995; 270(26):15671–4.

73. Schriner SE, Linford NJ, Martin GM, Treuting P, Ogburn CE, Emond M, Coskun PE, Ladiges W, Wolf N, Van Remmen H, Wallace DC, Rabinovitch PS. Extension of murine life span by overexpression of catalase targeted to mitochondria. *Science* 2005; 308(5730):1909–11.

74. Umanskaya A, Santulli G, Xie W, Andersson DC, Reiken SR, Marks AR. Genetically enhancing mitochondrial antioxidant activity improves muscle function in aging. *Proc Natl Acad Sci USA* 2014; 111(42):15250–5.

Chapter 10

Hydroxyl Radicals in Biology and Medicine

ABSTRACT | Hydroxyl radical (OH˙) is the most potent oxidizing reactive oxygen species (ROS) formed in biological systems. In cells and tissues, production of OH˙ occurs primarily as a result of the metal ion-catalyzed Haber-Weiss reaction and Fenton or Fenton-type reaction. This ROS may also be formed in biological systems upon exposure to ionizing radiation and ultraviolet light or following the reaction between superoxide and hypochlorous acid. In addition to the biological systems, OH˙ is also ubiquitously present in the environments, including the natural water, soils and deserts, the atmosphere, and indoor air. The high concentrations of OH˙ in the indoor air arise from solar photolysis of nitrous acid, which is abundant in the air. The high levels of OH˙ in the lower atmosphere as well as in the indoor air might also have an impact on animals and humans. Due to its extreme oxidizing potential, OH˙ reacts non-selectively with all cellular biomolecules that it encounters and is considered as one of the ultimate reactive species causing oxidative stress and tissue injury. On the other hand, controlled production of OH˙ by phagocytic cells is part of the innate immunity. Many antibiotic drugs might also employ this powerful ROS to exert bactericidal activity.

KEYWORDS | Antibiotic; Fenton reaction; Haber–Weiss reaction; Homolysis; Hydrogen peroxide; Hydroxyl radical; Hypochlorous acid; Immunity; Nitrous acid; Peroxynitrous acid; Radiation

CITATION | *Hopkins RZ and Li YR. Essentials of Free Radical Biology and Medicine. Cell Med Press, Raleigh, NC, USA. 2017. http://dx.doi.org/10.20455/efrbm.2017.10*

ABBREVIATIONS | GSH, reduced form of glutathione; IR, ionizing radiation; ME-3HB, methyl-esterified dimers and trimers of 3-hydroxybutyrate; ROS, reactive oxygen species; UV, ultraviolet

CHAPTER AT A GLANCE

1. OVERVIEW

Hydroxyl radical (OH') was first reported by Fritz Haber and Joseph Weiss in 1934, in a reaction, which is now known as the iron-catalyzed Haber–Weiss reaction [1]. The concentrations of OH' in the ambient air were measured in 1975 [2]. A series of studies in the 1970s also demonstrated the formation of this free radical in cellular systems, including phagocytes [3–5]. The ubiquitous occurrence of OH' in various types of entities, including natural waters, soils and deserts, the atmosphere, biological systems, and interstellar space is now well-established [6].

OH' is probably the most powerful oxidizing reactive oxygen species (ROS) in biology and medicine. Due to its extreme oxidizing potential, OH' reacts non-selectively with all cellular biomolecules that it encounters and is one of the ultimate reactive species causing oxidative stress and tissue injury. This chapter first examines the sources of OH' formation, emphasizing the chemical reactions that give rise to OH' in biological systems. It then discusses the basic chemistry and biochemistry of this highly reactive ROS and its cell and tissue defenses. Lastly, the chapter considers the involvement of OH' in biology and medicine, elaborating primarily on its role in innate immunity, drug action, and disease process.

2. SOURCES

2.1. Biological Sources

In biological systems, OH' occurs primarily as a result of the one electron reduction of hydrogen peroxide (H_2O_2) by transition metal ions (the so called Fenton reaction). In addition, there exist several other potential sources of OH' formation in biological systems (**Figure 10.1**).

2.1.1. Haber–Weiss Reaction and Fenton Reaction

Iron-catalyzed Haber–Weiss reaction is a major source of OH' formation in biological systems [7, 8]. As noted previously in Chapter 8, the iron ion-catalyzed Haber–Weiss reaction includes two sequential sub-reactions: (1) $O_2^{·-} + Fe^{3+} \rightarrow O_2 + Fe^{2+}$, and (2) $Fe^{2+} + H_2O_2 \rightarrow Fe^{3+} + OH' + OH^-$. The second sub-reaction is commonly referred to as the Fenton reaction. In addition to iron, other transition metals, such as copper and chromium, also react with H_2O_2, forming OH'. Due to the availability of transition metal ions, especially iron and copper in cells

and tissues and the constitutive production of cellular H_2O_2, the formation of OH' appears to be inevitable. In this context, chronic dietary iron loading generates OH' in vivo [9, 10]. In addition to free iron ions, iron-containing proteins, such as ferritin and aconitase may also be involved in OH' generation via releasing the iron ions [11, 12]. Likewise, copper-containing proteins, such as Cu,Zn superoxide dismutase (CuZnSOD) also generate OH' upon reaction with H_2O_2 or hydroquinone [13–15]. The beta-amyloid fibrils in Alzheimer disease, when bound to copper ions, can react with H_2O_2, forming OH' [16]. it is noteworthy that both copper and iron are mobilized following myocardial ischemia, which might participate in Fenton or Fenton-type reaction, giving rise to OH' to cause tissue injury [17].

2.1.2. Radiation-Induced Homolysis

Radiation includes ionizing radiation (e.g., X-ray, gamma-radiation) and non-ionizing radiation (e.g., ultraviolet light, microwave). Ionizing radiation induces homolytic cleavage of water to form OH' and hydrogen atom (H') (Reaction 1; IR denotes ionizing radiation) in biological systems. It is noteworthy that hydrogen atom is a free radical because it contains only one electron. Ultraviolet (UV) light-induced homolytic cleavage of H_2O_2 also yields OH' (Reaction 2; UV denotes ultraviolet light). In chemistry, the term homolyic cleavage (also known as homolytic fission or homolysis) refers to the cleavage of a bond so that each of the molecular fragments between which the bond is broken retains one of the bonding electrons. Thus, the products of homolysis are free radicals.

$$H_2O + IR \rightarrow H' + OH' \quad (1)$$

$$H_2O_2 + UV \rightarrow 2\,OH' \quad (2)$$

Formation of OH' by the above reactions as well as radiation-induced secondary ROS may contribute to ionizing radiation- and UV light-elicited oxidative cell and tissue injury [18].

2.1.3. Reaction of Hypochlorous Acid with Superoxide

Reaction of hypochlorous acid (HOCl) with superoxide produces OH' (Reaction 3). This reaction is particularly relevant to inflammation responses during which both hypochlorous acid and superoxide are formed [19]. In addition to HOCl, superoxide may

Iron-Catalyzed Haber–Weiss Reaction

$$O_2^{\cdot-} + H_2O_2 \xrightarrow{Fe^{3+}/Fe^{2+}} OH^{\cdot} + OH^- + O_2$$

Fenton or Fenton-Type Reaction

$$Fe^{2+} + H_2O_2 \rightarrow Fe^{3+} + OH^{\cdot} + OH^-$$
$$Cu^{1+} + H_2O_2 \rightarrow Cu^{2+} + OH^{\cdot} + OH^-$$

IR

UV

H_2O

$OH^{\cdot}$

H_2O_2

$HOCl + O_2^{\cdot-}$

ONOOH

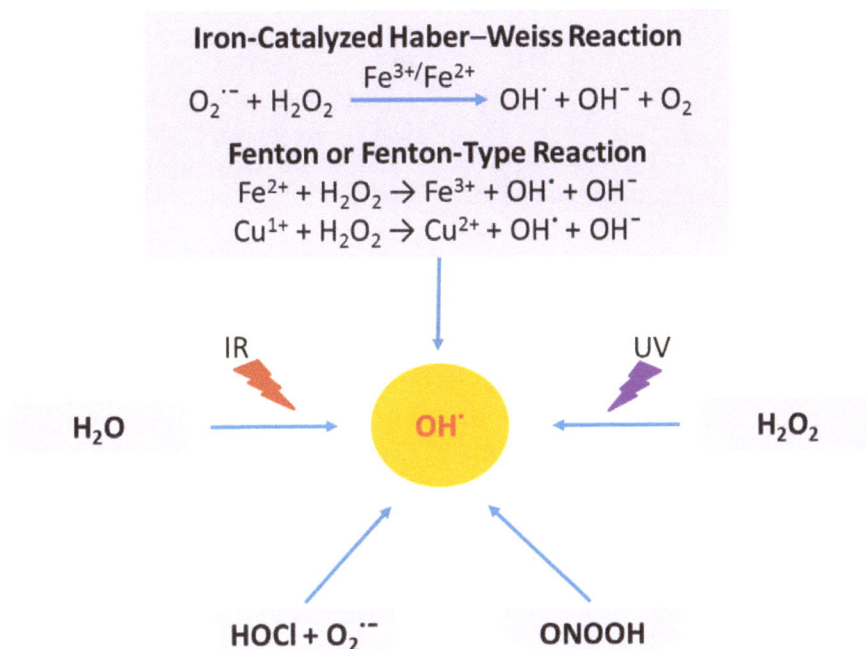

FIGURE 10.1. Hydroxyl radical (OH$^{\cdot}$) production in biological systems. As illustrated, iron-catalyzed Haber–Weiss reaction and Fenton or Fenton-type reaction are the primary sources of OH$^{\cdot}$ formation in cells and tissues. Other potential sources include ionizing radiation (IR)-induced homolysis of water, ultraviolet (UV) light-induced homolysis of H_2O_2, the reaction between superoxide ($O_2^{\cdot-}$) and hypochlorous acid (HOCl), and possibly the decomposition of peroxynitrous acid (ONOOH).

also react with other hypohalous acids to give rise to OH$^{\cdot}$ [20].

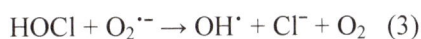

$$HOCl + O_2^{\cdot-} \rightarrow OH^{\cdot} + Cl^- + O_2 \quad (3)$$

2.1.4. Decomposition of Peroxynitrous Acid

Peroxynitrite anion (ONOO$^-$) becomes protonated to form peroxynitrous acid (ONOOH) (Reaction 4). Decomposition of peroxynitrous acid may produce OH$^{\cdot}$ and nitrogen dioxide radical (NO$_2^{\cdot}$) (Reaction 5) [21, 22]. However the significance of this route of OH$^{\cdot}$ formation in vivo is unclear (see Chapter 11).

$$ONOO^- + H^+ \rightarrow ONOOH \quad (4)$$

$$ONOOH \rightarrow OH^{\cdot} + NO_2^{\cdot} \quad (5)$$

2.2. Non-Biological Sources

As noted above, OH$^{\cdot}$ is also ubiquitously present in the environments, including the natural water, soils

and deserts, the atmosphere, and indoor air. The occurrence of this radical in the atmosphere and indoor air may also have important implications in biology and medicine.

2.2.1. Atmosphere

Reaction of electronically excited nitric dioxide (NO$_2$*) with water is reported to form OH$^{\cdot}$ via the following reaction: NO$_2$* + H$_2$O → OH$^{\cdot}$ + HONO. HONO is nitrous acid. The above reaction is considered a chemical mechanism of atmospheric OH$^{\cdot}$ production [23]. Notably, photolysis of nitrous acid also generates OH$^{\cdot}$ (HONO + hv → OH$^{\cdot}$ + NO$^{\cdot}$), and this reaction accounts for up to ~30% of the primary OH$^{\cdot}$ production in the lower atmosphere. Moreover, soil nitrite along with soil ammonia-oxidizing bacteria is an important source of atmospheric HONO, and fertilized soils with low pH appear to be particularly strong sources of HONO in the lower atmosphere [24, 25]. On the other hand, in the upper troposphere, OH$^{\cdot}$ formation occurs primarily via photolysis of ozone [6, 26]: $O_3 + h\nu \rightarrow O(^1D_2) + O_2$; $O(^1D_2) + H_2O \rightarrow 2\ OH^\cdot$, where $O(^1D_2)$ denotes excited state oxygen atom.

2.2.2. Indoor Air

The photolysis of HONO may also contribute to the $OH^\cdot$ production in the indoor air. In this regard, Alvarez et al. recently reported direct measurements of significant amount of $OH^\cdot$ of up to 1.8×10^6 molecules per cubic centimeter in a school classroom. This concentration is on the same order of magnitude of outdoor $OH^\cdot$ levels in the urban scenario. Direct solar irradiation inside the room results in high concentrations of $OH^\cdot$ via photolysis of HONO in the indoor air [27]. This finding may force a change in our understanding of indoor air quality and the impact of solar irradiation.

3. CHEMISTRY AND BIOCHEMISTRY

3.1. Reaction with Cellular Constituents

$OH^\cdot$ has a very high reduction potential (2.31 V for the redox couple of "$OH^\cdot$, H^+/H_2O"), and is known as the most powerful oxidizing species generated in biological systems. Due to its extreme high reduction potential, $OH^\cdot$ reacts with almost every type of biomolecules found in cells and tissues, including lipids, proteins, nucleic acids, amino acids, and carbohydrates. $OH^\cdot$ is believed to be one of the ultimate reactive species responsible for oxidative stress-induced tissue injury and disease process.

Besides causing oxidative damage, formation of $OH^\cdot$ might also be involved in redox signaling under specific conditions. The sensing of H_2O_2 is typically mediated by redox-active cysteines in sensors such as the bacterial OxyR, OhrR, and Hsp33 proteins, as well as eukaryotic signaling proteins (e.g., protein kinases/phosphatases, transcription factors). *Bacillus subtilis* PerR is the prototype for a widespread family of metal-dependent peroxide sensors that regulate inducible peroxide-defense genes. Sensing H_2O_2 by the iron-containing PerR may occur as a result of iron-catalyzed histidine oxidation via the formation of $OH^\cdot$ on the protein [28].

3.2. Half-Life, Diffusion, and Membrane Permeability

Due to its extremely high oxidizing capacity and extremely short half-life (1×10^{-9} s), $OH^\cdot$ reacts with the first biomolecule that it bumps into at a reaction rate constant very near the diffusion limit. Because of its very limited diffusion, damage of biomolecules typically occurs as a result of localized generation of $OH^\cdot$. This concept is also known as $OH^\cdot$-mediated site-specific damage. Because of its extreme short half-life, $OH^\cdot$ is unable to cross cell membranes.

4. CELL AND TISSUE DEFENSES

4.1. Non-Selective Defenses

$OH^\cdot$ reacts non-selectively with all cellular antioxidant compounds, including the reduced form of glutathione (GSH), ascorbic acid, and alpha-tocopherol. Hence, reaction of these antioxidant molecules or other non-vital biomolecules would protect the vital targets (e.g., DNA) from $OH^\cdot$ attack. However, it is also envisioned that $OH^\cdot$, if being generated on the vital target molecule, will readily cause damage to the target molecule, which would be unlikely or less effectively protected by nearby antioxidants.

4.2. Selective Defenses

It is noteworthy that some molecules may selectively react with $OH^\cdot$ and inhibit its toxicity. For example, molecular hydrogen (H_2) reacts with $OH^\cdot$ (Reaction 6), but not other ROS, and protects against oxidative injury in cultured cells. Inhalation of H_2 is also shown to protect against oxidative tissue injury in an animal model of cerebral ischemia-reperfusion injury [29, 30] (see Appendix B).

$$H_2 + OH^\cdot \rightarrow H_2O + H \quad (6)$$

A recent study shows that methyl-esterified dimers and trimers of 3-hydroxybutyrate (ME-3HB), produced by bacteria capable of polyhydroxybutyrate biosynthesis, have 3-fold greater $OH^\cdot$-scavenging activity than GSH and 11-fold higher activity than ascorbic acid or the monomer 3-hydroxybutyric acid. ME-3HB oligomers protect hypersensitive yeast deletion mutants lacking oxidative stress-response genes from $OH^\cdot$ stress [31].

In view of the extreme short half-life of $OH^\cdot$, it is generally believed that it is unlikely to have an enzymatic system for selective detoxification of $OH^\cdot$ in biological systems. In contrast to this notion, a study suggested that peroxiredoxin 1 from *Leishmania chagasi* might enzymatically detoxify $OH^\cdot$ [32] though the chemical mechanism remains unclear.

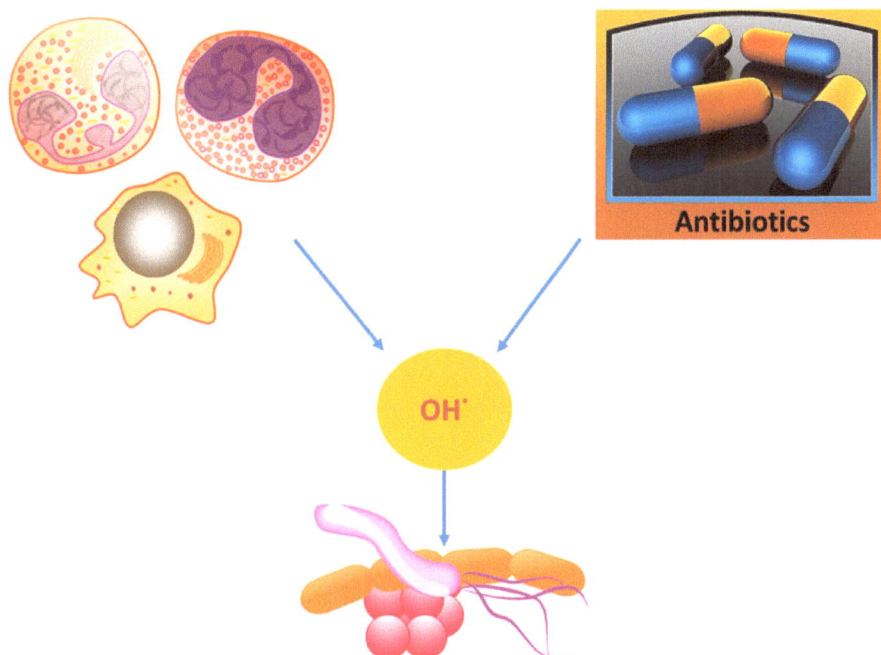

FIGURE 10.2. Involvement of hydroxyl radical (OH˙) formation in the killing of bacteria by phagocytes as well as antibiotic drugs. Interaction between invading bacteria and phagocytes causes phagocytic respiratory burst and formation of superoxide, hydrogen peroxide, and hypochlorous acid, as well as nitric oxide and peroxynitrite. Some of the reactive species can then react with each other to give rise to OH˙, the most powerful oxidizing species that causes killing of bacterial cells. Intriguingly, the three major classes of antibiotics (aminoglycosides, quinolones, and beta-lactams) are able to cause the formation of OH˙ via the Fenton reaction in the bacteria, which might be responsible, at least partly, for the bactericidal activity of these antibiotic drugs.

5. BIOLOGY AND MEDICINE

5.1. Immunity

As aforementioned, OH˙ is formed during phagocytic respiratory burst, a process leading to the formation of superoxide, and hydrogen peroxide, hypochlorous acid, as well as nitric oxide and peroxynitrite (see Figure 8.7 of Chapter 8). Although iron-catalyzed Haber-Weiss reaction is considered the chief source of phagocytic OH˙ production, the reaction between superoxide and hypochlorous acid as well as the decomposition of hypochlorous acid may also contribute to the OH˙ formation. The OH˙ not only is responsible for phagocyte-mediated killing of pathogens, but also might play a role in natural killer cell activity [33, 34]. Furthermore, as noted below, OH˙ production is also employed by drugs to kill target cells or microorganism (**Figure 10.2**).

5.2. Drug Action

Production of OH˙ in target cells might be an important mechanism of action of certain drugs, including anticancer drugs and antimicrobial agents [35–41]. In 2007, Kohanski et al. demonstrated for the first time that the three major classes of bactericidal antimicrobials (i.e., aminoglycosides, quinolones, and beta-lactams), regardless of drug-target interaction, stimulate the production of OH˙ in Gram-negative and Gram-positive bacteria, which ultimately contributes to cell death [36]. In contrast, bacteriostatic drugs do not produce OH˙. They further showed that the mechanism of OH˙ formation induced by bactericidal antibiotics is the end product of an oxidative damage cellular death pathway involving the tricarboxylic acid cycle, a transient depletion of nicotinamide adenine dinucleotide (NADH), destabilization of iron-sulfur clusters, and stimulation of the Fenton reaction [36]. Specifically, the common pathway model states that the primary drug-target interactions (aminoglycosides with the ribosome, quinolones with DNA gyrase, and beta-lactams with penicillin-binding proteins) stimulate oxidation of NADH via the electron transport chain that is dependent upon the tricarboxylic acid cycle in the bacteria. Hyperactivation of the electron transport chain stimulates superoxide formation, which in turn damages iron-sulfur clusters of proteins/enzymes, making ferrous iron available for oxidation by the Fenton reaction.

The Fenton reaction gives rise to $OH^{\cdot}$ formation, leading to oxidative damage to DNA, proteins, and lipids, which results in cell death [36]. This common pathway of antimicrobial-mediated cell death was supported by several subsequent studies [37–40, 42]. Notably, *Mycobacterium tuberculosis* is extremely sensitive to killing by $OH^{\cdot}$ derived from vitamin C-mediated Fenton reaction [41]. This finding highlights the potential to use $OH^{\cdot}$-generating modalities to treat infectious diseases that are difficult to treat with conventional antimicrobial drugs.

Despite its appeal, the above $OH^{\cdot}$-dependent model of antimicrobial lethality has been challenged by two studies reported in 2013, which found that antibiotic treatment did not promote the formation of ROS [43, 44]. In spite of these challenges, oxidative stress and redox alteration appear to be responsible, at least partly, for the killing of certain microorganisms by some antibiotics [45–47].

5.3. Disease Process

Although $OH^{\cdot}$, as discussed above, may be employed to achieve desirable effects as seen in innate immunity and antimicrobial therapy, uncontrolled production of, or prolonged exposure to, this free radical species inevitably causes oxidative damage to cellular constituents, leading to tissue injury and disease process. Indeed, $OH^{\cdot}$ is the most powerful ROS that readily causes DNA strand breaks and base modifications, protein oxidation, and lipid peroxidation. Reaction of $OH^{\cdot}$ with cellular constituents may result in the formation of secondary free radical and non-radical species, such as peroxyl radicals and reactive aldehydes. These secondary species, although less powerful than $OH^{\cdot}$, may also contribute to tissue injury and disease development. $OH^{\cdot}$ attack of vital cellular macromolecules not only causes structural damage, but also leads to malfunction of the molecules. For example, $OH^{\cdot}$-induced formation of 8-hydroxy-2′-deoxyguanosine (8-OH-dG) causes

base mispairing and mutations, which might contribute to cancer development [48–50]. Likewise, oxidative modifications of collagen type II by $OH^{\cdot}$ may increase its arthritogenicity and immunogenicity, contributing to the development of arthritic disorders [51].

The concept of $OH^{\cdot}$ as one of the major ultimate reactive species causing oxidative tissue injury and disease process has been around for decades, and this concept is in line with our current knowledge on the chemical and biochemical properties of this ROS. However, due to the lack of selective scavengers for $OH^{\cdot}$ as well as the lack of sensitive techniques to specifically detect in vivo $OH^{\cdot}$ production, the direct evidence for a causal role of $OH^{\cdot}$ in disease process is scarce. This also represents a general challenge for the entire field of free radical biology and medicine. Before techniques have become available to specifically detect and manipulate the levels of $OH^{\cdot}$ in biological systems, the exact causal role of this ROS in disease pathophysiology and development will remain largely speculated.

6. SUMMARY OF CHAPTER KEY POINTS

- $OH^{\cdot}$ was first reported by Fritz Haber and Joseph Weiss in 1934, in a reaction, which is now known as the iron-catalyzed Haber–Weiss reaction. The ubiquitous occurrence of $OH^{\cdot}$ in various types of entities, including natural waters, soils and deserts, the atmosphere, biological systems, and interstellar space is now well-established.

- In biological systems, $OH^{\cdot}$ occurs primarily as a result of the one electron reduction of H_2O_2 by transition metal ions via the so called Fenton or Fenton-type reaction.

- In addition, there are several other potential sources of $OH^{\cdot}$ formation in biological systems, including radiation-induced homolysis of cellular water or H_2O_2, the reaction between superoxide and hypochlorous acid, and possibly the decomposition of peroxynitrous acid.

- Due to its extreme high reduction potential, $OH^{\cdot}$ readily oxidizes almost every type of biomolecules found in cells and tissues, including lipids, proteins, nucleic acids, amino acids, and carbohydrates. Reactions between $OH^{\cdot}$ and cellular antioxidant compounds or other non-vital cellular molecules may protect vital molecular targets from $OH^{\cdot}$ attack.

- $OH^{\cdot}$ is formed by phagocytic cells and plays an important role in phagocyte-mediated killing of invading pathogens. OH˙ along with peroxynitrite and HOCl constitutes the chemical mechanism of pathogen-killing by innate immunity.

- Production of OH˙ in target cells might be an important mechanism of action of certain drugs, including anticancer drugs and antimicrobial agents. Production of OH˙ is considered a common mechanism of bactericidal antibiotics.

- Although OH˙ plays a desirable role in innate immunity and antimicrobial drug action, prolonged, uncontrolled production of this ROS inevitably causes oxidative cell and tissue injury, which might contribute to disease process.

- Due to the lack of selective scavengers for OH˙ as well as the lack of sensitive techniques to specifically detect in vivo OH˙ production, the direct evidence for a causal role of OH˙ in disease process remains scarce.

7. SELF-ASSESSMENT QUESTIONS

7.1. The term ROS refers to a group of oxygen-containing reactive chemical species. Which of the following ROS is considered the most powerful oxidizing species formed in biological systems?

A. Alkoxyl radical
B. Hydroxyl radical
C. Peroxyl radical
D. Singlet oxygen
E. Superoxide

7.2. A number of chemical reactions may contribute to the formation of hydroxyl radicals in cells and tissues. Which of the following is considered the major chemical reaction giving rise to hydroxyl radicals?

A. Decomposition of peroxynitrous acid
B. Homolysis of water
C. Iron-catalyzed Haber–Weiss reaction
D. Photolysis of nitrous acid
E. Photolysis of ozone

7.3. Hydroxyl radical has a very high reduction potential. Which of the following is the closest approximation of the reduction potential for the redox couple of "OH˙, H^+/H_2O" under a biologically relevant condition?

A. 150 mV
B. 282 mV

C. 320 mV
D. 2310 mV
E. 5700 mV

7.4. A series of recent studies suggest that certain antibiotics that belong to the major classes of antimicrobial drugs may kill bacteria via an oxidative stress mechanism. Which of the following ROS is most likely the ultimate reactive species responsible for the lethality?

A. Hydroxyl radical
B. Hypochlorous acid
C. Ozone
D. Peroxyl radical
E. Singlet oxygen

7.5. It is reported that high concentrations of hydroxyl radicals may occur in the indoor air. Which of the following reactions is most likely responsible for such high concentrations?

A. Fenton reaction
B. Haber–Weiss reaction
C. Homolysis of water vapor
D. Photolysis of nitrous acid
E. Photolysis of ozone

ANSWERS AND EXPLANATIONS

7.1. The answer is B. Hydroxyl radical is considered the most powerful oxidizing species formed in biological systems and it can oxidize nearly the entire spectrum of cellular molecules, including lipids, proteins, nucleic acids, and hydrocarbons.

7.2. The answer is C. Iron-catalyzed Haber–Weiss reaction is a major source of OH˙ formation in biological systems. This reaction consists of two sequential sub-reactions: (1) $O_2^{˙-} + Fe^{3+} \rightarrow O_2 + Fe^{2+}$, and (2) $Fe^{2+} + H_2O_2 \rightarrow Fe^{3+} + OH˙ + OH^-$. The second sub-reaction is commonly referred to as the Fenton reaction. The notion that iron-catalyzed Haber–Weiss reaction is a major source of cellular OH˙ is in line with the facts that both superoxide and hydrogen peroxide are constantly generated in aerobic cells that also contain iron and other redox metal ions.

7.3. The answer is D. Hydroxyl radical has a very high reduction potential (2.31 V for the redox couple of "OH˙, H^+/H_2O"), and is known as the most powerful oxidizing species generated in biological systems (refer to Table 5.1 of Chapter 5 for the standard reduction potential of common redox couples).

7.4. The answer is A. The Fenton reaction gives rise to hydroxyl radical formation, leading to oxidative damage to DNA, proteins, and lipids, which results in bacterial cell death.

7.5. The answer is D. A recent study reported direct measurements of significant amount of hydroxyl radicals of up to 1.8×10^6 molecules per cubic centimeter in a school classroom, and such high concentrations of hydroxyl radicals occur as a result of solar photolysis of nitrous acid in the indoor air: HONO + hv → OH· + NO·.

REFERENCES

1. Haber F, Weiss J, editors. The catalytic decomposition of hydrogen peroxide by iron salts. Proceedings of the Royal Society of London A: Mathematical, Physical and Engineering Sciences; 1934: The Royal Society.
2. Wang CC, Davis LI, Jr., Wu CH, Japar S, Niki H, Weinstock B. Hydroxyl radical concentrations measured in ambient air. *Science* 1975; 189(4205):797–800.
3. Weiss SJ, King GW, LoBuglio AF. Evidence for hydroxyl radical generation by human Monocytes. *J Clin Invest* 1977; 60(2):370–3.
4. Tauber AI, Babior BM. Evidence for hydroxyl radical production by human neutrophils. *J Clin Invest* 1977; 60(2):374–9.
5. Rosen H, Klebanoff SJ. Hydroxyl radical generation by polymorphonuclear leukocytes measured by electron spin resonance spectroscopy. *J Clin Invest* 1979; 64(6):1725–9.
6. Gligorovski S, Strekowski R, Barbati S, Vione D. Environmental Implications of Hydroxyl Radicals (·OH). *Chem Rev* 2015; 115(24):13051–92.
7. Starke PE, Farber JL. Ferric iron and superoxide ions are required for the killing of cultured hepatocytes by hydrogen peroxide: evidence for the participation of hydroxyl radicals formed by an iron-catalyzed Haber–Weiss reaction. *J Biol Chem* 1985; 260(18):10099–104.
8. Kehrer JP. The Haber–Weiss reaction and mechanisms of toxicity. *Toxicology* 2000; 149(1):43–50.
9. Kadiiska MB, Burkitt MJ, Xiang QH, Mason RP. Iron supplementation generates hydroxyl radical in vivo. An ESR spin-trapping investigation. *J Clin Invest* 1995; 96(3):1653–7.
10. Burkitt MJ, Mason RP. Direct evidence for in vivo hydroxyl-radical generation in experimental iron overload: an ESR spin-trapping investigation. *Proc Natl Acad Sci USA* 1991; 88(19):8440–4.
11. Thomas CE, Morehouse LA, Aust SD. Ferritin and superoxide-dependent lipid peroxidation. *J Biol Chem* 1985; 260(6):3275–80.
12. Vasquez-Vivar J, Kalyanaraman B, Kennedy MC. Mitochondrial aconitase is a source of hydroxyl radical: an electron spin resonance investigation. *J Biol Chem* 2000; 275(19):14064–9.
13. Yim MB, Chock PB, Stadtman ER. Copper, zinc superoxide dismutase catalyzes hydroxyl radical production from hydrogen peroxide. *Proc Natl Acad Sci USA* 1990; 87(13):5006–10.
14. Li Y, Kuppusamy P, Zweir JL, Trush MA. Role of Cu/Zn-superoxide dismutase in xenobiotic activation. II. Biological effects resulting from the Cu/Zn-superoxide dismutase-accelerated oxidation of the benzene metabolite 1,4-hydroquinone. *Mol Pharmacol* 1996; 49(3):412–21.
15. Sato K, Akaike T, Kohno M, Ando M, Maeda H. Hydroxyl radical production by H_2O_2 plus Cu,Zn-superoxide dismutase reflects the activity of free copper released from the oxidatively damaged enzyme. *J Biol Chem* 1992; 267(35):25371–7.
16. Mayes J, Tinker-Mill C, Kolosov O, Zhang H, Tabner BJ, Allsop D. Beta-Amyloid fibrils in Alzheimer disease are not inert when bound to copper ions but can degrade hydrogen peroxide and generate reactive oxygen species. *J Biol Chem* 2014; 289(17):12052–62.
17. Chevion M, Jiang Y, Har-El R, Berenshtein E, Uretzky G, Kitrossky N. Copper and iron are mobilized following myocardial ischemia: possible predictive criteria for tissue injury. *Proc Natl Acad Sci USA* 1993; 90(3):1102–6.
18. Halpern HJ, Yu C, Barth E, Peric M, Rosen GM. In situ detection, by spin trapping, of hydroxyl radical markers produced from ionizing radiation in the tumor of a living mouse. *Proc Natl Acad Sci USA* 1995; 92(3):796–800.
19. Candeias LP, Patel KB, Stratford MR, Wardman P. Free hydroxyl radicals are formed on reaction between the neutrophil-derived species superoxide anion and hypochlorous acid. *FEBS Lett* 1993; 333(1–2):151–3.

20. McCormick ML, Roeder TL, Railsback MA, Britigan BE. Eosinophil peroxidase-dependent hydroxyl radical generation by human eosinophils. *J Biol Chem* 1994; 269(45):27914–9.

21. Beckman JS, Beckman TW, Chen J, Marshall PA, Freeman BA. Apparent hydroxyl radical production by peroxynitrite: implications for endothelial injury from nitric oxide and superoxide. *Proc Natl Acad Sci USA* 1990; 87(4):1620–4.

22. Gerasimov OV, Lymar SV. The yield of hydroxyl radical from the decomposition of peroxynitrous acid. *Inorg Chem* 1999; 38(19):4317–21.

23. Li S, Matthews J, Sinha A. Atmospheric hydroxyl radical production from electronically excited NO_2 and H_2O. *Science* 2008; 319(5870):1657–60.

24. Su H, Cheng Y, Oswald R, Behrendt T, Trebs I, Meixner FX, Andreae MO, Cheng P, Zhang Y, Poschl U. Soil nitrite as a source of atmospheric HONO and OH radicals. *Science* 2011; 333(6049):1616–8.

25. Oswald R, Behrendt T, Ermel M, Wu D, Su H, Cheng Y, Breuninger C, Moravek A, Mougin E, Delon C, Loubet B, Pommerening-Roser A, et al. HONO emissions from soil bacteria as a major source of atmospheric reactive nitrogen. *Science* 2013; 341(6151):1233–5.

26. Rohrer F, Berresheim H. Strong correlation between levels of tropospheric hydroxyl radicals and solar ultraviolet radiation. *Nature* 2006; 442(7099):184–7.

27. Gomez Alvarez E, Amedro D, Afif C, Gligorovski S, Schoemaecker C, Fittschen C, Doussin JF, Wortham H. Unexpectedly high indoor hydroxyl radical concentrations associated with nitrous acid. *Proc Natl Acad Sci USA* 2013; 110(33):13294–9.

28. Lee JW, Helmann JD. The PerR transcription factor senses H_2O_2 by metal-catalysed histidine oxidation. *Nature* 2006; 440(7082):363–7.

29. Christensen H, Sehested K. Reaction of hydroxyl radicals with hydrogen at elevated temperatures. Determination of the activation energy. *J Phys Chem* 1983; 87(1):118–20.

30. Ohsawa I, Ishikawa M, Takahashi K, Watanabe M, Nishimaki K, Yamagata K, Katsura K, Katayama Y, Asoh S, Ohta S. Hydrogen acts as a therapeutic antioxidant by selectively reducing cytotoxic oxygen radicals. *Nat Med* 2007; 13(6):688–94.

31. Koskimaki JJ, Kajula M, Hokkanen J, Ihantola EL, Kim JH, Hautajarvi H, Hankala E, Suokas M, Pohjanen J, Podolich O, Kozyrovska N, Turpeinen A, et al. Methyl-esterified 3-hydroxybutyrate oligomers protect bacteria from hydroxyl radicals. *Nat Chem Biol* 2016; 12(5):332–8.

32. Barr SD, Gedamu L. Cloning and characterization of three differentially expressed peroxidoxin genes from *Leishmania chagasi*: evidence for an enzymatic detoxification of hydroxyl radicals. *J Biol Chem* 2001; 276(36):34279–87.

33. Suthanthiran M, Solomon SD, Williams PS, Rubin AL, Novogrodsky A, Stenzel KH. Hydroxyl radical scavengers inhibit human natural killer cell activity. *Nature* 1984; 307(5948):276–8.

34. Duwe AK, Werkmeister J, Roder JC, Lauzon R, Payne U. Natural killer cell-mediated lysis involves an hydroxyl radical-dependent step. *J Immunol* 1985; 134(4):2637–44.

35. Doroshow JH. Role of hydrogen peroxide and hydroxyl radical formation in the killing of Ehrlich tumor cells by anticancer quinones. *Proc Natl Acad Sci USA* 1986; 83(12):4514–8.

36. Kohanski MA, Dwyer DJ, Hayete B, Lawrence CA, Collins JJ. A common mechanism of cellular death induced by bactericidal antibiotics. *Cell* 2007; 130(5):797–810.

37. Kohanski MA, Dwyer DJ, Wierzbowski J, Cottarel G, Collins JJ. Mistranslation of membrane proteins and two-component system activation trigger antibiotic-mediated cell death. *Cell* 2008; 135(4):679–90.

38. Davies BW, Kohanski MA, Simmons LA, Winkler JA, Collins JJ, Walker GC. Hydroxyurea induces hydroxyl radical-mediated cell death in Escherichia coli. *Mol Cell* 2009; 36(5):845–60.

39. Kashyap DR, Wang M, Liu LH, Boons GJ, Gupta D, Dziarski R. Peptidoglycan recognition proteins kill bacteria by activating protein-sensing two-component systems. *Nat Med* 2011; 17(6):676–83.

40. Grant SS, Kaufmann BB, Chand NS, Haseley N, Hung DT. Eradication of bacterial persisters with antibiotic-generated hydroxyl radicals. *Proc Natl Acad Sci USA* 2012; 109(30):12147–52.

41. Vilcheze C, Hartman T, Weinrick B, Jacobs WR, Jr. *Mycobacterium tuberculosis* is extraordinarily sensitive to killing by a vitamin C-induced Fenton reaction. *Nat Commun* 2013;

4:1881.

42. Foti JJ, Devadoss B, Winkler JA, Collins JJ, Walker GC. Oxidation of the guanine nucleotide pool underlies cell death by bactericidal antibiotics. *Science* 2012; 336(6079):315–9.

43. Keren I, Wu Y, Inocencio J, Mulcahy LR, Lewis K. Killing by bactericidal antibiotics does not depend on reactive oxygen species. *Science* 2013; 339(6124):1213–6.

44. Liu Y, Imlay JA. Cell death from antibiotics without the involvement of reactive oxygen species. *Science* 2013; 339(6124):1210–3.

45. Dwyer DJ, Belenky PA, Yang JH, MacDonald IC, Martell JD, Takahashi N, Chan CT, Lobritz MA, Braff D, Schwarz EG, Ye JD, Pati M, et al. Antibiotics induce redox-related physiological alterations as part of their lethality. *Proc Natl Acad Sci USA* 2014; 111(20):E2100–9.

46. Belenky P, Ye JD, Porter CB, Cohen NR, Lobritz MA, Ferrante T, Jain S, Korry BJ, Schwarz EG, Walker GC, Collins JJ. Bactericidal antibiotics induce toxic metabolic perturbations that lead to cellular damage. *Cell Rep* 2015; 13(5):968–80.

47. Dwyer DJ, Collins JJ, Walker GC. Unraveling the physiological complexities of antibiotic lethality. *Annu Rev Pharmacol Toxicol* 2015; 55:313–32.

48. Cheng KC, Cahill DS, Kasai H, Nishimura S, Loeb LA. 8-Hydroxyguanine, an abundant form of oxidative DNA damage, causes G–T and A–C substitutions. *J Biol Chem* 1992; 267(1):166–72.

49. Kuchino Y, Mori F, Kasai H, Inoue H, Iwai S, Miura K, Ohtsuka E, Nishimura S. Misreading of DNA templates containing 8-hydroxydeoxyguanosine at the modified base and at adjacent residues. *Nature* 1987; 327(6117):77–9.

50. Malins DC, Polissar NL, Gunselman SJ. Progression of human breast cancers to the metastatic state is linked to hydroxyl radical-induced DNA damage. *Proc Natl Acad Sci USA* 1996; 93(6):2557–63.

51. Shahab U, Ahmad S, Moinuddin, Dixit K, Habib S, Alam K, Ali A. Hydroxyl radical modification of collagen type II increases its arthritogenicity and immunogenicity. *PLoS One* 2012; 7(2):e31199.

Chapter 11

Peroxynitrite in Biology and Medicine

ABSTRACT | Since the demonstration of peroxynitrite as a biological oxidant in the early 1990s, substantial studies over the past two decades have established peroxynitrite as a major reactive oxygen species in biology and medicine. In biological systems, the diffusion-limited reaction between superoxide and nitric oxide is the chief source of peroxynitrite formation. Peroxynitrite possesses high one- and two-electron reduction potentials and causes oxidation of cellular biomolecules, including lipids, proteins, and DNA either directly or indirectly via forming secondary reactive species. Peroxynitrite reacts with metal centers, sulfhydryl groups, and tyrosine residues of proteins, causing protein damage and dysfunction. Attack of lipids by peroxynitrite induces lipid peroxidation. Interaction between peroxynitrite and DNA elicits DNA base modifications and strand breaks. These adverse effects of peroxynitrite are affected by cell and tissue defenses that scavenge or decompose this reactive species. These include reduced form of glutathione (GSH), glutathione peroxidase, and peroxiredoxin. While uncontrolled production of peroxynitrite results in oxidative and nitrative stress, leading to cell and tissue injury, controlled production of peroxynitrite may fulfil important physiological functions. These include participating in killing the invading pathogens by innate immunity and potentially acting as a second messenger in cell signal transduction.

KEYWORDS | Cell signaling; Disease process; Glutathione peroxidase; Innate immunity; Nitration; Nitric oxide; 3-Nitrotyrosine; Peroxiredoxin; Peroxynitrite; Peroxynitrous acid; Redox modulation; Superoxide

CITATION | Hopkins RZ and Li YR. *Essentials of Free Radical Biology and Medicine. Cell Med Press, Raleigh, NC, USA. 2017. http://dx.doi.org/10.20455/efrbm.2017.11*

ABBREVIATIONS | CBS, cystathionine β-synthase; GSH, reduced form of glutathione; MDSC, myeloid-derived suppressor cell; NOS, nitric oxide synthase; NOX, NADPH oxidase; PARP, poly(ADP-ribose) polymerase; ROS, reactive oxygen species; SERCA, sarco-endoplasmic reticulum Ca^{2+} ATPase; TCR, T cell receptor

CHAPTER AT A GLANCE

1. OVERVIEW

The possible formation of peroxynitrite ($ONOO^-$) (also known as peroxynitrite anion) was first suggested in 1901 by Adolf Baeyer (1835–1917) and Victor Villiger (1868–1934) in their studies on the reactions between nitrites and hydrogen peroxide [1]. Both were German Chemists, and A. Baeyer was awarded the Nobel Prize for Chemistry in 1905 for his work on organic dyes and hydroaromatic compounds. In 1935, peroxynitrite was reported to be synthesized from the reaction of hydrogen peroxide and nitrite at a low pH [2]. However, the chemistry of peroxynitrite was not thoroughly investigated until 1970, when several studies demonstrated the decomposition of peroxynitrite to form nitric dioxide and hydroxyl radical (see refs in [3]). In a 1985 paper, Neil V. Blough and Oliver C. Zafiriou for the first time demonstrated the reaction of superoxide with nitric oxide to form peroxynitrite (then called peroxonitrite) in an alkaline aqueous solution [4]. This was an important observation that was followed by a number of studies in the early 1990s showing peroxynitrite as a biologically relevant oxidant capable of reacting with cellular constituents [5–8]. Since then, substantial studies over the past two decades have established peroxynitrite as an important reactive oxygen species (ROS) in biology and medicine. This chapter first provides an overview on the biological sources of peroxynitrite, discussing the major chemical reactions that give rise to this ROS. The chapter then considers the chemistry and biochemistry of peroxynitrite, and its major cell and tissue defenses. Lastly, the chapter examines the roles of peroxynitrite in biology and medicine, elaborating primarily on its involvement in innate immunity, cell signaling, and disease process.

2. SOURCES

2.1. Reaction between Superoxide and Nitric Oxide

Both superoxide ($O_2^{\cdot-}$) and nitric oxide ($NO^\cdot$) (see Chapter 12 for nitric oxide and related nitrogen oxides) are formed constitutively in biological systems. The reaction between these two radical species is considered the primary source of biological peroxynitrite (**Figure 11.1**). Because both superoxide and nitric oxide are free radicals, the above reaction is a bi-radical reaction. This bi-radical reaction occurs at a diffusion-limited rate ($k = 4–16 \times 10^9$ $M^{-1}s^{-1}$) which is much higher than that of superoxide dismutase-catalyzed dismutation of superoxide ($k = 1–2 \times 10^9$ $M^{-1}s^{-1}$). As such, peroxynitrite forms upon the simultaneous occurrence of superoxide and nitric oxide in a biological system.

2.2. Other Reactions

In addition to the above classic pathway ($O_2^{\cdot-}$ + $NO^\cdot \rightarrow ONOO^-$), other reactions might also contribute to the formation of peroxynitrite in biological systems. For example, nitroxyl (NO^-) reacts with molecular oxygen forming peroxynitrite (NO^- + O_2 $\rightarrow ONOO^-$) [9, 10]. Since nitroxyl may be released endogenously by a variety of biomolecules, this reaction might generate a significant amount of peroxynitrite in biological systems.

Cystathionine β-synthase (CBS) is a pyridoxal phosphate-dependent heme-containing enzyme that catalyzes the condensation of homocysteine with serine or with cysteine to form cystathionine and either water or hydrogen sulfide, respectively. Recently, CBS has been shown to catalyze the reduction of nitrite (NO_2^-) to form peroxynitrite [11]. This might constitute a previously unrecognized cellular source of peroxynitrite.

3. CHEMISTRY AND BIOCHEMISTRY

3.1. General Chemical Properties

Although it is a non-radical, peroxynitrite is much more reactive than its precursors, namely, superoxide and nitric oxide. Peroxynitrite possesses high one-electron and two-electron reduction potentials, being 1400 mV ($ONOO^-$, 2 $H^+/NO_2^\cdot$, H_2O) and 1200 mV ($ONOO^-$, 2 H^+/NO_2^-, H_2O), respectively [12]. As such, peroxynitrite acts as a potent biological oxidant capable of reacting with a wide range of cellular constituents, including lipids, proteins, and nucleic acids.

In addition to its direct reaction with biomolecules, peroxynitrite may also give rise to secondary reactive species that cause biological damage. For example, decomposition of peroxynitrous acid (ONOOH, the

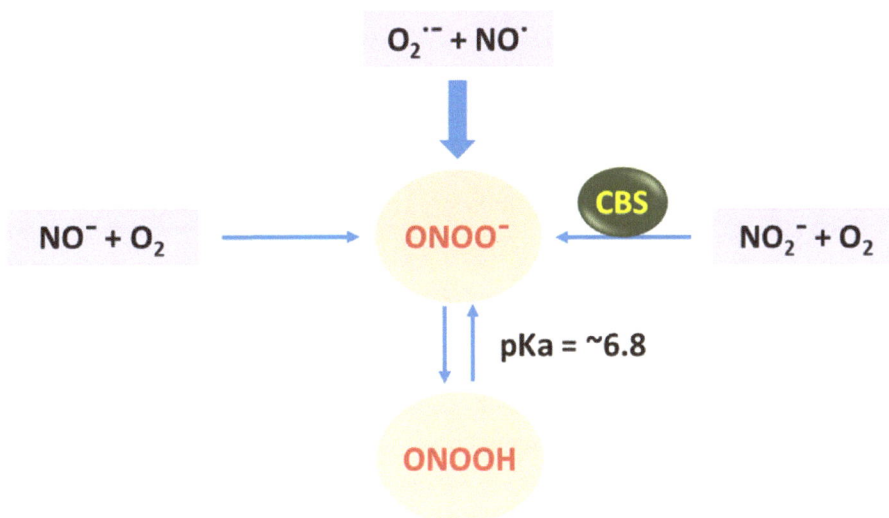

FIGURE 11.1. Peroxynitrite (ONOO⁻) production in biological systems. As illustrated, the diffusion-limited reaction between superoxide ($O_2^{\cdot-}$) and nitric oxide ($NO^\cdot$) is the primary source of ONOO⁻ formation in cells and tissues. Other potential sources include the reaction of nitroxyl (NO^-) with molecular oxygen as well as the cystathionine β-synthase (CBS)-catalyzed reduction of nitrite (NO_2^-). As also depicted in the figure, peroxynitrite exists in equilibrium with its protonated form (ONOOH) (pka = ~6.8)

protonated form of peroxynitrite) (see Section 3.3 below) forms hydroxyl radical ($OH^\cdot$) and nitrogen dioxide ($NO_2^\cdot$) (Reaction 1) [5], both being highly reactive species capable of damaging biomolecules. It is noteworthy that nitrogen dioxide, like nitric oxide ($NO^\cdot$), is a free radical and the superscript dot indicates the unpaired electron. Like nitric oxide being frequently written as NO with the superscript dot omitted, nitrogen dioxide is also written as NO_2. Thus, $NO_2^\cdot$ and NO_2 refer to the same chemical species.

$$ONOOH \rightarrow OH^\cdot + NO_2^\cdot \quad (1)$$

Peroxynitrite also reacts with carbon dioxide (CO_2), resulting in the formation of carbonate radical ($CO_3^{\cdot-}$) and nitrogen dioxide via an unstable intermediate nitrosoperoxycarbonate ($ONOOCO_2^-$) (Reaction 2) [13, 14].

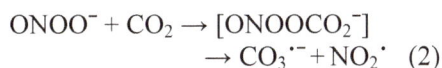

$$ONOO^- + CO_2 \rightarrow [ONOOCO_2^-]$$
$$\rightarrow CO_3^{\cdot-} + NO_2^\cdot \quad (2)$$

The $CO_3^{\cdot-}$ formed from Reaction 2 is a potent oxidant capable of oxidizing biomolecules. Due to the presence of high levels of CO_2 in cells and tissues, the above reaction pathway is believed to play a ma-

jor role in peroxynitrite-induced biological injury in vivo. On the contrary, the decomposition of peroxynitrous acid to form hydroxyl radical and nitrogen dioxide (Reaction 1) is believed to be insignificant in vivo [3]. **Figure 11.2** illustrates the chemical mechanisms involved in peroxynitrite-mediated adverse effects in biological systems.

3.2. Reaction with Cellular Constituents

3.2.1. Proteins

Peroxynitrite reacts readily with iron-sulfur clusters of several enzymes, including mitochondrial aconitase and the enzyme complexes of the mitochondrial electron transport chain, leading to enzyme inactivation [15–17]. Peroxynitrite causes oxidation of the zinc-thiolate complex of the endothelial nitric oxide synthase (eNOS), leading to increased eNOS uncoupling and generation of superoxide [18]. Peroxynitrite is also able to oxidize the sulfhydryl groups of proteins, causing protein dysfunction and enzyme inactivation [6]. Exposure to peroxynitrite results in tyrosine nitration of proteins in tissues.

Protein tyrosine nitration refers to the addition of a nitroso (-NO₂) group adjacent to the hydroxyl group on the aromatic ring of the tyrosine residue. Upon

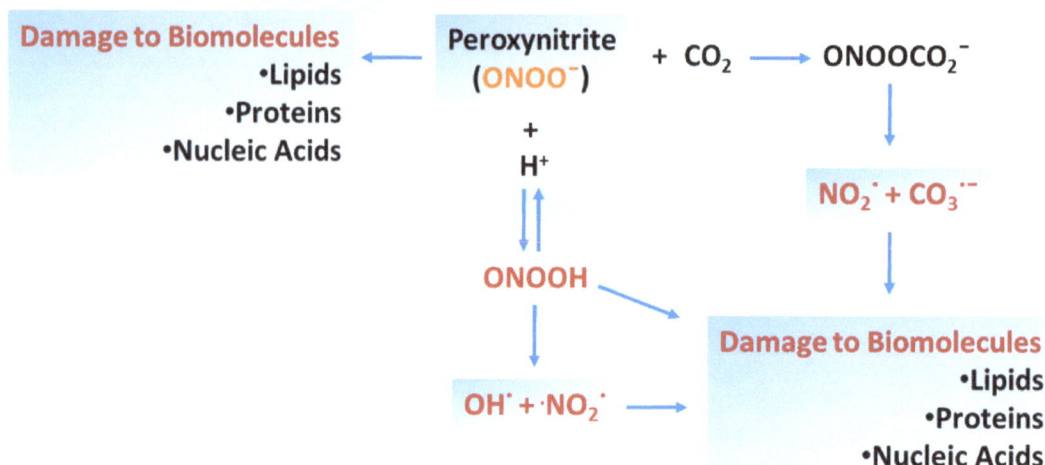

FIGURE 11.2. Chemical and biochemical reactivity of peroxynitrite (ONOO⁻) in biological systems. As depicted, peroxynitrite may directly react with cellular constituents, including lipids, proteins, and nucleic acid, causing damage to these biomolecules. More importantly, reaction of peroxynitrite with carbon dioxide forms nitrosoperoxycarbonate ($ONOOCO_2^-$), an unstable intermediate giving rise to carbonate radical ($CO_3^{\cdot-}$) and nitrogen dioxide ($NO_2^\cdot$), which are also highly reactive and able to cause damage to biomolecules. Less importantly, decomposition of peroxynitrous acid (ONOOH) may lead to the formation of hydroxyl radical ($OH^\cdot$) and nitrogen dioxide. In addition, peroxynitrous acid may also directly cause damage to biomolecules.

exposure to peroxynitrite, tyrosine nitration in tissues occurs in a two-step reaction in which the peroxynitrite-derived $CO_3^{\cdot-}$ abstracts a hydrogen atom from the tyrosine residue, generating a tyrosine radical. This tyrosine radical then reacts with the peroxynitrite-derived $NO_2^\cdot$, giving rise to 3-nitrotyrosine (**Figure 11.3**).

3-Nitrotyrosine is an indicator of peroxynitrite formation in biological systems. 3-Nitrotyrosine can, however, also be formed from the interaction of other reactive species with tyrosine residue. Thus, 3-nitrotyrosine is not a specific biomarker for peroxynitrite formation in cells or tissues. Regardless of the reactive species involved in the formation of 3-nitrotyrosine, tyrosine nitration modifies protein function and has been identified in a number of pathophysiological conditions. For example, nitration of the pro-survival chaperone heat shock protein 90 (Hsp90) in positions 33 and 56 induces motor neuron

death through a toxic gain-of-function mechanism [19].

It is necessary to define a few terms and symbols related to the discussion in this chapter. The anion NO_3^- as in $NaNO_3$ is called nitrate anion, whereas NO_2^- as in $NaNO_2$ is called nitrite anion. The chemical group $-NO_2$ is a nitro group, whereas $-NO$ is a nitroso group. The term nitration refers to addition of a nitro ($-NO_2$) group to a compound, whereas nitrosation refers to the addition of a nitroso ($-NO$) group to a thiol. The covalent attachment of an $-NO$ group to a thiol group of a protein is called S-nitrosation (or more commonly, but less accurately, called S-nitrosylation). S-Nitrosylation is an important mechanism of post-translational regulation of protein functions. It conveys a large part of the ubiquitous influence of nitric oxide on cell signaling and provides a mechanism of redox-based physiological regulation in mammals. Dysregulation of protein S-

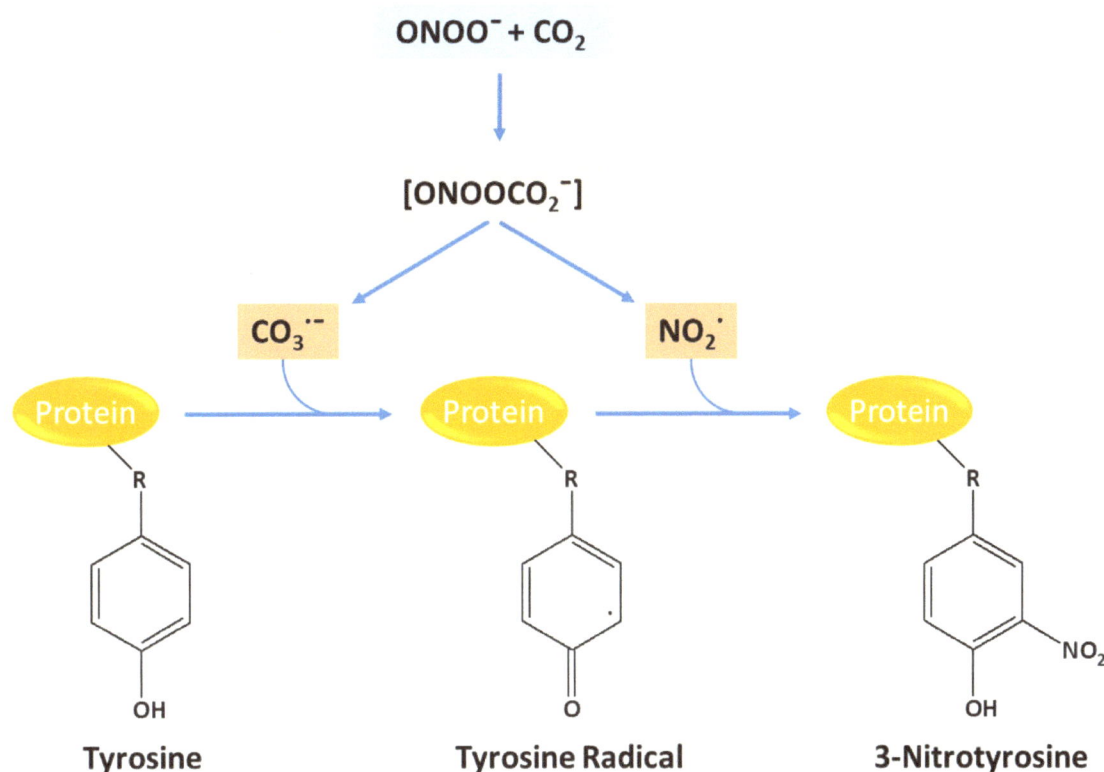

FIGURE 11.3. Formation of 3-nitrotyrosine following exposure to peroxynitrite (ONOO⁻). As shown, peroxynitrite reacts with carbon dioxide present in cells or tissues to form carbonate radical ($CO_3^{•-}$) and nitrogen dioxide ($NO_2^{•}$) via an unstable intermediate, nitrosoperoxycarbonate ($ONOOCO_2^{-}$). The carbonate radical is a potent oxidant and abstracts a hydrogen atom from a protein tyrosine residue, generating a tyrosine radical. This tyrosine radical then reacts with the peroxynitrite-derived nitrogen dioxide, giving rise to 3-nitrotyrosine.

nitrosylation is associated with a growing list of pathophysiological conditions [20].

3.2.2. Lipids

Peroxynitrite can cause lipid peroxidation in biomembranes and lipoproteins by abstracting a hydrogen atom from polyunsaturated fatty acids. This occurs likely via the formation of secondary reactive radical species from peroxynitrite [7]. Interaction of peroxynitrite with membrane lipids also leads to the formation of various nitrated lipids [21]. Nitrated lipids may act as mediators of cell signal transduction [22, 23].

3.2.3. Nucleic Acids

Peroxynitrite can damage DNA by introducing oxidative modifications in both bases and sugar-phosphate backbone. Among the four bases, guanine base is most reactive to peroxynitrite due to its low reduction potential. The major product of guanine oxidation is 8-hydroxyguanine [24]. Peroxynitrite can also nitrate guanine, yielding 8-nitroguanine [25]. Attack on the sugar-phosphate backbone by peroxynitrite causes DNA strand breaks, which may trigger the activation of the nuclear enzyme poly(ADP-ribose) polymerase (PARP). Sustained activation of PARP can lead to cell death and tissue inflammatory response [26].

3.3. Half-Life, Diffusion, and Membrane Permeability

The half-life of peroxynitrite at a physiological pH is estimated to be $\sim 1 \times 10^{-2}$ s. Despite its short half-life, peroxynitrite is able to cross cell membranes and likely diffuse $\sim$5–20 µm [27–29]. Peroxynitrite

(ONOO⁻) exists in equilibrium with its protonated form (ONOOH) (pKa = ~6.8): $ONOO^- + H^+ \leftrightarrow ONOOH$. Hence, both forms exist in biological systems under physiologically relevant conditions, and the ratios depend on local pH. For example, at a physiological pH of 7.4, the ratio of ONOO⁻ to ONOOH is ~80:20, and the anion form predominates. On the other hand, at an acidic pH of 6.2, the ratio of ONOO⁻ to ONOOH is ~20:80, and the protonated form predominates.

4. CELL AND TISSUE DEFENSES

The reduced form of glutathione (GSH) is the most important antioxidant molecule for the detoxification of peroxynitrite in mammalian cells and tissues. Both glutathione peroxidase and peroxiredoxin (see Appendix B) are able to catalyze the conversion of peroxynitrite to nitrite in vitro [30–34]. However, the exact role of these two enzymes in protecting against peroxynitrite toxicity in vivo remains to be further established.

In addition to glutathione peroxidase and peroxiredoxin, phagocytic myeloperoxidase also scavenges peroxynitrite, which may overcome the uncontrolled production of peroxynitrite and the resulting tissue injury associated with inflammation [35]. Multiple non-peroxiredoxin proteins or enzymes, such as organic hydroperoxide resistance (Ohr) enzymes in bacteria may also constitute antioxidant defenses against peroxynitrite toxicity [36, 37]. These bacterial defenses against peroxynitrite may counteract the innate immunity. In this context, as discussed below, phagocytic cell-derived peroxynitrite plays an important role in killing the invading pathogens.

5. BIOLOGY AND MEDICINE

5.1. Immunity

Interaction between pathogens and immune cells, especially phagocytic cells results in the production of superoxide and nitric oxide from the activation of NADPH oxidase (NOX) and inducible nitric oxide synthase (iNOS), respectively. Due to the extremely high reaction rate constant between superoxide and nitric oxide, peroxynitrite formation is inevitable. Indeed, phagocytic peroxynitrite formation constitutes an important mechanism of bacterium- and parasite-eradicating activity of the innate immunity [8, 38–41]. Peroxynitrite may also play a role in control-

ling viral infections. For example, peroxynitrite inhibits Coxsackievirus infection by prevention of viral RNA entry into the host cell [42].

5.2. Redox Modulation and Cell Signaling

Like other ROS, peroxynitrite affects a number of cell signaling molecules, including growth factor receptors (e.g., epidermal growth factor receptor), protein kinase cascades (e.g., mitogen-activated protein kinases), and transcription factors (e.g., nuclear factor kappaB) (see refs in [3]). Modulation of the above signaling pathways may contribute to peroxynitrite-induced alterations in cell function as well as cell viability.

Unlike its precursor nitric oxide which is a well-established second messenger in cell signal transduction leading to physiological responses, the role of peroxynitrite as a potential second messenger remains largely unknown. Nevertheless, a recent study demonstrated that peroxynitrite (generated from neuronal NOS-derived nitric oxide and NOX4-derived superoxide) acts as a mediator (second messenger) that converts a mechanical load into an intracellular signaling pathway, resulting in skeletal muscle hypertrophy [43]. Augmentation of this peroxynitrite-mediated hypertrophy-inducing signaling might be a potential strategy for treating muscle atrophy that occurs in aging and pathological conditions.

It is well-known that nitric oxide is able to physiologically stimulate the sarco-endoplasmic reticulum Ca²⁺ATPase (SERCA) to decrease intracellular Ca²⁺ concentrations and relax cardiac, skeletal, and vascular smooth muscle. Nitric oxide-derived peroxynitrite also directly increases SERCA activity by S-glutathiolation of the cysteine residue 674, suggesting that peroxynitrite might be an intracellular mediator of nitric oxide-induced vasodilation [44]. This effect is in line with the observation that peroxynitrite at physiologically relevant concentrations may mediate cardioprotection against myocardial ischemic injury [45, 46].

Peroxynitrite may also act as an intermediate involved in the regulation of T cell tolerance. In this regard, antigen-specific CD8⁺ T cell tolerance is induced by myeloid-derived suppressor cells (MDSCs). The direct interaction between MDSCs and CD8⁺ T cells leads to the production of peroxynitrite which in turn causes nitration of tyrosines in a T cell receptor (TCR)-CD8 complex, making CD8-expressing T cells unable to bind to specific peptide–major histocompatibility complex, thereby leading to T cell tolerance [47].

5.3. Disease Process

The involvement of peroxynitrite in the pathophysiology of a wide variety of disease processes has been extensively investigated over the past decades. This has also been a topic of extensive literature review [3, 29]. Although the exact causal role of peroxynitrite in disease process remains to be established, substantial evidence suggests a potential contribution of uncontrolled production of peroxynitrite to disease conditions ranging from cardiovascular disorders and diabetes [48–51] to neurodegeneration and cancer development [47, 52–55].

With regard to cancer development, peroxynitrite-induced DNA damage, gene mutations, and tumor suppressor gene inactivation apparently play a role [56]. Epigenetic mechanisms, such as suppression of cancer immunosurveillance, may play an even more important part in cancer development associated with overproduction of peroxynitrite. In this context, peroxynitrite released by the myeloid-derived suppressor cells causes CD8$^+$ T cell tolerance in cancer via nitration of tyrosines in a TCR-CD8 complex, leading to tumor cell escape and consequent cancer progression [47, 55].

Determination of the role of peroxynitrite in disease pathophysiology has been largely based on the use of biomarkers for peroxynitrite (e.g., 3-nitrotyrosine; also see **Figure 11.3**) as well as peroxynitrite decomposition catalysts (e.g., FeTMPyP). As noted earlier, while 3-nitrotyrosine is widely used as a biomarker for biological peroxynitrite formation, ROS other than peroxynitrite can also give rise to 3-nitrotyrosine. A number of iron and manganese metalloporphyrin compounds have been developed over the past decades showing catalytic activity toward peroxynitrite decomposition. Many of these so called peroxynitrite decomposition catalysts have been used extensively as experimental modalities to protect against peroxynitrite toxicity, and the protection mediated by these compounds in a biological system is frequently interpreted as evidence for peroxynitrite formation as well as its causal involvement in disease pathophysiology.

As with other ROS scavengers, currently available peroxynitrite decomposition catalysts (although they are claimed to be peroxynitrite-specific) are not exclusively specific for scavenging peroxynitrite [57]. As such, while the protection by these compounds may suggest a role for peroxynitrite in a disease process, the possible involvement of other ROS cannot be excluded solely based on the use of these peroxynitrite scavengers. In this context, development of

compounds that only scavenge peroxynitrite will certainly facilitate the investigation of the causal involvement of peroxynitrite in disease process.

6. SUMMARY OF CHAPTER KEY POINTS

- The possible formation of peroxynitrite was first suggested in 1901 by A. Baeyer and V. Villiger in their studies on the reactions between nitrites and hydrogen peroxide.
- In a 1985 paper, N. Blough and O. Zafiriou for the first time demonstrated the reaction of superoxide with nitric oxide to form peroxynitrite in an alkaline aqueous solution. This was followed by studies in the early 1990s showing peroxynitrite as a biologically relevant oxidant capable of reacting with cellular constituents.
- The diffusion-limited reaction between superoxide and nitric oxide is considered the primary source of biological peroxynitrite formation. Other sources of biological relevance include the reaction between nitroxyl and molecular oxygen as well as the CBS-catalyzed reduction of nitrite.
- Peroxynitrite possesses high one-electron and two-electron reduction potentials and as such is capable of reacting with a wide range of cellular constituents, including lipids, proteins, and nucleic acids.
- In addition to its direct reaction with biomolecules, peroxynitrite also gives rise to secondary reactive species such as carbonate radicals, nitrogen dioxide, and possible hydroxyl radical. Hence, both direct and indirect chemical mechanisms underlie peroxynitrite-induced biological effects.
- Peroxynitrite reacts with metal ion centers, thiol groups, and tyrosine residues of proteins and enzymes, causing enzyme inhibition or dysfunction. Formation of 3-nitrotyrosine is a commonly used biomarker of peroxynitrite production in biological systems.
- Peroxynitrite causes lipid peroxidation in biomembranes and lipoproteins by abstracting a hydrogen atom from polyunsaturated fatty acids. It damages DNA by introducing oxidative modifications in both bases and sugar-phosphate backbone. Oxidation and nitration of DNA guanine base lead to the formation of 8-hydroxyguanine and 8-nitroguanine, respectively.
- Peroxynitrite has a relatively short half-life (~1 $\times10^{-2}$ s), but can cross cell membranes and likely diffuse ~5–20 μm in cells and tissues depending on the availability and levels of surrounding antioxidant molecules. The major cellular defenses of

peroxynitrite include GSH, glutathione peroxidase, and peroxiredoxin.

- Due to its unique chemical and biochemical properties, peroxynitrite has been implicated in biology and medicine. Peroxynitrite constitutes an important part of the innate immunity against invading pathogens.
- Although it is well established that peroxynitrite, like other ROS, can cause redox modulation of a number of cell signaling molecules, its role as a potential second messenger in cell signal transduction remains to be established.
- Excessive oxidation of cellular constituents and redox modulation of cell signaling pathways are the underlying biochemical basis of peroxynitrite overproduction-mediated pathophysiology in a number of disease processes. These include cardiovascular disorders, diabetes, neurodegeneration, and cancer, among many others.

7. SELF-ASSESSMENT QUESTIONS

7.1. Although the reaction between superoxide and nitric oxide is the primary source of biological peroxynitrite formation, other reactions may also contribute to the production of this reactive species in biological systems. Which of the following enzymes has recently been shown to catalyze the reduction of nitrite to peroxynitrite?

A. Catalase
B. Cystathionine β-synthase
C. Cytochrome P450 2E1
D. Glutathione peroxidase
E. Superoxide dismutase

7.2. The high one-electron reduction potential of peroxynitrite makes it a potent biological oxidant. Which of the following is the estimated standard one-electron reduction potential of peroxynitrite?

A. 160 mV
B. 480 mV
C. 920 mV
D. 1400 mV
E. 2300 mV

7.3. 3-Nitrotyrosine is widely used as a biomarker for peroxynitrite formation in biological systems. It is known that the formation of 3-nitrotyrosine upon exposure to peroxynitrite under physiologically relevant conditions occurs via a tyrosine free radical in-

termediate. Which of the following species is most likely responsible for the formation of the above tyrosine radical?

A. Carbonate radical
B. Hydrogen peroxide
C. Nitric dioxide
D. Nitric oxide
E. Superoxide

7.4. Which of the following enzymes is most likely to be able to catalyze the conversion of peroxynitrite to nitrite under a biologically relevant condition?

A. Catalase
B. Cystathionine β-synthase
C. Glutathione peroxidase
D. NADPH:quinone oxidoreductase 1
E. Superoxide dismutase

7.5. Mitochondrial aconitase is an iron-sulfur cluster-containing enzyme that has been shown to be susceptible to superoxide-mediated inhibition. Which of the following species is also most likely to cause inactivation of this enzyme?

A. Carbon dioxide
B. Hydrogen peroxide
C. Nitric oxide
D. Nitrite
E. Peroxynitrite

ANSWERS AND EXPLANATIONS

7.1. The answer is B. Cystathionine β-synthase catalyzes the condensation of homocysteine with serine or with cysteine to form cystathionine and either water or hydrogen sulfide, respectively. This enzyme is shown to also catalyze the reduction of nitrite to form peroxynitrite.

7.2. The answer is D. Peroxynitrite possesses very high one-electron and two-electron reduction potentials, which are 1400 mV ($ONOO^-$, 2 H^+/$NO_2^·$, H_2O) and 1200 mV ($ONOO^-$, 2 H^+/NO_2^-, H_2O), respectively, under a pH of 7.0.

7.3. The answer is A. Upon exposure to peroxynitrite, tyrosine nitration in cells and tissues occurs in a two-step reaction in which the peroxynitrite-derived $CO_3^{·-}$ abstracts a hydrogen atom from the tyrosine residue, generating a tyrosine radical. This tyrosine radical then reacts with the peroxynitrite-derived nitric dioxide, forming 3-nitrotyrosine.

7.4. The answer is C. Both glutathione peroxidase and peroxiredoxin are able to catalyze the conversion of peroxynitrite to nitrite in vitro.

7.5. The answer is E. Peroxynitrite reacts readily with iron-sulfur clusters of several enzymes, including mitochondrial aconitase and the enzyme complexes of the mitochondrial electron transport chain, leading to enzyme inactivation.

REFERENCES

1. Baeyer A, Villiger V. Ueber die salpetrige Säure. *Berichte der deutschen chemischen Gesellschaft* 1901; 34(1):755–62.

2. Glau K, Hubold R. Die Einwirkung von Wasserstoffsuperoxyd auf salpetrige Säure. Persalpetrige Säure. II. *Zeitschrift für anorganische und allgemeine Chemie* 1935; 223(4):305–17.

3. Pacher P, Beckman JS, Liaudet L. Nitric oxide and peroxynitrite in health and disease. *Physiol Rev* 2007; 87(1):315–424.

4. Blough NV, Zafiriou OC. Reaction of superoxide with nitric oxide to form peroxonitrite in alkaline aqueous solution. *Inorg Chem* 1985; 24(22):3502–4.

5. Beckman JS, Beckman TW, Chen J, Marshall PA, Freeman BA. Apparent hydroxyl radical production by peroxynitrite: implications for endothelial injury from nitric oxide and superoxide. *Proc Natl Acad Sci USA* 1990; 87(4):1620–4.

6. Radi R, Beckman JS, Bush KM, Freeman BA. Peroxynitrite oxidation of sulfhydryls: the cytotoxic potential of superoxide and nitric oxide. *J Biol Chem* 1991; 266(7):4244–50.

7. Radi R, Beckman JS, Bush KM, Freeman BA. Peroxynitrite-induced membrane lipid peroxidation: the cytotoxic potential of superoxide and nitric oxide. *Arch Biochem Biophys* 1991; 288(2):481–7.

8. Ischiropoulos H, Zhu L, Beckman JS. Peroxynitrite formation from macrophage-derived nitric oxide. *Arch Biochem Biophys* 1992; 298(2):446–51.

9. Kirsch M, de Groot H. Formation of peroxynitrite from reaction of nitroxyl anion with molecular oxygen. *J Biol Chem* 2002; 277(16):13379–88.

10. Smulik R, Debski D, Zielonka J, Michalowski B, Adamus J, Marcinek A, Kalyanaraman B, Sikora A. Nitroxyl (HNO) reacts with molecular oxygen and forms peroxynitrite at physiological pH: biological Implications. *J Biol Chem* 2014; 289(51):35570–81.

11. Carballal S, Cuevasanta E, Yadav PK, Gherasim C, Ballou DP, Alvarez B, Banerjee R. Kinetics of nitrite reduction and peroxynitrite formation by ferrous heme in human cystathionine beta-synthase. *J Biol Chem* 2016; 291(15):8004–13.

12. Koppenol WH, Moreno JJ, Pryor WA, Ischiropoulos H, Beckman JS. Peroxynitrite, a cloaked oxidant formed by nitric oxide and superoxide. *Chem Res Toxicol* 1992; 5(6):834–42.

13. Denicola A, Freeman BA, Trujillo M, Radi R. Peroxynitrite reaction with carbon dioxide/bicarbonate: kinetics and influence on peroxynitrite-mediated oxidations. *Arch Biochem Biophys* 1996; 333(1):49–58.

14. Bonini MG, Radi R, Ferrer-Sueta G, Ferreira AM, Augusto O. Direct EPR detection of the carbonate radical anion produced from peroxynitrite and carbon dioxide. *J Biol Chem* 1999; 274(16):10802–6.

15. Hausladen A, Fridovich I. Superoxide and peroxynitrite inactivate aconitases, but nitric oxide does not. *J Biol Chem* 1994; 269(47):29405–8.

16. Castro L, Rodriguez M, Radi R. Aconitase is readily inactivated by peroxynitrite, but not by its precursor, nitric oxide. *J Biol Chem* 1994; 269(47):29409–15.

17. Murray J, Taylor SW, Zhang B, Ghosh SS, Capaldi RA. Oxidative damage to mitochondrial complex I due to peroxynitrite: identification of reactive tyrosines by mass spectrometry. *J Biol Chem* 2003; 278(39):37223–30.

18. Zou MH, Shi C, Cohen RA. Oxidation of the zinc-thiolate complex and uncoupling of endothelial nitric oxide synthase by peroxynitrite. *J Clin Invest* 2002; 109(6):817–26.

19. Franco MC, Ye Y, Refakis CA, Feldman JL, Stokes AL, Basso M, Melero Fernandez de Mera RM, Sparrow NA, Calingasan NY, Kiaei M, Rhoads TW, Ma TC, et al. Nitration of Hsp90 induces cell death. *Proc Natl Acad Sci USA* 2013; 110(12):E1102–11.

20. Hess DT, Matsumoto A, Kim SO, Marshall HE, Stamler JS. Protein S-nitrosylation: purview and parameters. *Nat Rev Mol Cell Biol* 2005;

6(2):150–66.

21. O'Donnell VB, Eiserich JP, Chumley PH, Jablonsky MJ, Krishna NR, Kirk M, Barnes S, Darley-Usmar VM, Freeman BA. Nitration of unsaturated fatty acids by nitric oxide-derived reactive nitrogen species peroxynitrite, nitrous acid, nitrogen dioxide, and nitronium ion. *Chem Res Toxicol* 1999; 12(1):83–92.

22. Li Y, Zhang J, Schopfer FJ, Martynowski D, Garcia-Barrio MT, Kovach A, Suino-Powell K, Baker PR, Freeman BA, Chen YE, Xu HE. Molecular recognition of nitrated fatty acids by PPAR gamma. *Nat Struct Mol Biol* 2008; 15(8):865–7.

23. Wright MM, Schopfer FJ, Baker PR, Vidyasagar V, Powell P, Chumley P, Iles KE, Freeman BA, Agarwal A. Fatty acid transduction of nitric oxide signaling: nitrolinoleic acid potently activates endothelial heme oxygenase 1 expression. *Proc Natl Acad Sci USA* 2006; 103(11):4299–304.

24. Epe B, Ballmaier D, Roussyn I, Briviba K, Sies H. DNA damage by peroxynitrite characterized with DNA repair enzymes. *Nucleic Acids Res* 1996; 24(21):4105–10.

25. Yermilov V, Rubio J, Becchi M, Friesen MD, Pignatelli B, Ohshima H. Formation of 8-nitroguanine by the reaction of guanine with peroxynitrite in vitro. *Carcinogenesis* 1995; 16(9):2045–50.

26. Szabo C, Zingarelli B, O'Connor M, Salzman AL. DNA strand breakage, activation of poly (ADP-ribose) synthetase, and cellular energy depletion are involved in the cytotoxicity of macrophages and smooth muscle cells exposed to peroxynitrite. *Proc Natl Acad Sci USA* 1996; 93(5):1753–8.

27. Marla SS, Lee J, Groves JT. Peroxynitrite rapidly permeates phospholipid membranes. *Proc Natl Acad Sci USA* 1997; 94(26):14243–8.

28. Denicola A, Souza JM, Radi R. Diffusion of peroxynitrite across erythrocyte membranes. *Proc Natl Acad Sci USA* 1998; 95(7):3566–71.

29. Szabo C, Ischiropoulos H, Radi R. Peroxynitrite: biochemistry, pathophysiology and development of therapeutics. *Nat Rev Drug Discov* 2007; 6(8):662–80.

30. Sies H, Sharov VS, Klotz LO, Briviba K. Glutathione peroxidase protects against peroxynitrite-mediated oxidations: a new function for selenoproteins as peroxynitrite reductase. *J Biol Chem* 1997; 272(44):27812–7.

31. Briviba K, Kissner R, Koppenol WH, Sies H.

Kinetic study of the reaction of glutathione peroxidase with peroxynitrite. *Chem Res Toxicol* 1998; 11(12):1398–401.

32. Bryk R, Griffin P, Nathan C. Peroxynitrite reductase activity of bacterial peroxiredoxins. *Nature* 2000; 407(6801):211–5.

33. Trujillo M, Ferrer-Sueta G, Radi R. Kinetic studies on peroxynitrite reduction by peroxiredoxins. *Methods Enzymol* 2008; 441:173–96.

34. Selles B, Hugo M, Trujillo M, Srivastava V, Wingsle G, Jacquot JP, Radi R, Rouhier N. Hydroperoxide and peroxynitrite reductase activity of poplar thioredoxin-dependent glutathione peroxidase 5: kinetics, catalytic mechanism and oxidative inactivation. *Biochem J* 2012; 442(2):369–80.

35. Koyani CN, Flemmig J, Malle E, Arnhold J. Myeloperoxidase scavenges peroxynitrite: A novel anti-inflammatory action of the heme enzyme. *Arch Biochem Biophys* 2015; 571:1–9.

36. Bryk R, Lima CD, Erdjument-Bromage H, Tempst P, Nathan C. Metabolic enzymes of mycobacteria linked to antioxidant defense by a thioredoxin-like protein. *Science* 2002; 295(5557):1073–7.

37. Alegria TG, Meireles DA, Cussiol JR, Hugo M, Trujillo M, de Oliveira MA, Miyamoto S, Queiroz RF, Valadares NF, Garratt RC, Radi R, Di Mascio P, et al. Ohr plays a central role in bacterial responses against fatty acid hydroperoxides and peroxynitrite. *Proc Natl Acad Sci USA* 2017; 114(2):E132-41.

38. Zhu L, Gunn C, Beckman JS. Bactericidal activity of peroxynitrite. *Arch Biochem Biophys* 1992; 298(2):452–7.

39. Denicola A, Rubbo H, Rodriguez D, Radi R. Peroxynitrite-mediated cytotoxicity to *Trypanosoma cruzi*. *Arch Biochem Biophys* 1993; 304(1):279–86.

40. Alvarez MN, Piacenza L, Irigoin F, Peluffo G, Radi R. Macrophage-derived peroxynitrite diffusion and toxicity to *Trypanosoma cruzi*. *Arch Biochem Biophys* 2004; 432(2):222–32.

41. Alvarez MN, Peluffo G, Piacenza L, Radi R. Intraphagosomal peroxynitrite as a macrophage-derived cytotoxin against internalized *Trypanosoma cruzi*: consequences for oxidative killing and role of microbial peroxiredoxins in infectivity. *J Biol Chem* 2011; 286(8):6627–40.

42. Padalko E, Ohnishi T, Matsushita K, Sun H, Fox-Talbot K, Bao C, Baldwin WM, 3rd, Lowenstein CJ. Peroxynitrite inhibition of

Coxsackievirus infection by prevention of viral RNA entry. *Proc Natl Acad Sci USA* 2004; 101(32):11731–6.

43. Ito N, Ruegg UT, Kudo A, Miyagoe-Suzuki Y, Takeda S. Activation of calcium signaling through Trpv1 by nNOS and peroxynitrite as a key trigger of skeletal muscle hypertrophy. *Nat Med* 2013; 19(1):101–6.

44. Adachi T, Weisbrod RM, Pimentel DR, Ying J, Sharov VS, Schoneich C, Cohen RA. S-Glutathiolation by peroxynitrite activates SERCA during arterial relaxation by nitric oxide. *Nat Med* 2004; 10(11):1200–7.

45. Nossuli TO, Hayward R, Scalia R, Lefer AM. Peroxynitrite reduces myocardial infarct size and preserves coronary endothelium after ischemia and reperfusion in cats. *Circulation* 1997; 96(7):2317–24.

46. Li J, Loukili N, Rosenblatt-Velin N, Pacher P, Feihl F, Waeber B, Liaudet L. Peroxynitrite is a key mediator of the cardioprotection afforded by ischemic postconditioning in vivo. *PLoS One* 2013; 8(7):e70331.

47. Nagaraj S, Gupta K, Pisarev V, Kinarsky L, Sherman S, Kang L, Herber DL, Schneck J, Gabrilovich DI. Altered recognition of antigen is a mechanism of CD8$^+$ T cell tolerance in cancer. *Nat Med* 2007; 13(7):828–35.

48. White CR, Brock TA, Chang LY, Crapo J, Briscoe P, Ku D, Bradley WA, Gianturco SH, Gore J, Freeman BA, et al. Superoxide and peroxynitrite in atherosclerosis. *Proc Natl Acad Sci USA* 1994; 91(3):1044–8.

49. Cabassi A, Binno SM, Tedeschi S, Ruzicka V, Dancelli S, Rocco R, Vicini V, Coghi P, Regolisti G, Montanari A, Fiaccadori E, Govoni P, et al. Low serum ferroxidase I activity is associated with mortality in heart failure and related to both peroxynitrite-induced cysteine oxidation and tyrosine nitration of ceruloplasmin. *Circ Res* 2014; 114(11):1723–32.

50. Cassuto J, Dou H, Czikora I, Szabo A, Patel VS, Kamath V, Belin de Chantemele E, Feher A, Romero MJ, Bagi Z. Peroxynitrite disrupts endothelial caveolae leading to eNOS uncoupling and diminished flow-mediated dilation in coronary arterioles of diabetic patients. *Diabetes* 2014; 63(4):1381–93.

51. Seimetz M, Parajuli N, Pichl A, Veit F, Kwapiszewska G, Weisel FC, Milger K, Egemnazarov B, Turowska A, Fuchs B, Nikam S, Roth M, et al. Inducible NOS inhibition reverses tobacco-smoke-induced emphysema and pulmonary hypertension in mice. *Cell* 2011; 147(2):293–305.

52. Guix FX, Wahle T, Vennekens K, Snellinx A, Chavez-Gutierrez L, Ill-Raga G, Ramos-Fernandez E, Guardia-Laguarta C, Lleo A, Arimon M, Berezovska O, Munoz FJ, et al. Modification of gamma-secretase by nitrosative stress links neuronal ageing to sporadic Alzheimer's disease. *EMBO Mol Med* 2012; 4(7):660–73.

53. Park L, Wang G, Moore J, Girouard H, Zhou P, Anrather J, Iadecola C. The key role of transient receptor potential melastatin-2 channels in amyloid-beta-induced neurovascular dysfunction. *Nat Commun* 2014; 5:5318.

54. Yemisci M, Gursoy-Ozdemir Y, Vural A, Can A, Topalkara K, Dalkara T. Pericyte contraction induced by oxidative-nitrative stress impairs capillary reflow despite successful opening of an occluded cerebral artery. *Nat Med* 2009; 15(9):1031–7.

55. Lu T, Ramakrishnan R, Altiok S, Youn JI, Cheng P, Celis E, Pisarev V, Sherman S, Sporn MB, Gabrilovich D. Tumor-infiltrating myeloid cells induce tumor cell resistance to cytotoxic T cells in mice. *J Clin Invest* 2011; 121(10):4015–29.

56. Cobbs CS, Whisenhunt TR, Wesemann DR, Harkins LE, Van Meir EG, Samanta M. Inactivation of wild-type p53 protein function by reactive oxygen and nitrogen species in malignant glioma cells. *Cancer Res* 2003; 63(24):8670–3.

57. Slosky LM, Vanderah TW. Therapeutic potential of peroxynitrite decomposition catalysts: a patent review. *Expert Opin Ther Pat* 2015; 25(4):443–66.

Chapter 12

Nitric Oxide in Biology and Medicine

ABSTRACT | Nitric oxide (NO) is one of the most important free radical species in biology and medicine. In biological systems, NO is generated via pathways including the enzymatic action of the nitric oxide synthases (NOS) and the nonenzymatic nitrate-nitrite-NO pathway. NO is both a poor reductant and a poor oxidant, and its direct reaction with most cellular biomolecules is much limited. However, NO potently activates soluble guanylate cyclase via quick and high affinity binding to the heme iron of the enzyme. This serves as the primary molecular basis of NO signaling in biological systems. In addition to heme iron, NO also reacts with superoxide as well as other radical species (including molecular oxygen, a di-radical), leading to the formation of more reactive species capable of causing biological damage. Hence, NO, like a double-edged sword, can cause both physiological and pathophysiological responses. On the one hand, NO, when its production is well-controlled, acts as a signaling molecule responsible for physiological homeostasis, including cardiovascular function, neurotransmission, and immunity, among many others. On the other hand, overproduction of NO may cause tissue injury and contribute to disease pathogenesis via, primarily, the formation of the secondary NO-derived reactive species, such as peroxynitrite.

KEYWORDS | Cell signaling; Disease process; Heme iron; Immunity; Nitric oxide; Nitrosation; Nitrosylation; Peroxynitrite; Superoxide

CITATION | Hopkins RZ and Li YR. Essentials of Free Radical Biology and Medicine. Cell Med Press, Raleigh, NC, USA. 2017. http://dx.doi.org/10.20455/efrbm.2017.12

ABBREVIATIONS | cGMP, cyclic guanosine monophosphate; EDRF, endothelium-derived relaxing factor; eNOS (NOS3), endothelial NOS; HO-1, heme oxygenase-1; iNOS (NOS2), inducible NOS; mARC, mitochondrial amidoxime reducing component; METC, mitochondrial electron transport chain; nNOS (NOS1), neuronal NOS; NO, nitric oxide; NOS, nitric oxide synthase; Nrf2, nuclear factor E2-related factor 2; RBC, red blood cell; sGC, soluble guanylate cyclase

CHAPTER AT A GLANCE

1. OVERVIEW

Nitric oxide (also called nitric monoxide) was first identified as a gas in 1772 by Joseph Priestly who is also credited with the discovery of oxygen in 1774 (see Section 4 of Chapter 1). Nitric oxide (NO) is a simple molecule consisting of just one atom of oxygen and one atom of nitrogen. Because it contains one unpaired electron, nitric oxide is also a free radical and written as NO˙. For simplicity, in this chapter, NO is used to denote nitric oxide.

For much of the time since its discovery, NO has been thought of simply as an air pollutant. In 1977, Ferid Murad and associates discovered the release of NO from nitroglycerin (a drug that has been used for over a century) and its action on vascular smooth muscle [1, 2]. Just three years after the discovery of the vasodilatory effects of NO, Robert F. Furchgott and John V. Zawadski demonstrated the importance of the endothelium in acetylcholine-induced vasorelaxation in 1980 and called the endothelium-derived vasodilatory substance endothelium-derived relaxing factor (EDRF) [3]. Subsequently, in 1987 Louis J. Ignarro (and associates) and Salvador Moncada (and associates) independently identified EDRF as NO [4–6].

Given the realization that NO could be made by endothelium, the following decade witnessed the discovery of the enzymatic machineries (i.e., nitric oxide synthases) for NO biosynthesis [7]. Because of the importance of NO in biology and medicine, this biological free radical was named "Molecule of the Year" by the Science magazine in 1992 [8]. Six years later in 1998, R.F. Furchgott, L.J. Ignarro, and F. Murad were awarded the Nobel Prize in Physiology or Medicine for their discoveries concerning nitric oxide as a signaling molecule in the cardiovascular system. This Nobel Prize has caused great excitement in the research field of NO. Indeed, the past two decades have witnessed the explosion of the knowledge on NO in biology and medicine. A Pub-Med searching using nitric oxide as the keyword in title/abstract resulted in 127,149 entries on January 2, 2017, highlighting the vast amounts of information on this molecule. This chapter provides an overview of the key findings on NO with regard to its biological sources, chemistry and biochemistry, and its roles in biology and medicine.

2. SOURCES

Nitric oxide is formed in biological systems by two general pathways. They are (1) nitric oxide synthase-dependent pathway and (2) nitrate-nitrite-nitric oxide pathway (**Figure 12.1**).

2.1. Nitric Oxide Synthase-Dependent Pathway

Nitric oxide synthase (NOS) catalyzes the formation of nitric oxide from L-arginine. There are three isoforms of nitric oxide synthase, i.e., NOS1, NOS2, and NOS3 [9–11]. These isoforms differ in their cell and tissue distribution and mode of regulation. NOS1 is also called neuronal NOS (nNOS), and was originally identified in neurons. NOS1 is also expressed in many other types of tissues, such as skeletal muscle, cardiac tissue, and endothelium. NOS2 is also called inducible NOS (iNOS), and was first identified in macrophages. NOS2 is expressed in multiple types of cells and tissues. NOS3 is also called endothelial NOS (eNOS) and is expressed in endothelium as well as other types of cells and tissues, including the brain. NOS1 and NOS3 are constitutively expressed. NOS2, as the name indicates, is highly inducible and capable of generating large amounts of nitric oxide under conditions such as dysregulated inflammation. NOS2 is also constitutively expressed in certain tissues, such as lung epithelium. NOS1 and NOS3 are regulated by Ca^{2+}/calmodulin, whereas NOS2 is Ca^{2+}-independent.

2.2. Nitrate-Nitrite-Nitric Oxide Pathway

Both diet and metabolism of endogenous nitric oxide contribute to the nitrate (NO_3^-) and nitrite (NO_2^-) pool in the body. These inorganic anions can be recycled in vivo to form nitric oxide, representing an alternative source of nitric oxide to the classical L-arginine-NOS pathway. The L-arginine-NOS pathway is oxygen-dependent whereas the nitrate-nitrite-nitric oxide pathway is gradually activated as oxygen tension falls. Thus, this NOS-independent pathway can be viewed as a backup system to ensure sufficient nitric oxide formation when oxygen supply is limited.

The nitrate in mammals including humans is reduced to nitrite by commensal bacteria in the gastro-

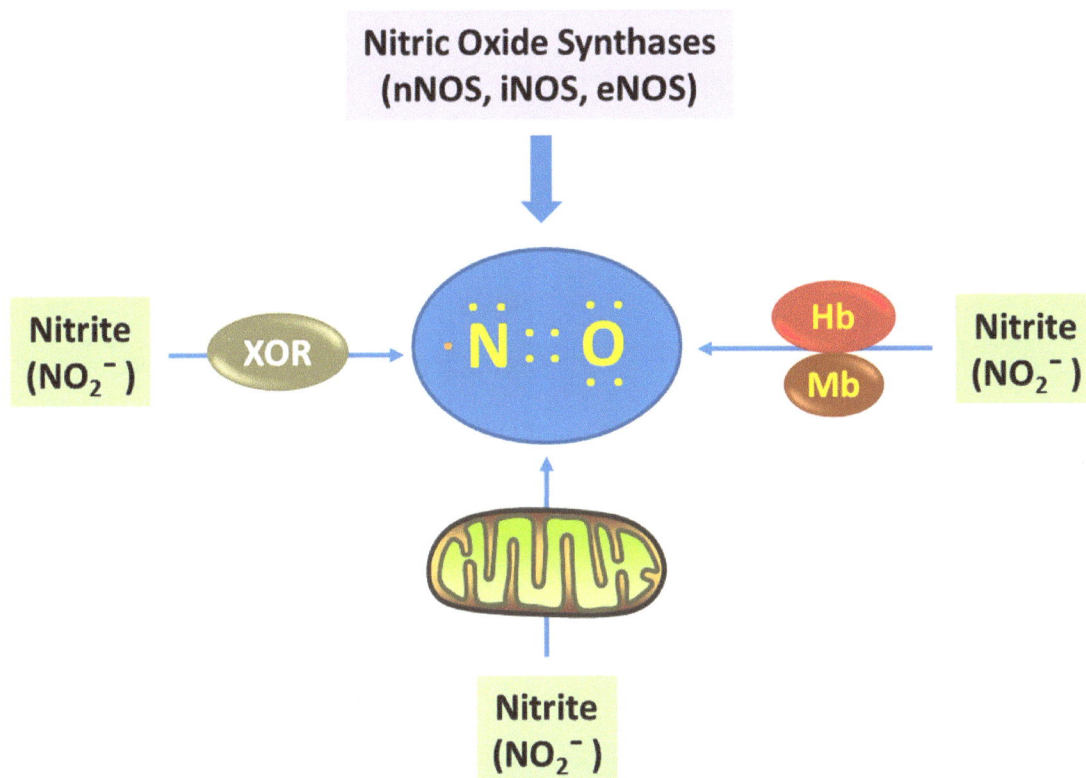

FIGURE 12.1. Nitric oxide (NO) production in biological systems. As illustrated, nitric oxide synthases (NOS) are the primary machineries for NO biosynthesis. In addition to this classical pathway, a number of NOS-independent mechanisms may operate under certain conditions such as low oxygen tension to reduce nitrite to form NO. These include xanthine oxidoreductase (XOR), hemoglobin (Hb) and myoglobin (Mb), as well as mitochondrial electron transport chain (mainly complex IV) and mitochondrial amidoxime reducing component.

intestinal tract and on body surfaces. There are several pathways in the body for further reduction of nitrite to nitric oxide. These include hemoglobin and myoglobin, acidic reduction, xanthine oxidoreductase, mitochondrial electron transport chain (cytochrome c oxidase, also known as complex IV) and others [12].

2.2.1. Hemoglobin and Myoglobin

Nitrite reacts with ferrous deoxyhemoglobin ($HbFe^{2+}$) and a proton (H^+) to form NO and methemoglobin ($HbFe^{3+}$) (Reaction 1) [13, 14]. Deoxymyoglobin also rapidly reduces nitrite to form nitric oxide [15, 16]. Hence, under hypoxic conditions, hemoglobin and myoglobin can be converted from NO scavengers to NO producers. During the process, methemoglobin and metmyoglobin are formed.

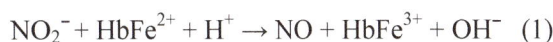

$$NO_2^- + HbFe^{2+} + H^+ \rightarrow NO + HbFe^{3+} + OH^- \quad (1)$$

2.2.2. Acidic Reduction

Under acidic conditions, nitrite is protonated to form nitrous acid (HNO_2), which then decomposes to form NO and other nitrogen oxides, such as nitrogen dioxide (NO_2) and dinitrogen trioxide (N_2O_3) (Reactions 2–5) [17]. Both NO_2 and N_2O_3 are reactive species capable of modifying biomolecules.

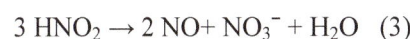

$$NO_2^- + H^+ \rightarrow HNO_2 \quad (2)$$

$$3\,HNO_2 \rightarrow 2\,NO + NO_3^- + H_2O \quad (3)$$

$$2\,HNO_2 \rightarrow N_2O_3 + H_2O \quad (4)$$

$$N_2O_3 \rightarrow NO + NO_2 \quad (5)$$

2.2.3. Xanthine Oxidoreductase

Xanthine oxidoreductase is known to reduce molecular oxygen to superoxide and hydrogen peroxide. At low oxygen tensions and pH values, this enzyme can also reduce nitrite to NO at the molybdenum (Mo) site of the enzyme (Reaction 7) [18, 19].

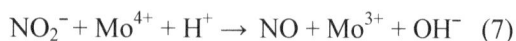

$$NO_2^- + Mo^{4+} + H^+ \rightarrow NO + Mo^{3+} + OH^- \quad (7)$$

2.2.4. Mitochondria

On the one hand, mitochondrial electron transport chain (METC) enzyme complexes, especially complex V (cytochrome c oxidase) can be inhibited by NO at physiological concentrations (see Section 3.2 below), resulting in suppression of respiration. On the other hand, under hypoxic conditions, mitochondrial cytochrome c oxidase may reduce nitrite to form NO and employ this as a mechanism of mitochondria-mediated hypoxic signaling [20, 21].

In addition to the METC, other enzymes in mitochondria may also play a role in reducing nitrite to NO. In this regard, mitochondrial amidoxime reducing component (mARC) proteins are molybdopterin-containing enzymes of unclear physiological function. Both human isoforms mARC-1 and mARC-2 are able to catalyze the reduction of nitrite to NO through reaction with the molybdenum cofactor. Mitochondria may thus represent a new pathway for nicotinamide adenine dinucleotide (NADH)-dependent hypoxic NO production [22].

2.2.5. Others

NO is produced in the skin, a hypoxic tissue enriched in nitrites wherein NO has important roles in wound healing and other biological processes. A recent study shows that activation of TRPV3, a heat-activated transient receptor potential ion channel expressed in keratinocytes, induces NO production via a nitrite-dependent pathway [23].

It has been suggested that eNOS may be present on red blood cells (RBCs). The RBC-associated eNOS is shown to be able to reduce nitrite to NO under hypoxic conditions [24].

In addition to mammalian hemoglobin and myoglobin, globin X (a protein found in fish, amphibians, and reptiles that diverged from a common ancestor of mammalian hemoglobins and myoglobins) has been shown to be much more potent than mammalian hemoglobin and myoglobin in reducing nitrite to NO [25].

3. CHEMISTRY AND BIOCHEMISTRY

3.1. General Chemical Properties

The one-electron reduction potential for NO (NO/NO$^-$) is estimated to be about –0.8 V. Because of this very low reduction potential, direct one-electron reduction of NO to NO$^-$ is biologically inaccessible [26]. On the other hand, oxidation of NO is also difficult in biological systems due to the high redox potential of 1.2 V for the redox couple of NO/NO$^+$ [27]. Hence, chemically NO is both a poor oxidant and a poor reductant in biological systems though it is a free radical. Indeed, spin pairing with other species containing unpaired electrons, such as other free radicals and transition metal ion-containing proteins provides the only known rapid reactions of NO with biological components and intermediates. This selectivity of reactions is crucial for NO to act as a biological signaling molecule [27].

3.2. Reaction with Cellular Constituents

As noted earlier, the direct reactions of NO with most biomolecules, including proteins (except for certain transition metal ion-containing proteins), lipids, and nucleic acids are very limited. However, NO is a unique ligand for heme groups of various proteins (**Figure 12.2**). The vasodilatory effects of nitric oxide result from the activation of soluble guanylate cyclase, a heme-containing enzyme. Nitric oxide binds to the heme iron of the enzyme, leading to its activation. Activated guanylate cyclase catalyzes the conversion of guanosine triphosphate (GTP) to cyclic guanosine monophosphate (cGMP). cGMP governs cellular pathways, eventually leading to vascular smooth muscle relaxation. This is a well-established signaling pathway underlying nitric oxide-mediated physiological effects [28].

The high affinity and rapid binding of NO to heme iron in mitochondrial cytochrome c oxidase (complex IV) is a major chemical basis for NO regulation of mitochondrial respiration [29–31]. NO regulation of mitochondrial respiration may play an important role in both physiology and pathophysiology [29–31]. In addition, NO is also shown to regulate mitochondrial biogenesis [32], implicating a possible role for NO signaling in promoting lifespan [33].

Although interaction with heme iron of proteins is a major mechanism of action for nitric oxide, other nonheme iron-dependent pathways (e.g., iron-sulfur clusters of proteins) are also involved in nitric oxide-mediated physiological processes [34, 35].

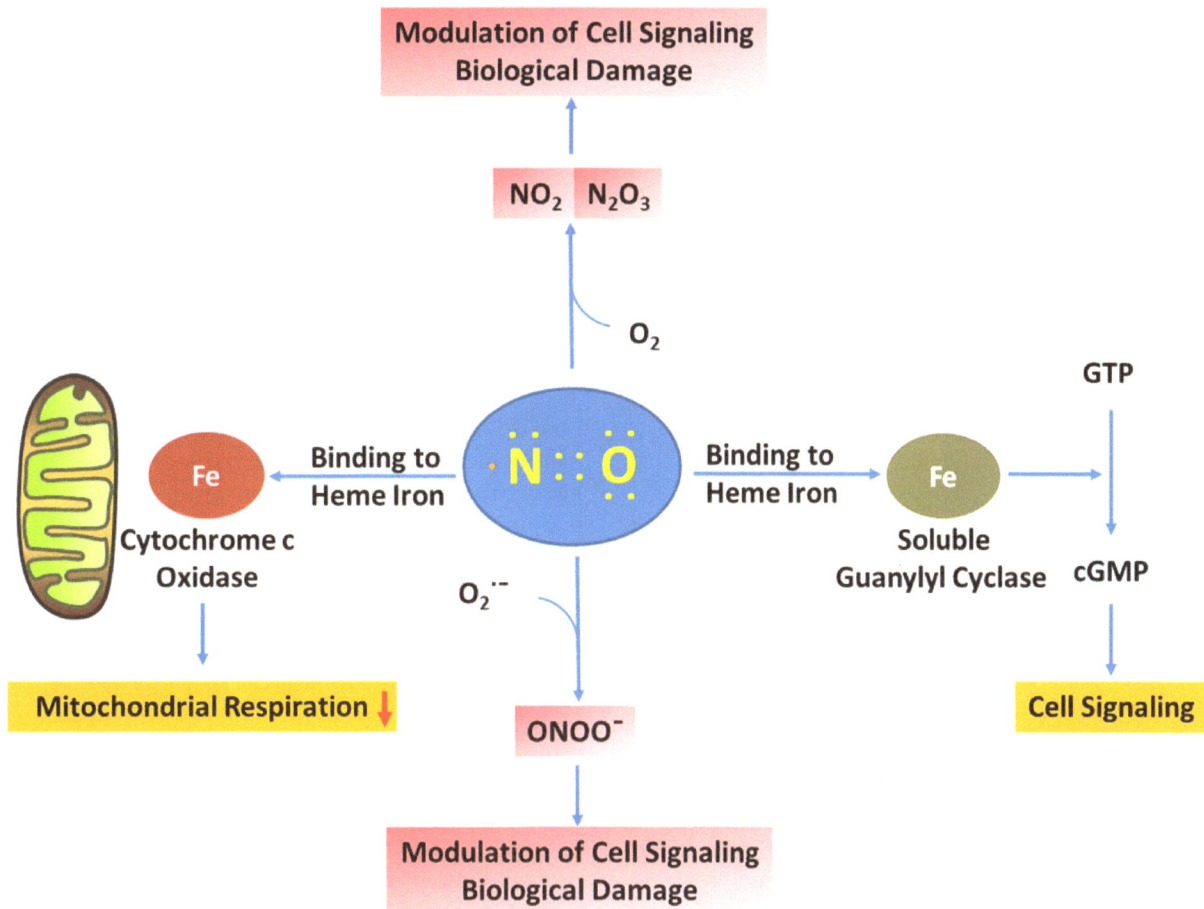

FIGURE 12.2. Chemical and biochemical reactivity of nitric oxide (NO) in biological systems. As depicted, quick and high affinity binding of NO to heme iron of soluble guanylyl cyclase causes the activation of the enzyme, resulting in the formation of cyclic guanosine monophosphate (cGMP) and the subsequent cCMP-dependent signal transduction. NO also binds to the heme iron of mitochondrial cytochrome c oxidase, causing its inhibition and the subsequent decreased mitochondrial respiration. Hence, via binding to heme iron NO at physiological levels mediates cell signaling and regulates mitochondrial respiration. NO also reacts with molecular oxygen (O_2) and superoxide ($O_2^{\cdot-}$) to form more reactive species, including nitrogen dioxide (NO_2), dinitrogen trioxide (N_2O_3), and peroxynitrite ($ONOO^-$). These reactive species can modulate cell signaling and damage biomolecules, especially under the conditions where both NO and superoxide are overproduced.

It is imperative to emphasize the difference between nitrosation and nitrosylation. Nitrosation involves the nitroso group (R–NO, where R denotes typically an organic molecule such as an amino acid residue) and the type of the bond to R is covalent. On the other hand, nitrosylation involves the non-covalent association between NO and a metal ion (such as heme ferric ion): M + NO ↔ MNO (where M denotes a transition metal ion and MNO denotes a coordinate complex of NO with the transition metal ion). NO typically has a higher affinity for a given transition metal ion than molecular oxygen and carbon monoxide and has a higher affinity for ferrous iron (Fe^{2+}) than for ferric iron (Fe^{3+}) [27].

3.3. Reaction with Other Free Radical Species

3.3.1. Reaction with Superoxide

As described in Chapters 8 and 11, NO reacts with superoxide at a diffusion-limited rate to form peroxynitrite, a potent oxidant capable of reacting with a wide range of biomolecules. Formation of peroxynitrite appears to be a major mechanism responsible for the deleterious effects associated with NO over-production (see Section 5 below).

3.3.2. Reaction with Lipid Radicals

NO may inhibit lipid peroxidation. This occurs by chain-breaking termination reactions of NO with lipid alkoxyl radical (LO$^\bullet$) and peroxyl radical (LOO$^\bullet$) (Reactions 8 and 9).

$$LO^\bullet + NO \rightarrow LONO \quad (8)$$

$$LOO^\bullet + NO \rightarrow LOONO \quad (9)$$

LONO is relatively stable, whereas LOONO (lipid peroxynitrite) can decompose to form NO_2 and LO$^\bullet$. The majority of these two free radicals formed rapidly recombine to yield nonreactive alkyl nitrate ($LONO_2$) (Reaction 10) [36].

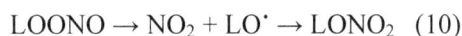

$$LOONO \rightarrow NO_2 + LO^\bullet \rightarrow LONO_2 \quad (10)$$

As lipid radicals (LO$^\bullet$, LOO$^\bullet$) propagate the chain reaction of lipid peroxidation (see Section 2.1 of Chapter 7), NO readily reacts with LO$^\bullet$ and LOO$^\bullet$ leading to the eventual formation of less reactive non-radical species and thereby the termination of the chain reactions of lipid peroxidation. This may explain, at least partially, the antioxidant properties of NO observed in biological systems, especially its protection against oxidation of low-density lipoprotein (LDL) [37, 38]. Oxidation of LDL is a major mechanism of atherosclerotic cardiovascular injury.

3.3.3. Reaction with Molecular Oxygen

Molecular oxygen (O_2) is a di-radical with two un-paired electrons (see Figure 2.1 of Chapter 2). This feature makes it reactive with other species containing unpaired electrons, including NO. The overall interaction between NO and O_2 in biological milieu may proceed via the following reactions (Reactions 11–13) [27]. The resultant NO_2 and N_2O_3 are reactive species capable of causing nitrosation reactions as well as other deleterious effects.

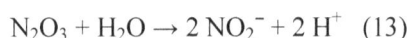

$$2\,NO + O_2 \rightarrow 2\,NO_2 \quad (11)$$

$$NO + NO_2 \leftrightarrow N_2O_3 \quad (12)$$

$$N_2O_3 + H_2O \rightarrow 2\,NO_2^- + 2\,H^+ \quad (13)$$

3.4. Half-Life, Diffusion, and Membrane Permeability

Due to its limited reactivity to most biomolecules, the half-life of NO in a biological system can be up to a few seconds depending on the surrounding environment, especially the levels of heme-containing proteins. In this regard, hemoglobin in RBCs may be a factor affecting the half-life and concentrations of NO in the circulation [39]. The RBC membrane or other intrinsic structures, however, may present a barrier for the uptake of NO [40, 41]. Nevertheless, as an uncharged molecule with high solubility in lipid environments NO may freely diffuse across cell membranes in most, if not all, types of cells, and signal many cell diameters distant from its site of generation [10].

4. CELL AND TISSUE DEFENSES

NO typically does not directly cause damage to cellular constituents due to its limited reactivity to lipids, proteins, and nucleic acid. Under pathophysiological conditions, excessive production of NO, especially in the presence of simultaneously increased formation of superoxide, may lead to tissue injury and disease process. Indeed, the deleterious effects of NO in biological systems are generally mediated by the formation of peroxynitrite as well as the secondary radical species derived from peroxynitrite, including nitrogen dioxide and carbonate radicals. Cell and tissue antioxidants that react with these oxidants and radical species derived from NO protect other vital biomolecules from being damaged. In this context, the reduced form of glutathione (GSH) and glutathione peroxidase and peroxiredoxin are crucial cellular factors in the detoxification of peroxynitrite (see Section 4 of Chapter 11).

5. BIOLOGY AND MEDICINE

5.1. Cell Signaling

NO is the first gaseous species identified as an endogenously generated signaling molecule. As a signaling molecule, NO plays important roles in wide range of physiological processes, including cardiovascular homeostasis, neurotransmission and neurodevelopment, and host defense, among others [28]. Notably, NO is also responsible for regulating neuronal developmental remodeling as well as the de-

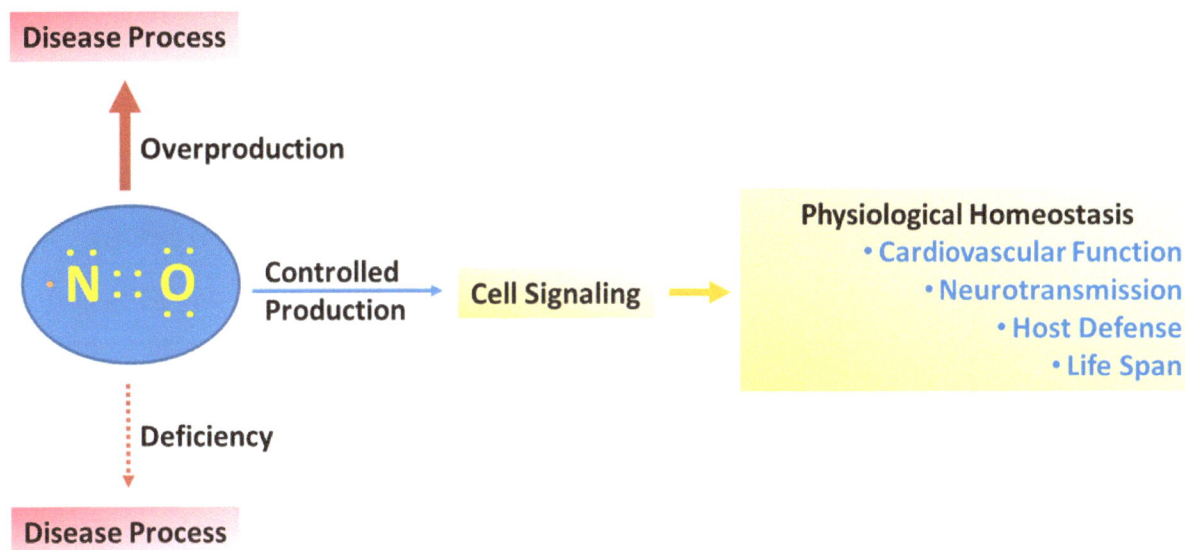

FIGURE 12.3. Nitric oxide (NO) in physiology and disease process. NO may act as a double-edged sword. On the one hand, NO, when its production is well-controlled, acts as a signaling molecule responsible for maintaining physiological homeostasis, including cardiovascular function, neurotransmission, host defense, and possibly lifespan. NO deficiency may compromise the NO-regulated physiological homeostasis, leading to disease process. On the other hand, overproduction of NO under certain pathophysiological conditions (e.g., chronic inflammation) may lead to the increased formation of more reactive species (e.g., peroxynitrite) that cause damage to cellular biomolecules, resulting in tissue injury and disease development.

velopment of excitatory synapses involved in learning [42, 43] (**Figure 12.3**).

The physiological functions of NO are primarily mediated by its high affinity and rapid binding to heme iron of soluble guanylate cyclase (sGC) and the subsequent activation of the sGC-cGMP-dependent signal pathways. NO-dependent modifications of protein thiols and low-molecular weight thiols occur in cells likely via the secondary reactive species derived from the reaction of NO with molecular oxygen (see Section 3.3.2), such as NO_2 and N_2O_3 that are capable of causing S-nitrosation. Increasing evidence also supports a role for S-nitrosation in NO signaling and NO-mediated disease protection [44–46].

5.2. Immunity

NO is one of the most versatile players in the immune system. It is involved in (1) the control of infectious diseases, (2) regulation of T and B cells, (3) cancer immunosurveillance, and (4) inflammatory disorders, among others. As noted earlier, the biological effects of NO may involve its direct interaction

with molecular targets (e.g., heme iron) and indirect actions via the formation of secondary reactive species (e.g., peroxynitrite, NO_2, N_2O_3). Hence, an NO-dependent biological effect may not necessarily result from the direct reaction of NO with its targets. As described next, this notion is particularly relevant with regard to the involvement of NO in innate immunity against invading pathogens. Accordingly, wherever indicated, NO/peroxynitrite is used in the discussion of NO-dependent immune responses in this section.

5.2.1. Phagocytic Defenses against Pathogens

Interactions of phagocytes with invading pathogens cause increased formation of NO (primarily from iNOS) and superoxide (primarily from NADPH oxidase), leading to the production of peroxynitrite, a potent oxidant capable of killing invading pathogens (also see Chapter 11). Substantial evidence supports a critical role for NO/peroxynitrite in phagocytic eradication of invading pathogens, including bacteria [47–49] and parasites [50–52]. Notably, the diffusion of NO between cells promotes equally effective pathogen killing in NO-producing and bystander cells. This cooperative mechanism of collective production of NO by numerous phagocytes generates an effective antimicrobial milieu that provides the basis for pathogen containment at the tissue level [53].

In addition to exerting killing activity toward pathogens, NO may also reduce the metabolic activity of intracellular parasites, thereby adding a chronic pressure on pathogen proliferation [54]. Notably, iNOS-derived NO may upregulate ferroportin-1, a major cellular iron exporter, in macrophages via a nuclear factor E2-related factor 2 (Nrf2)-dependent mechanism. The resultant decrease in cellular iron levels augments macrophage-mediated control of Salmonella infection [55]. NO/peroxynitrite not only is involved in the eradication of invading bacteria and parasites, but also may contribute to immunity against fungal and viral infections [56–58]. Besides phagocytes, other types of cells such as endothelial cells and B cells may also be able to kill pathogens via releasing NO [59, 60].

5.2.2. Cancer Immunity

Similar to killing of invading pathogens, phagocytes may also employ NO/peroxynitrite to achieve tumoricidal activity [61, 62]. So do dendritic cells [63]. Effective immune cell-based cancer cell killing requires overcoming immunosuppressive tumor microenvironments. In this context, a recent study shows that local NO production by tumor-infiltrating myeloid cells is important for adoptively transferred CD8$^+$ cytotoxic T cells to destroy tumors. These myeloid cells express iNOS that causes activation of CD40-CD40L, leading to tumor killing [64].

5.2.3. Regulation of T and B Cells

As important players of cell-mediated immunity, both T and B lymphocytes, especially T cells are subject to NO-mediated regulation. T cells express both iNOS and eNOS. The NOS-derived NO regulates T cell receptor signaling, T cell death, and T cell memory [65, 66]. NO also plays a role in controlling T cell proliferation and expansion [67, 68]. The NO-mediated suppression of T cell expansion may play a role in protecting against experimental autoimmune myocarditis [69]. T helper 17 (Th17) cells are associated with autoimmune diseases. NO derived from iNOS in activated T cells is involved in switching off Th17 cell differentiation and thereby controlling Th17 cell-associated colitis [70]. T cell activation is involved in cerebral malaria. NO sup-

presses the pathogenesis of cerebral malaria via suppressing both CD4$^+$ and CD8$^+$ T cell activation in response to Plasmodium infection. This suppression occurs as a result of NO-mediated activation of Nrf2, induction of heme oxygenase-1 (HO-1), and HO-1-derived carbon monoxide [71]. Hence, NO may regulate T cells via different mechanisms and pathways in protecting against disease processes associated with dysregulated immune responses.

Studies on NO regulation of B cells are not as extensive as those on T cells. Nevertheless, multiple groups reported the role of iNOS-derived NO in regulating antibody production by B cells as well as supporting the survival of plasma cells [72–74].
NO-mediated regulation of lymphocytes may also cause detrimental effects. In this context, iNOS-derived NO enhances T helper 9 (Th9) cell differentiation and Th9 cell-induced airway inflammation [75]. Indeed, as discussed below (Section 5.2.4), dysregulated production of NO is an important mechanism of inflammatory disorders.

5.2.4. Inflammation

Like other ROS, NO may also act as a double-edged sword. In this regard, deregulated production of NO/peroxynitrite along with the formation of other secondary reactive species during immune responses may directly cause tissue injury contributing to the pathogenesis of inflammatory disorders. For example, iNOS-derived NO and secondary reactive species are responsible, at least partly, for experimental endotoxemia-induced mortality [76]. In contrast, transgenic mice overexpressing eNOS are resistant to endotoxin shock [77], but nNOS-derived NO promotes nuclear factor kappaB (NF-κB) transcriptional activity and inflammatory cytokine gene expression [78], collectively pointing to the complexity of NO in inflammation.

Besides acting through the formation of peroxynitrite or other secondary reactive species, NO may regulate immune cells in a way to exaggerate immune responses causing tissue injury [75]. Moreover, iNOS-derived NO is shown to increase the susceptibility of toll-like receptor-activated macrophages to spreading *Listeria monocytogenes* and promote the pathogen spread during systemic in vivo infection [79]. Regardless of the mechanisms involved, dysregulated NO-dependent inflammatory response appears to be primarily responsible for the disease processes associated with NO production. In this context, dysregulated inflammation is a fundamental pathophysiological mechanism of many diseases.

5.3. Disease Process

5.3.1. NO Deficiency Contributes to Disease Process

No is a physiological signaling molecule and plays important roles in physiological homeostasis, including cardiovascular physiology, endocrine and metabolic regulation, neurotransmission and neuron development, and immune regulation, among others. Thus, deficiency of NO bioavailability either due to decreased production (e.g., diminished NOS activity) or increased consumption (e.g., reaction with superoxide or other free radicals) compromises physiological homeostasis, contributing to the development of cardiovascular disorders (e.g., myocardial infarction, atrial fibrillation) [80–83], metabolic syndrome and diabetes [84–86], neurological disorders (e.g., Alzheimer's disease, depression) [87–89], compromised immunity [70, 72], sexual dysfunction [90], and aging [33, 91], to name a few.

5.3.2. NO Overproduction Contributes to Disease Process

Overproduction of NO may contribute to disease pathophysiology via either its direct effects on molecular targets or indirectly through the generation of NO-derived secondary reactive species such as peroxynitrite. Because NO possesses limited reactivity to cellular biomolecules in general, most of the deleterious effects associated with NO overproduction may be primarily mediated by peroxynitrite and other secondary reactive species. Hence, discussion of NO toxicity frequently involves the use of the compound term of NO/peroxynitrite. Because of the inevitable reaction between NO and superoxide as well as between NO and molecular oxygen to form peroxynitrite and other reactive species in biological milieu, it is often time difficult, if not impossible, to attribute the adverse effects to a specific reactive species.

The pathophysiological effects associated with NO overproduction are influenced by various factors, including the sources (e.g., iNOS, eNOS, nNOS), levels, duration, and locations of NO production, the concomitantly increased production of superoxide or other free radical species, and the levels of surrounding antioxidant defenses. As both NO and superoxide are overproduced simultaneously by immune cells during inflammation, especially prolonged inflammation, much of the pathophysiological process of inflammatory disorder may be attributed to the un-

controlled formation of peroxynitrite. In this context, as mentioned earlier, chronic inflammation is a common pathophysiological mechanism of many human diseases.

The involvement of NO/peroxynitrite in disease pathophysiology has been extensively investigated over the past decades and a topic of extensive reviews [9, 92] (also see Section 5.3 of Chapter 11). The disease conditions associated with NO overproduction range from sepsis and autoimmune disorders to neurodegeneration and cancer development [9, 92]. Multistage tumorigenesis is a notable example of NO/peroxynitrite-associated pathophysiological conditions, for which chronic inflammation is both a major risk factor and a key tumor microenvironmental characteristic. Tumorigenesis associated with NO overproduction may result from the following effects elicited by NO/peroxynitrite: (1) gene mutations, Ras activation, and inactivation of the tumor suppressor p53 [93–95]; (2) suppression of cancer immunosurveillance leading to tumor escape [96, 97]; and (3) epigenetic modifications leading to dysregulated cell signaling, which eventually results in uncontrolled cell proliferation and tumor expansion and metastasis [98–101].

6. SUMMARY OF CHAPTER KEY POINTS

- NO was first identified as a gas in 1772 by Joseph Priestly who also discovered oxygen in 1774. More than two centuries later, R.F. Furchgott, L.J. Ignarro, and F. Murad were awarded the 1998 Nobel Prize in Physiology or Medicine for their discoveries concerning NO as a signaling molecule in the cardiovascular system.
- In biological systems NO is formed by two general pathways: nitric oxide synthase-dependent pathway and nitrate-nitrite-nitric oxide pathway. There are three isoforms of nitric oxide synthase, namely, nNOS or NOS1, iNOS or NOS2, and eNOS or NOS3.
- Multiple NOS-independent mechanisms are involved in the reduction of nitrite to NO. These include hemoglobin and myoglobin, acidic reduction, xanthine oxidoreductase, and mitochondria, among others.
- NO has a very low one-electron reduction potential and a very high one-electron oxidation potential. As such, NO is both a poor oxidant and a poor reductant in biological systems though it is a free radical. Indeed, the direct reactions of NO with most biomolecules, including proteins (except for

certain transition metal ion-containing proteins), lipids, and nucleic acids are very limited.

- NO is a unique ligand for heme groups of various proteins. The high affinity and rapid binding of NO to heme iron of sGC causes its activation and the subsequent formation of cGMP. This is a well-established signaling pathway underlying NO-mediated physiological effects. On the other hand, the high affinity and rapid binding of NO to heme iron in mitochondrial cytochrome c oxidase is a major chemical basis for NO regulation of mitochondrial respiration.

- NO reacts with lipid radicals, leading to the termination of lipid peroxidation. This may partly explain the antioxidant properties of NO observed in biological systems.

- NO reacts with superoxide at a diffusion-limited rate to form peroxynitrite, a potent oxidant capable of reacting with a wide range of biomolecules. NO also reacts with molecular oxygen, giving rise to secondary reactive species, such as NO_2 and N_2O_3. These reactive species may largely be responsible for injury associated with NO overproduction.

- NO is one of the most important free radical species in biology and medicine. It is the first gaseous species identified as an endogenously generated signaling molecule. As a signaling molecule, NO is crucial for physiological homeostasis, including cardiovascular function, neurotransmission, and host defense. Deficiency of NO is associated with the pathogenesis of many human disorders.

- NO is like a double-edged sword. Its overproduction under pathophysiological conditions may contribute to the development of a number of human diseases. Because NO possesses limited reactivity to cellular biomolecules in general, most of the deleterious effects associated with NO overproduction may be primarily mediated by NO-derived reactive species, such as peroxynitrite.

7. SELF-ASSESSMENT QUESTIONS

7.1. Biological signaling molecules are instrumental in maintaining cellular physiological homeostasis. Which of the following is the first gaseous signaling molecule identified in biological systems?

A. CO
B. H_2
C. H_2S
D. NO
E. NO_2

7.2. R.F. Furchgott, L.J. Ignarro, and F. Murad were awarded the 1998 Nobel Prize in Physiology or Medicine for their discoveries concerning nitric oxide as which of the following?

A. A mediator of neuronal remodeling
B. A precursor of peroxynitrite formation
C. A signaling molecule in plants
D. A signaling molecule in the cardiovascular system
E. A toxic species in cardiovascular disease

7.3. Formation of NO in biological systems may occur via both NOS-dependent or -independent pathways. In this regard, which of the following enzymes has been shown to reduce nitrite to form NO under biologically relevant conditions?

A. Catalase
B. Glutathione peroxidase
C. Monoamine oxidase
D. Superoxide dismutase
E. Xanthine oxidoreductase

7.4. Due to its unique chemical properties, NO selectively reacts with certain molecular targets in biological systems. Which of the following enzymes is most likely to be inhibited by NO at a physiologically relevant concentration?

A. Ca^{2+}-ATPase
B. Cytochrome c oxidase
C. Glutathione reductase
D. NADPH:quinone oxidoreductase
E. Peroxiredoxin

7.5. Reaction of NO with which of the following species may explain the antioxidant activity of this free radical species in inhibiting lipid peroxidation?

A. Hydrogen peroxide
B. Lipid peroxyl radical
C. Molecular oxygen
D. Peroxynitrite
E. Superoxide

ANSWERS AND EXPLANATIONS

7.1. The answer is D. NO is the first gaseous species identified as an endogenously generated signaling molecule. Both H_2S and CO also act as biological signaling molecules.

7.2. The answer is D. In 1998, R.F. Furchgott, L.J. Ignarro, and F. Murad were awarded the Nobel Prize in Physiology or Medicine for their discoveries concerning nitric oxide as a signaling molecule in the cardiovascular system.

7.3. The answer is E. At low oxygen tensions and pH values, xanthine oxidoreductase is able to reduce nitrite to NO at the molybdenum (Mo) site of the enzyme via the following reaction: $NO_2^- + Mo^{4+} + H^+ \rightarrow NO + Mo^{3+} + OH^-$.

7.4. The answer is B. The high affinity and rapid binding of NO to heme iron in mitochondrial cytochrome c oxidase is a major chemical basis for NO regulation of mitochondrial respiration.

7.5. The answer is B. NO may inhibit lipid peroxidation. This occurs by a chain-breaking termination reaction of NO with lipid peroxyl radical (LOO˙), leading to the eventual formation of less reactive non-radical species. The reaction occurs as following: $LOO˙ + NO \rightarrow LOONO \rightarrow NO_2 + LO˙ \rightarrow LONO_2$.

REFERENCES

1. Katsuki S, Arnold W, Mittal C, Murad F. Stimulation of guanylate cyclase by sodium nitroprusside, nitroglycerin and nitric oxide in various tissue preparations and comparison to the effects of sodium azide and hydroxylamine. *J Cyclic Nucleotide Res* 1977; 3(1):23–35.
2. Arnold WP, Mittal CK, Katsuki S, Murad F. Nitric oxide activates guanylate cyclase and increases guanosine 3':5'-cyclic monophosphate levels in various tissue preparations. *Proc Natl Acad Sci USA* 1977; 74(8):3203–7.
3. Furchgott RF, Zawadzki JV. The obligatory role of endothelial cells in the relaxation of arterial smooth muscle by acetylcholine. *Nature* 1980; 288(5789):373–6.
4. Ignarro LJ, Byrns RE, Buga GM, Wood KS. Endothelium-derived relaxing factor from pulmonary artery and vein possesses pharmacologic and chemical properties identical to those of nitric oxide radical. *Circ Res* 1987; 61(6):866–79.
5. Ignarro LJ, Buga GM, Wood KS, Byrns RE, Chaudhuri G. Endothelium-derived relaxing factor produced and released from artery and vein is nitric oxide. *Proc Natl Acad Sci USA* 1987; 84(24):9265–9.
6. Palmer RM, Ferrige AG, Moncada S. Nitric oxide release accounts for the biological activity of endothelium-derived relaxing factor. *Nature* 1987; 327(6122):524–6.
7. Steinhorn BS, Loscalzo J, Michel T. Nitroglycerin and Nitric oxide--a rondo of themes in cardiovascular therapeutics. *N Engl J Med* 2015; 373(3):277–80.
8. Koshland DE, Jr. The molecule of the year. *Science* 1992; 258(5090):1861.
9. Pacher P, Beckman JS, Liaudet L. Nitric oxide and peroxynitrite in health and disease. *Physiol Rev* 2007; 87(1):315–424.
10. Hill BG, Dranka BP, Bailey SM, Lancaster JR, Jr., Darley-Usmar VM. What part of NO don't you understand? Some answers to the cardinal questions in nitric oxide biology. *J Biol Chem* 2010; 285(26):19699–704.
11. Vanhoutte PM, Zhao Y, Xu A, Leung SW. Thirty years of saying NO: sources, fate, actions, and misfortunes of the endothelium-derived vasodilator mediator. *Circ Res* 2016; 119(2):375–96.
12. Lundberg JO, Weitzberg E, Gladwin MT. The nitrate-nitrite-nitric oxide pathway in physiology and therapeutics. *Nat Rev Drug Discov* 2008; 7(2):156–67.
13. Nagababu E, Ramasamy S, Abernethy DR, Rifkind JM. Active nitric oxide produced in the red cell under hypoxic conditions by deoxyhemoglobin-mediated nitrite reduction. *J Biol Chem* 2003; 278(47):46349–56.
14. Cosby K, Partovi KS, Crawford JH, Patel RP, Reiter CD, Martyr S, Yang BK, Waclawiw MA, Zalos G, Xu X, Huang KT, Shields H, et al. Nitrite reduction to nitric oxide by deoxyhemoglobin vasodilates the human circulation. *Nat Med* 2003; 9(12):1498–505.
15. Shiva S, Huang Z, Grubina R, Sun J, Ringwood LA, MacArthur PH, Xu X, Murphy E, Darley-Usmar VM, Gladwin MT. Deoxymyoglobin is a nitrite reductase that generates nitric oxide and regulates mitochondrial respiration. *Circ Res* 2007; 100(5):654–61.
16. Hendgen-Cotta UB, Merx MW, Shiva S, Schmitz J, Becher S, Klare JP, Steinhoff HJ, Goedecke A, Schrader J, Gladwin MT, Kelm M, Rassaf T. Nitrite reductase activity of myoglobin regulates respiration and cellular viability in myocardial ischemia-reperfusion injury. *Proc Natl Acad Sci USA* 2008; 105(29):10256–61.
17. McKnight GM, Smith LM, Drummond RS, Duncan CW, Golden M, Benjamin N. Chemical

synthesis of nitric oxide in the stomach from dietary nitrate in humans. *Gut* 1997; 40(2):211–4.

18. Godber BL, Doel JJ, Sapkota GP, Blake DR, Stevens CR, Eisenthal R, Harrison R. Reduction of nitrite to nitric oxide catalyzed by xanthine oxidoreductase. *J Biol Chem* 2000; 275(11):7757–63.

19. Baliga RS, Milsom AB, Ghosh SM, Trinder SL, Macallister RJ, Ahluwalia A, Hobbs AJ. Dietary nitrate ameliorates pulmonary hypertension: cytoprotective role for endothelial nitric oxide synthase and xanthine oxidoreductase. *Circulation* 2012; 125(23):2922–32.

20. Castello PR, David PS, McClure T, Crook Z, Poyton RO. Mitochondrial cytochrome oxidase produces nitric oxide under hypoxic conditions: implications for oxygen sensing and hypoxic signaling in eukaryotes. *Cell Metab* 2006; 3(4):277–87.

21. Castello PR, Woo DK, Ball K, Wojcik J, Liu L, Poyton RO. Oxygen-regulated isoforms of cytochrome c oxidase have differential effects on its nitric oxide production and on hypoxic signaling. *Proc Natl Acad Sci USA* 2008; 105(24):8203–8.

22. Sparacino-Watkins CE, Tejero J, Sun B, Gauthier MC, Thomas J, Ragireddy V, Merchant BA, Wang J, Azarov I, Basu P, Gladwin MT. Nitrite reductase and nitric-oxide synthase activity of the mitochondrial molybdopterin enzymes mARC1 and mARC2. *J Biol Chem* 2014; 289(15):10345–58.

23. Miyamoto T, Petrus MJ, Dubin AE, Patapoutian A. TRPV3 regulates nitric oxide synthase-independent nitric oxide synthesis in the skin. *Nat Commun* 2011; 2:369.

24. Webb AJ, Milsom AB, Rathod KS, Chu WL, Qureshi S, Lovell MJ, Lecomte FM, Perrett D, Raimondo C, Khoshbin E, Ahmed Z, Uppal R, et al. Mechanisms underlying erythrocyte and endothelial nitrite reduction to nitric oxide in hypoxia: role for xanthine oxidoreductase and endothelial nitric oxide synthase. *Circ Res* 2008; 103(9):957–64.

25. Corti P, Xue J, Tejero J, Wajih N, Sun M, Stolz DB, Tsang M, Kim-Shapiro DB, Gladwin MT. Globin X is a six-coordinate globin that reduces nitrite to nitric oxide in fish red blood cells. *Proc Natl Acad Sci USA* 2016; 113(30):8538–43.

26. Bartberger MD, Liu W, Ford E, Miranda KM, Switzer C, Fukuto JM, Farmer PJ, Wink DA, Houk KN. The reduction potential of nitric oxide (NO) and its importance to NO biochemistry.

Proc Natl Acad Sci USA 2002; 99(17):10958–63.

27. Toledo JC, Jr., Augusto O. Connecting the chemical and biological properties of nitric oxide. *Chem Res Toxicol* 2012; 25(5):975–89.

28. Murad F. Shattuck Lecture. Nitric oxide and cyclic GMP in cell signaling and drug development. *N Engl J Med* 2006; 355(19):2003–11.

29. Xu W, Charles IG, Moncada S. Nitric oxide: orchestrating hypoxia regulation through mitochondrial respiration and the endoplasmic reticulum stress response. *Cell Res* 2005; 15(1):63–5.

30. Antunes F, Boveris A, Cadenas E. On the mechanism and biology of cytochrome oxidase inhibition by nitric oxide. *Proc Natl Acad Sci USA* 2004; 101(48):16774–9.

31. Husain M, Bourret TJ, McCollister BD, Jones-Carson J, Laughlin J, Vazquez-Torres A. Nitric oxide evokes an adaptive response to oxidative stress by arresting respiration. *J Biol Chem* 2008; 283(12):7682–9.

32. Nisoli E, Clementi E, Paolucci C, Cozzi V, Tonello C, Sciorati C, Bracale R, Valerio A, Francolini M, Moncada S, Carruba MO. Mitochondrial biogenesis in mammals: the role of endogenous nitric oxide. *Science* 2003; 299(5608):896–9.

33. Nisoli E, Tonello C, Cardile A, Cozzi V, Bracale R, Tedesco L, Falcone S, Valerio A, Cantoni O, Clementi E, Moncada S, Carruba MO. Calorie restriction promotes mitochondrial biogenesis by inducing the expression of eNOS. *Science* 2005; 310(5746):314–7.

34. Ding H, Demple B. Direct nitric oxide signal transduction via nitrosylation of iron-sulfur centers in the SoxR transcription activator. *Proc Natl Acad Sci USA* 2000; 97(10):5146–50.

35. Crack JC, Stapleton MR, Green J, Thomson AJ, Le Brun NE. Mechanism of [4Fe-4S](Cys)4 cluster nitrosylation is conserved among NO-responsive regulators. *J Biol Chem* 2013; 288(16):11492–502.

36. Pryor WA, Houk KN, Foote CS, Fukuto JM, Ignarro LJ, Squadrito GL, Davies KJ. Free radical biology and medicine: it's a gas, man! *Am J Physiol Regul Integr Comp Physiol* 2006; 291(3):R491–511.

37. Rubbo H, Radi R, Anselmi D, Kirk M, Barnes S, Butler J, Eiserich JP, Freeman BA. Nitric oxide reaction with lipid peroxyl radicals spares alpha-tocopherol during lipid peroxidation: greater oxidant protection from the pair nitric

oxide/alpha-tocopherol than alpha-tocopherol/ascorbate. *J Biol Chem* 2000; 275(15):10812–8.

38. Kotamraju S, Hogg N, Joseph J, Keefer LK, Kalyanaraman B. Inhibition of oxidized low-density lipoprotein-induced apoptosis in endothelial cells by nitric oxide: peroxyl radical scavenging as an antiapoptotic mechanism. *J Biol Chem* 2001; 276(20):17316–23.

39. Gow AJ, Stamler JS. Reactions between nitric oxide and haemoglobin under physiological conditions. *Nature* 1998; 391(6663):169–73.

40. Vaughn MW, Huang KT, Kuo L, Liao JC. Erythrocytes possess an intrinsic barrier to nitric oxide consumption. *J Biol Chem* 2000; 275(4):2342–8.

41. Huang KT, Han TH, Hyduke DR, Vaughn MW, Van Herle H, Hein TW, Zhang C, Kuo L, Liao JC. Modulation of nitric oxide bioavailability by erythrocytes. *Proc Natl Acad Sci USA* 2001; 98(20):11771–6.

42. Nikonenko I, Nikonenko A, Mendez P, Michurina TV, Enikolopov G, Muller D. Nitric oxide mediates local activity-dependent excitatory synapse development. *Proc Natl Acad Sci USA* 2013; 110(44):E4142–51.

43. Rabinovich D, Yaniv SP, Alyagor I, Schuldiner O. Nitric Oxide as a Switching Mechanism between Axon Degeneration and Regrowth during Developmental Remodeling. *Cell* 2016; 164(1–2):170–82.

44. Thibeault S, Rautureau Y, Oubaha M, Faubert D, Wilkes BC, Delisle C, Gratton JP. S-Nitrosylation of beta-catenin by eNOS-derived NO promotes VEGF-induced endothelial cell permeability. *Mol Cell* 2010; 39(3):468–76.

45. Marin N, Zamorano P, Carrasco R, Mujica P, Gonzalez FG, Quezada C, Meininger CJ, Boric MP, Duran WN, Sanchez FA. S-Nitrosation of beta-catenin and p120 catenin: a novel regulatory mechanism in endothelial hyperpermeability. *Circ Res* 2012; 111(5):553–63.

46. Chouchani ET, Methner C, Nadtochiy SM, Logan A, Pell VR, Ding S, James AM, Cocheme HM, Reinhold J, Lilley KS, Partridge L, Fearnley IM, et al. Cardioprotection by S-nitrosation of a cysteine switch on mitochondrial complex I. *Nat Med* 2013; 19(6):753–9.

47. Evans TJ, Buttery LD, Carpenter A, Springall DR, Polak JM, Cohen J. Cytokine-treated human neutrophils contain inducible nitric oxide synthase that produces nitration of ingested bacteria. *Proc Natl Acad Sci USA* 1996; 93(18):9553–8.

48. Foley E, O'Farrell PH. Nitric oxide contributes to induction of innate immune responses to gram-negative bacteria in Drosophila. *Genes Dev* 2003; 17(1):115–25.

49. Lee WB, Kang JS, Choi WY, Zhang Q, Kim CH, Choi UY, Kim-Ha J, Kim YJ. Mincle-mediated translational regulation is required for strong nitric oxide production and inflammation resolution. *Nat Commun* 2016; 7:11322.

50. Vouldoukis I, Riveros-Moreno V, Dugas B, Ouaaz F, Becherel P, Debre P, Moncada S, Mossalayi MD. The killing of Leishmania major by human macrophages is mediated by nitric oxide induced after ligation of the Fc epsilon RII/CD23 surface antigen. *Proc Natl Acad Sci USA* 1995; 92(17):7804–8.

51. Hobbs MR, Udhayakumar V, Levesque MC, Booth J, Roberts JM, Tkachuk AN, Pole A, Coon H, Kariuki S, Nahlen BL, Mwaikambo ED, Lal AL, et al. A new NOS2 promoter polymorphism associated with increased nitric oxide production and protection from severe malaria in Tanzanian and Kenyan children. *Lancet* 2002; 360(9344):1468–75.

52. Lima-Junior DS, Costa DL, Carregaro V, Cunha LD, Silva AL, Mineo TW, Gutierrez FR, Bellio M, Bortoluci KR, Flavell RA, Bozza MT, Silva JS, et al. Inflammasome-derived IL-1beta production induces nitric oxide-mediated resistance to Leishmania. *Nat Med* 2013; 19(7):909–15.

53. Olekhnovitch R, Ryffel B, Muller AJ, Bousso P. Collective nitric oxide production provides tissue-wide immunity during Leishmania infection. *J Clin Invest* 2014; 124(4):1711–22.

54. Muller AJ, Aeschlimann S, Olekhnovitch R, Dacher M, Spath GF, Bousso P. Photoconvertible pathogen labeling reveals nitric oxide control of *Leishmania major* infection in vivo via dampening of parasite metabolism. *Cell Host Microbe* 2013; 14(4):460–7.

55. Nairz M, Schleicher U, Schroll A, Sonnweber T, Theurl I, Ludwiczek S, Talasz H, Brandacher G, Moser PL, Muckenthaler MU, Fang FC, Bogdan C, et al. Nitric oxide-mediated regulation of ferroportin-1 controls macrophage iron homeostasis and immune function in Salmonella infection. *J Exp Med* 2013; 210(5):855–73.

56. Jones-Carson J, Vazquez-Torres A, van der Heyde HC, Warner T, Wagner RD, Balish E. Gamma delta T cell-induced nitric oxide

production enhances resistance to mucosal candidiasis. *Nat Med* 1995; 1(6):552–7.

57. Saura M, Zaragoza C, McMillan A, Quick RA, Hohenadl C, Lowenstein JM, Lowenstein CJ. An antiviral mechanism of nitric oxide: inhibition of a viral protease. *Immunity* 1999; 10(1):21–8.

58. Zaragoza C, Ocampo C, Saura M, Leppo M, Wei XQ, Quick R, Moncada S, Liew FY, Lowenstein CJ. The role of inducible nitric oxide synthase in the host response to *Coxsackievirus myocarditis*. *Proc Natl Acad Sci USA* 1998; 95(5):2469–74.

59. Oswald IP, Eltoum I, Wynn TA, Schwartz B, Caspar P, Paulin D, Sher A, James SL. Endothelial cells are activated by cytokine treatment to kill an intravascular parasite, *Schistosoma mansoni*, through the production of nitric oxide. *Proc Natl Acad Sci USA* 1994; 91(3):999–1003.

60. Mannick JB, Asano K, Izumi K, Kieff E, Stamler JS. Nitric oxide produced by human B lymphocytes inhibits apoptosis and Epstein-Barr virus reactivation. *Cell* 1994; 79(7):1137–46.

61. Dinapoli MR, Calderon CL, Lopez DM. The altered tumoricidal capacity of macrophages isolated from tumor-bearing mice is related to reduce expression of the inducible nitric oxide synthase gene. *J Exp Med* 1996; 183(4):1323–9.

62. Zhao X, Mohaupt M, Jiang J, Liu S, Li B, Qin Z. Tumor necrosis factor receptor 2-mediated tumor suppression is nitric oxide dependent and involves angiostasis. *Cancer Res* 2007; 67(9):4443–50.

63. Huang J, Tatsumi T, Pizzoferrato E, Vujanovic N, Storkus WJ. Nitric oxide sensitizes tumor cells to dendritic cell-mediated apoptosis, uptake, and cross-presentation. *Cancer Res* 2005; 65(18):8461–70.

64. Marigo I, Zilio S, Desantis G, Mlecnik B, Agnellini AH, Ugel S, Sasso MS, Qualls JE, Kratochvill F, Zanovello P, Molon B, Ries CH, et al. T cell cancer therapy requires CD40-CD40L activation of tumor necrosis factor and inducible nitric-oxide-synthase-producing dendritic cells. *Cancer Cell* 2016; 30(3):377–90.

65. Vig M, Srivastava S, Kandpal U, Sade H, Lewis V, Sarin A, George A, Bal V, Durdik JM, Rath S. Inducible nitric oxide synthase in T cells regulates T cell death and immune memory. *J Clin Invest* 2004; 113(12):1734–42.

66. Ibiza S, Victor VM, Bosca I, Ortega A, Urzainqui A, O'Connor JE, Sanchez-Madrid F, Esplugues JV, Serrador JM. Endothelial nitric

oxide synthase regulates T cell receptor signaling at the immunological synapse. *Immunity* 2006; 24(6):753–65.

67. Sato K, Ozaki K, Oh I, Meguro A, Hatanaka K, Nagai T, Muroi K, Ozawa K. Nitric oxide plays a critical role in suppression of T-cell proliferation by mesenchymal stem cells. *Blood* 2007; 109(1):228–34.

68. Lukacs-Kornek V, Malhotra D, Fletcher AL, Acton SE, Elpek KG, Tayalia P, Collier AR, Turley SJ. Regulated release of nitric oxide by nonhematopoietic stroma controls expansion of the activated T cell pool in lymph nodes. *Nat Immunol* 2011; 12(11):1096–104.

69. Kania G, Siegert S, Behnke S, Prados-Rosales R, Casadevall A, Luscher TF, Luther SA, Kopf M, Eriksson U, Blyszczuk P. Innate signaling promotes formation of regulatory nitric oxide-producing dendritic cells limiting T-cell expansion in experimental autoimmune myocarditis. *Circulation* 2013; 127(23):2285–94.

70. Jianjun Y, Zhang R, Lu G, Shen Y, Peng L, Zhu C, Cui M, Wang W, Arnaboldi P, Tang M, Gupta M, Qi CF, et al. T cell-derived inducible nitric oxide synthase switches off Th17 cell differentiation. *J Exp Med* 2013; 210(7):1447–62.

71. Jeney V, Ramos S, Bergman ML, Bechmann I, Tischer J, Ferreira A, Oliveira-Marques V, Janse CJ, Rebelo S, Cardoso S, Soares MP. Control of disease tolerance to malaria by nitric oxide and carbon monoxide. *Cell Rep* 2014; 8(1):126–36.

72. Tezuka H, Abe Y, Iwata M, Takeuchi H, Ishikawa H, Matsushita M, Shiohara T, Akira S, Ohteki T. Regulation of IgA production by naturally occurring TNF/iNOS-producing dendritic cells. *Nature* 2007; 448(7156):929–33.

73. Fritz JH, Rojas OL, Simard N, McCarthy DD, Hapfelmeier S, Rubino S, Robertson SJ, Larijani M, Gosselin J, Ivanov, II, Martin A, Casellas R, et al. Acquisition of a multifunctional IgA⁺ plasma cell phenotype in the gut. *Nature* 2011; 481(7380):199–203.

74. Saini AS, Shenoy GN, Rath S, Bal V, George A. Inducible nitric oxide synthase is a major intermediate in signaling pathways for the survival of plasma cells. *Nat Immunol* 2014; 15(3):275–82.

75. Niedbala W, Besnard AG, Nascimento DC, Donate PB, Sonego F, Yip E, Guabiraba R, Chang HD, Fukada SY, Salmond RJ, Schmitt E, Bopp T, et al. Nitric oxide enhances Th9 cell differentiation and airway inflammation. *Nat*

Commun 2014; 5:4575.

76. Wei XQ, Charles IG, Smith A, Ure J, Feng GJ, Huang FP, Xu D, Muller W, Moncada S, Liew FY. Altered immune responses in mice lacking inducible nitric oxide synthase. *Nature* 1995; 375(6530):408–11.

77. Yamashita T, Kawashima S, Ohashi Y, Ozaki M, Ueyama T, Ishida T, Inoue N, Hirata K, Akita H, Yokoyama M. Resistance to endotoxin shock in transgenic mice overexpressing endothelial nitric oxide synthase. *Circulation* 2000; 101(8):931–7.

78. Baig MS, Zaichick SV, Mao M, de Abreu AL, Bakhshi FR, Hart PC, Saqib U, Deng J, Chatterjee S, Block ML, Vogel SM, Malik AB, et al. NOS1-derived nitric oxide promotes NF-kappaB transcriptional activity through inhibition of suppressor of cytokine signaling-1. *J Exp Med* 2015; 212(10):1725–38.

79. Cole C, Thomas S, Filak H, Henson PM, Lenz LL. Nitric oxide increases susceptibility of Toll-like receptor-activated macrophages to spreading Listeria monocytogenes. *Immunity* 2012; 36(5):807–20.

80. Erdmann J, Stark K, Esslinger UB, Rumpf PM, Koesling D, de Wit C, Kaiser FJ, Braunholz D, Medack A, Fischer M, Zimmermann ME, Tennstedt S, et al. Dysfunctional nitric oxide signalling increases risk of myocardial infarction. *Nature* 2013; 504(7480):432–6.

81. Belge C, Hammond J, Dubois-Deruy E, Manoury B, Hamelet J, Beauloye C, Markl A, Pouleur AC, Bertrand L, Esfahani H, Jnaoui K, Gotz KR, et al. Enhanced expression of beta3-adrenoceptors in cardiac myocytes attenuates neurohormone-induced hypertrophic remodeling through nitric oxide synthase. *Circulation* 2014; 129(4):451–62.

82. Reilly SN, Liu X, Carnicer R, Recalde A, Muszkiewicz A, Jayaram R, Carena MC, Wijesurendra R, Stefanini M, Surdo NC, Lomas O, Ratnatunga C, et al. Up-regulation of miR-31 in human atrial fibrillation begets the arrhythmia by depleting dystrophin and neuronal nitric oxide synthase. *Sci Transl Med* 2016; 8(340):340ra74.

83. Reilly S, Liu X, Carnicer R, Rajakumar T, Sayeed R, Krasopoulos G, Verheule S, Fulga T, Schotten U, Casadei B. Evaluation of the role of miR-31-dependent reduction in dystrophin and nNOS on atrial-fibrillation-induced electrical remodelling in man. *Lancet* 2015; 385 Suppl 1:S82.

84. Carlstrom M, Larsen FJ, Nystrom T, Hezel M, Borniquel S, Weitzberg E, Lundberg JO. Dietary inorganic nitrate reverses features of metabolic syndrome in endothelial nitric oxide synthase-deficient mice. *Proc Natl Acad Sci USA* 2010; 107(41):17716–20.

85. Sansbury BE, Cummins TD, Tang Y, Hellmann J, Holden CR, Harbeson MA, Chen Y, Patel RP, Spite M, Bhatnagar A, Hill BG. Overexpression of endothelial nitric oxide synthase prevents diet-induced obesity and regulates adipocyte phenotype. *Circ Res* 2012; 111(9):1176–89.

86. Trevellin E, Scorzeto M, Olivieri M, Granzotto M, Valerio A, Tedesco L, Fabris R, Serra R, Quarta M, Reggiani C, Nisoli E, Vettor R. Exercise training induces mitochondrial biogenesis and glucose uptake in subcutaneous adipose tissue through eNOS-dependent mechanisms. *Diabetes* 2014; 63(8):2800–11.

87. Hu Y, Wu DL, Luo CX, Zhu LJ, Zhang J, Wu HY, Zhu DY. Hippocampal nitric oxide contributes to sex difference in affective behaviors. *Proc Natl Acad Sci USA* 2012; 109(35):14224–9.

88. Morairty SR, Dittrich L, Pasumarthi RK, Valladao D, Heiss JE, Gerashchenko D, Kilduff TS. A role for cortical nNOS/NK1 neurons in coupling homeostatic sleep drive to EEG slow wave activity. *Proc Natl Acad Sci USA* 2013; 110(50):20272–7.

89. Austin SA, Katusic ZS. Loss of Endothelial nitric oxide synthase promotes p25 generation and Tau phosphorylation in a murine model of Alzheimer's disease. *Circ Res* 2016; 119(10):1128–34.

90. Hurt KJ, Sezen SF, Lagoda GF, Musicki B, Rameau GA, Snyder SH, Burnett AL. Cyclic AMP-dependent phosphorylation of neuronal nitric oxide synthase mediates penile erection. *Proc Natl Acad Sci USA* 2012; 109(41):16624–9.

91. Gusarov I, Gautier L, Smolentseva O, Shamovsky I, Eremina S, Mironov A, Nudler E. Bacterial nitric oxide extends the lifespan of *C. elegans*. *Cell* 2013; 152(4):818–30.

92. Szabo C, Ischiropoulos H, Radi R. Peroxynitrite: biochemistry, pathophysiology and development of therapeutics. *Nat Rev Drug Discov* 2007; 6(8):662–80.

93. Wink DA, Kasprzak KS, Maragos CM, Elespuru RK, Misra M, Dunams TM, Cebula TA, Koch WH, Andrews AW, Allen JS, et al. DNA deaminating ability and genotoxicity of nitric oxide and its progenitors. *Science* 1991; 254(5034):1001–3.

94. Calmels S, Hainaut P, Ohshima H. Nitric oxide induces conformational and functional modifications of wild-type p53 tumor suppressor protein. *Cancer Res* 1997; 57(16):3365–9.

95. Lim KH, Ancrile BB, Kashatus DF, Counter CM. Tumour maintenance is mediated by eNOS. *Nature* 2008; 452(7187):646–9.

96. Nagaraj S, Gupta K, Pisarev V, Kinarsky L, Sherman S, Kang L, Herber DL, Schneck J, Gabrilovich DI. Altered recognition of antigen is a mechanism of CD8[+] T cell tolerance in cancer. *Nat Med* 2007; 13(7):828–35.

97. Lu T, Ramakrishnan R, Altiok S, Youn JI, Cheng P, Celis E, Pisarev V, Sherman S, Sporn MB, Gabrilovich D. Tumor-infiltrating myeloid cells induce tumor cell resistance to cytotoxic T cells in mice. *J Clin Invest* 2011; 121(10):4015–29.

98. Shen X, Burguillos MA, Osman AM, Frijhoff J, Carrillo-Jimenez A, Kanatani S, Augsten M, Saidi D, Rodhe J, Kavanagh E, Rongvaux A, Rraklli V, et al. Glioma-induced inhibition of caspase-3 in microglia promotes a tumor-supportive phenotype. *Nat Immunol* 2016; 17(11):1282–90.

99. Heinecke JL, Ridnour LA, Cheng RY, Switzer CH, Lizardo MM, Khanna C, Glynn SA, Hussain SP, Young HA, Ambs S, Wink DA. Tumor microenvironment-based feed-forward regulation of NOS2 in breast cancer progression. *Proc Natl Acad Sci USA* 2014; 111(17):6323–8.

100. Dave B, Granados-Principal S, Zhu R, Benz S, Rabizadeh S, Soon-Shiong P, Yu KD, Shao Z, Li X, Gilcrease M, Lai Z, Chen Y, et al. Targeting RPL39 and MLF2 reduces tumor initiation and metastasis in breast cancer by inhibiting nitric oxide synthase signaling. *Proc Natl Acad Sci USA* 2014; 111(24):8838–43.

101. Lopez-Rivera E, Jayaraman P, Parikh F, Davies MA, Ekmekcioglu S, Izadmehr S, Milton DR, Chipuk JE, Grimm EA, Estrada Y, Aguirre-Ghiso J, Sikora AG. Inducible nitric oxide synthase drives mTOR pathway activation and proliferation of human melanoma by reversible nitrosylation of TSC2. *Cancer Res* 2014; 74(4):1067–78.

Chapter 13

Hypochlorous Acid in Biology and Medicine

ABSTRACT | Hypochlorous acid (HOCl), the active ingredient of bleach, has long been used as a disinfectant. In biological systems, HOCl is generated via two pathways, namely, the myeloperoxidase (MPO)-H_2O_2-chloride and the vascular peroxidase 1 (VPO1)-H_2O_2-chloride pathways, with the former being much better characterized. HOCl is a weak acid, and under a physiological pH HOCl and hypochlorite (OCl^-) are approximately at equal concentrations. HOCl is a potent oxidant capable of reacting with and causing damage to cellular constituents, including lipids, proteins, and nucleic acids. HOCl also reacts with other reactive oxygen species, such as superoxide and hydroperoxides to form secondary reactive radical species (e.g., hydroxyl radical and singlet oxygen). Currently, there is no known enzyme capable of directly catalyzing the detoxification of HOCl. The reduced form of glutathione (GSH) appears to be the chief antioxidant defense against HOCl toxicity in mammalian cells. As a biologically formed reactive species, HOCl is implicated in biology and medicine. The controlled production of HOCl by phagocytic cells during respiratory burst is an integral part of the host defense against invading pathogens. However, under certain conditions such as chronic inflammation, overproduction of HOCl along with other reactive species may cause damage to host cellular biomolecules, leading to cell and tissue injury. Overproduction of HOCl has been suggested to contribute to the pathophysiology of various disease processes, especially atherosclerotic cardiovascular injury.

KEYWORDS | Atherosclerosis; Hydrogen peroxide; Hypochlorite; Hypochlorous acid; Immunity; Myeloperoxidase; Reactive chlorine species; Redox signaling; Vascular peroxidase 1

CITATION | *Hopkins RZ and Li YR. Essentials of Free Radical Biology and Medicine. Cell Med Press, Raleigh, NC, USA. 2017. http://dx.doi.org/10.20455/efrbm.2017.13*

ABBREVIATIONS | ABCA1, ATP-binding cassette A1; ApoA-I, apolipoprotein A-I; eNOS, endothelial nitric oxide synthase; GSH, reduced form of glutathione; HDL, high-density lipoprotein; HOSCN, hypothiocyanous acid; LDL, low-density lipoprotein; MPO, myeloperoxidase; Msr, methionine sulfoxide reductase; Nrf2, nuclear factor E2-related factor 2; SR-B1, scavenger receptor B1; VPO, vascular peroxidase; VWF, von Willebrand factor

CHAPTER AT A GLANCE

1. OVERVIEW

Hypochlorous acid (HOCl) is a weak acid and its deprotonated form is called hypochlorite ion (OCl$^-$). The salts of HOCl are known as hypochlorites (e.g., sodium hypochlorite, NaOCl; potassium hypochlorite, KOCl). In this chapter, the above terms are used interchangeably and as the prototype of reactive chlorine species (RCS) (also see Section 3.5 of Chapter 2).

HOCl and its salts were described centuries ago and also have a long history of use as the active ingredient of bleach and disinfectants. The effectiveness of HOCl as an antiseptic agent in treating wounds and gas gangrene was first reported in a prestigious medical journal in 1915 [1, 2], and the topical HOCl solution is still presently used in the management of disease conditions including wounds [3], skin and soft tissue infections [4], and chronic sinusitis [5].

Although HOCl and its salts have been used as disinfectants for over 100 years, detailed biological studies on HOCl were not witnessed until after the demonstration of the production of this acid in biologically relevant systems in the 1970s. In 1976, John E. Harrison and Julius Schultz reported the formation of HOCl from myeloperoxidase (MPO)-catalyzed peroxidation of chloride ion in the presence of hydrogen peroxide (H$_2$O$_2$) [6]. It is noteworthy that this observation was made at a time when MPO-containing leukocytes had already been found to produce superoxide and H$_2$O$_2$ [7]. Subsequent studies in the early 1980s with leukocytes as well as under simulated conditions of phagosomes confirmed the formation of HOCl by granulocytes and monocytes via the MPO-H$_2$O$_2$-chloride pathway, and the potential role of HOCl in host defense was also suggested [8–12].

It is now known that leukocyte production of HOCl along with other reactive species is an important mechanism of innate immunity against invading microorganisms [13]. As a reactive species, HOCl, like a double-edged sword, is not only toxic to invading pathogens, but also can cause host cell and tissue injury when it is overproduced under certain conditions, such as dysregulated inflammation. This chapter first considers the biological sources of HOCl production, and then discusses the chemical and biochemical properties of this biologically generated acid. Lastly, the chapter surveys the roles of HOCl in biology and medicine, focusing primarily on its involvement in immunity, redox modulation, and disease pathophysiology.

2. SOURCES

Currently, two major pathways have been identified to contribute to the formation of HOCl in biological systems. They are MPO-H$_2$O$_2$-chloride and vascular peroxidase 1 (VPO1)-H$_2$O$_2$-chloride pathways (**Figure 13.1**). The former is restricted to leukocytes and the latter to cardiovascular tissues.

2.1. MPO-H$_2$O$_2$-Chloride Pathway

The MPO-H$_2$O$_2$-chloride pathway is generally considered the primary source of biological HOCl production and has also been most extensively investigated. MPO is a heme enzyme that is released from intracellular granules by activated phagocytic cells, mainly neutrophils [14]. Activation of these cells results in the formation of superoxide by NADPH oxidase during respiratory burst. Dismutation of superoxide forms H$_2$O$_2$. MPO utilizes H$_2$O$_2$ derived from NADPH oxidase as well as other potential sources to oxidize chloride to yield HOCl. MPO also utilizes H$_2$O$_2$ to oxidize bromide (Br$^-$) and thiocyanate (SCN$^-$) to generate two other potent oxidants hypobromous acid (HOBr) and hypothiocyanous acid (HOSCN), respectively, though they are minor products as compared to HOCl [13]. Likewise, due to the relative low number of eosinophils the production of HOCl via eosinophil peroxidase (EPO)-catalyzed peroxidation of chloride represents a minor contribution to the total HOCl load in biological systems. However, EPO-mediated formation of HOCl or other reactive species may become significant under conditions where eosinophils accumulate, such as asthma [15].

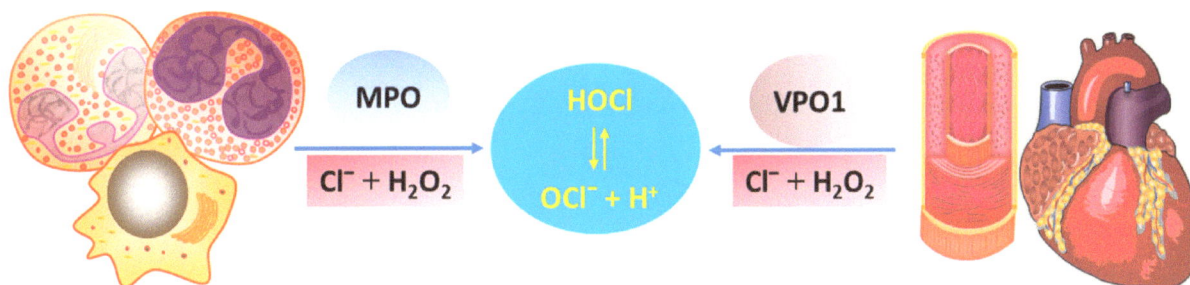

FIGURE 13.1. Hypochlorous acid (HOCl) production in biological systems. As illustrated, myeloperoxidase (MPO)-H_2O_2-chloride pathway is the primary machinery for HOCl biosynthesis in leukocytes, including granulocytes and monocytes. In addition to this classical pathway, vascular peroxidase 1 (VPO1), a newly characterized peroxidase in cardiovascular tissues, also catalyzes the formation of HOCl from H_2O_2 and chloride ion. This VPO1-H_2O_2-chloride pathway is independent of leukocytes. Both the physiological function and the pathophysiological role of the VPO1-H_2O_2-chloride pathway in mammalian systems remain to be further elucidated.

2.2. VPO1-H_2O_2-Chloride Pathway

Recently, two novel heme-containing peroxidases, known as vascular peroxidases (VPO), have been identified. VPO1 is highly expressed in both the heart and the vascular wall, whereas VPO2 is highly expressed only in the heart [16]. Although the exact physiological function of VPO1 remains unclear, studies suggest that VPO1, possibly like MPO, can catalyze the peroxidation of chloride to form HOCl in the presence of H_2O_2 derived from NADPH oxidases (also known as NOXs) [17]. NOXs are expressed in cardiovascular tissues and are upregulated under various pathophysiological conditions (see Section 2.1 of Chapter 6 for more details on NOXs).

3. CHEMISTRY AND BIOCHEMISTRY

3.1. General Chemical Properties

HOCl is a weak acid with a pKa of ~7.5. As such, in physiologically relevant milieu, HOCl and its deprotonated form OCl$^-$ are approximately at equal concentrations. HOCl is a potent oxidant and the standard redox potential for the redox couple of "HOCl, H$^+$/Cl$^-$, H_2O" is estimated to be ~1.5 V. Indeed, HOCl is the major reactive species made by neutrophils to kill invading pathogens. The high redox potential also makes HOCl a potent oxidizing species towards cellular constituents, including lipids, proteins, and nucleic acids (**Figure 13.2**).

3.2. Reaction with Cellular Constituents

3.2.1. Lipids

HOCl, especially at relatively high concentrations, can react with phospholipids at either the lipid head groups or the unsaturated fatty acid side-chains. Reaction of HOCl with the double-bond of the unsaturated fatty acid side-chains results in the formation of chlorohydrins [18] (**Figure 13.2**). Formation of chlorohydrins may disrupt membrane structure leading to cell injury. HOCl also oxidizes low-density lipoprotein (LDL) causing aggregation of the LDL particles. This, however, occurs via oxidation of the protein lysine residues rather than lipid peroxidation [19]. Indeed, HOCl does not seem to act directly to cause lipid peroxidation.

3.2.2. Proteins

HOCl oxidizes the sulfur-containing amino acid residues (e.g., cysteine and methionine) of proteins. Chlorination of the tyrosine residue by HOCl leads to the formation of 3-chlorotyrosine, which serves as a biomarker for HOCl formation in tissues [20]. Further reactions between 3-chlorotyrosine with HOCl may lead to the formation of aldehydic products [21]. Amine groups of amino acid side-chains of proteins and the α-amino groups of free amino acids react with HOCl yielding chloramines, which are also reactive to biomolecules and capable of causing cell injury [22, 23].

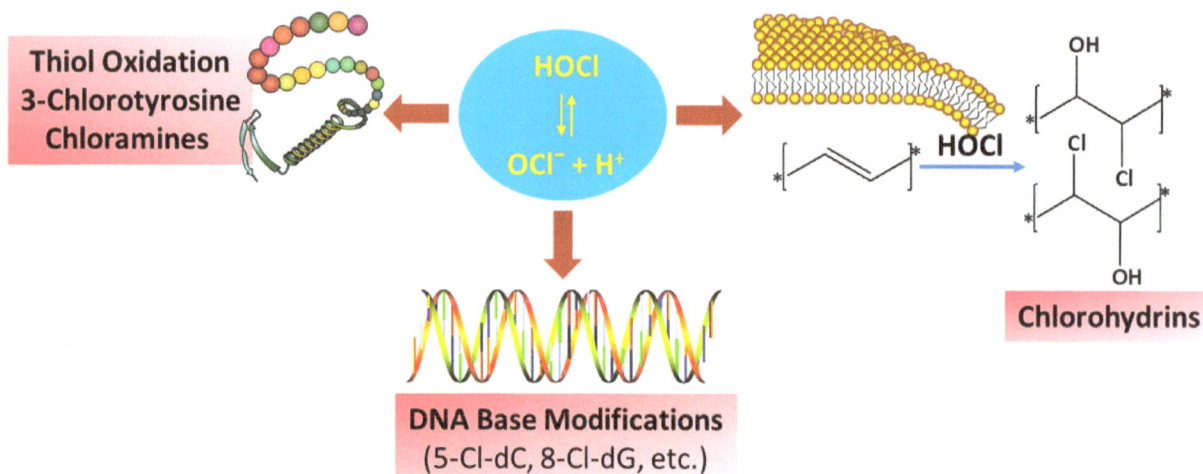

FIGURE 13.2. Reaction of hypochlorous acid (HOCl) with cellular constituents. As depicted, HOCl, as a potent oxidizing species, can react with lipids, proteins, and nucleic acid. Reaction of HOCl with the double-bond of polyunsaturated fatty acids results in the formation of chlorohydrins. Reaction of HOCl with proteins may cause thiol oxidation as well as the formation of 3-chlorotyrosine and chloramines. Reaction of HOCl with DNA causes base modifications, leading to the formation of 5-chloro-2′-deoxycytidine (5-Cl-dC) and 8-chloro-2′-deoxyguanosine (8-Cl-dG), among others. Collectively, the above reactions are the chemical and biochemical basis underling the biological effects caused by HOCl, including cell and tissue injury, and possibly, tumorigenesis.

3.2.3. Nucleic Acids

HOCl reacts readily with nucleobases, nucleosides, and nucleotides, as well as related compounds such as nicotinamide adenine dinucleotide (NADH) and nicotinamide adenine dinucleotide phosphate (NADPH) via either reacting with the available nitrogen atoms or adduction to the aromatic ring. Reaction of HOCl with DNA causes base modifications, leading to the formation of 5-chloro-2′-deoxycytidine (5-Cl-dC) and 8-chloro-2′-deoxyguanosine (8-Cl-dG), among others [24, 25]. Chlorination of DNA bases by HOCl may cause gene mutations, contributing to tumorigenesis associated with inflammation [25].

3.3. Reaction with Other Reactive Oxygen Species

Several secondary oxidizing species can be derived from the reaction between HOCl and other reactive oxygen species (ROS). For example, HOCl reacts with superoxide to form hydroxyl radical (Reaction 2). In addition, singlet oxygen can be formed from the reaction of HOCl with H_2O_2 (Reaction 3). HOCl also reacts with lipid hydroperoxides (e.g., linoleic acid hydroperoxide) generating singlet oxygen [26].

Formation of these secondary reactive species may contribute to the biological effects of HOCl.

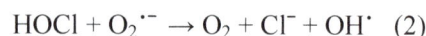

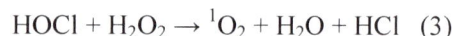

$$HOCl + O_2^{\cdot -} \rightarrow O_2 + Cl^- + OH^{\cdot} \quad (2)$$

$$HOCl + H_2O_2 \rightarrow {}^1O_2 + H_2O + HCl \quad (3)$$

3.4. Half-Life, Diffusion, and Membrane Permeability

The half-life of HOCl in biological systems may range from seconds to minutes, depending on the availability and levels of surrounding antioxidant molecules (especially the reduced form of glutathione [GSH]) and cellular constituents [27]. HOCl penetrates cell membranes and may diffuse across several cell diameters [28].

4. CELL AND TISSUE DEFENSES

4.1. Non-Enzymatic Defense System

HOCl reacts with cellular and tissue antioxidants and other small molecules, including GSH, NADH,

NADPH, urate, vitamin C, and vitamin E. GSH is a major cellular defense in the detoxification of HOCl [28, 29]. The reaction between cellular GSH and HOCl results in the formation of glutathione sulfonamide as a major product rather than glutathione disulfide [29]. HOCl also reacts with the sulfonate amino acid taurine to form a much less reactive chloramine product. Taurine is present at high concentrations in neutrophils, and may act to detoxify HOCl. Nitrite (NO_2^-), a product that accumulates at sites of chronic inflammation, is found to react with HOCl to form nitryl chloride (NO_2Cl), which is less toxic to the cells [30]. Nitrite may also decrease the formation of HOCl by inhibiting MPO [31]. Recently, ceruloplasmin, a major copper-carrying protein in the blood, is shown to bind to and inhibit MPO and MPO-catalyzed HOCl formation [32].

4.2. Enzymatic Defense System

Currently, there is no known enzyme capable of directly catalyzing the detoxification of HOCl in mammalian systems. As noted earlier, leukocytes also produce HOSCN though the amount of its formation is much less than that of HOCl. HOSCN also inhibits and kills invading pathogens, but paradoxically is well tolerated by mammalian host tissue. A recent study demonstrates that mammalian thioredoxin reductase (see Chapter 19) is able to catalyze the metabolism of HOSCN, but not HOCl and protect against HOSCN toxicity to human cells [33].

While there is no known specific enzymatic machinery for the metabolism of HOCl, nuclear factor E2-related factor 2 (Nrf2)-regulated antioxidative defenses may be involved in the detoxification of HOCl in cells. In this regard, HOCl at low, non-cytotoxic concentrations can cause Nrf2 activation, leading to increased production of cellular antioxidant enzymes, including the enzymatic machinery for synthesizing GSH [34], a major defense against HOCl toxicity (see Section 4.1 above). Activation of Nrf2 by low concentrations of HOCl makes the cells more resistant to cytotoxicity induced by high concentrations of HOCl [34] as well as other oxidative species.

5. BIOLOGY AND MEDICINE

5.1. Immunity and Redox Signaling

The involvement of HOCl in immunity is two-fold, namely, pathogen killing and pathogen resistance.

5.1.1. Host Defense against Pathogens

Formation of HOCl by phagocytic cells (mainly neutrophils) during respiratory burst plays an integral part in the innate immune defense. HOCl along with other oxidizing species produced by phagocytic cells, including peroxynitrite and hydroxyl radicals contributes to the killing of invading microorganisms [13]. The chemical reactivity of HOCl with biomolecules underlies the pathogen-killing activity of HOCl formed in the phagosomes, where the locally formed HOCl may reach high concentrations. One key mechanism of bactericidal activity of HOCl is to cause oxidative protein damage and aggregation in bacteria [35].

5.1.2. Pathogen Defense against HOCl

The pathogen-killing activity of phagocytic cell-produced HOCl also depends on other factors, such as the intrinsic defenses in the microorganisms. In this context, several mechanisms operate in bacteria to protect them from HOCl-induced killing. For example, as a defense mechanism, bacteria use the redox-regulated chaperone heat shock protein 33 (Hsp33), which responds to HOCl exposure with the reversible oxidative unfolding of its C-terminal redox switch domain. HOCl-mediated unfolding turns inactive Hsp33 into a highly active chaperone holdase, which protects essential *Escherichia coli* proteins against HOCl-induced oxidative aggregation and thereby increases bacterial resistance to HOCl [35]. *E. Coli* also express an enzyme system known as MsrPQ (a novel member of the methionine sulfoxide reductase [Msr] family), which is responsible for repairing proteins containing methionine sulfoxide in the bacterial cell envelope. MsrPQ uses electrons from the respiratory chain and is highly inducible by HOCl [36]. Likewise, *Mycobacterium tuberculosis* expresses MsrA and MsrB that protect them from killing by HOCl [37]. These findings support an essential role for methionine oxidation in HOCl-induced bactericidal activity.

5.1.3. Redox Signaling of Pathogen Resistance to HOCl

Several transcription factors in *Escherichia coli* have been shown to be selectively responsive to HOCl, resulting in increased expression of genes whose products are involved in the detoxification of electrophiles, including HOCl. These transcription factors include (1) RclR (reactive chlorine-specific transcriptional regulator, formerly known as YkgD), a member of the AraC family, sensing HOCl via cysteine oxidation [38]; (2) HypT (hypochlorite-responsive transcription factor), sensing HOCl via methionine oxidation [39]; and (3) NemR, sensing HOCl via cysteine oxidation [40]. Hence, bacteria have evolved specific transcriptional mechanisms to defend against HOCl toxicity.

5.2. Disease Process

While HOCl production is an integral part of the innate immunity machinery, under certain conditions such as chronic inflammation, overproduction of HOCl along with other reactive species may also attack host cellular biomolecules, leading to cell and tissue injury. In this context, HOCl is implicated in the pathogenesis of various human diseases, including cancer [25, 41], cardiovascular diseases [42, 43], diabetes [44, 45], pulmonary disorders [46, 47], and neurodegeneration [48, 49]. In particular, the role of HOCl in atherosclerosis has been most extensively investigated. Hence, this section surveys the molecular and cellular basis of atherosclerotic cardiovascular injury associated with HOCl overproduction (**Figure 13.3**).

5.2.1. Presence of HOCl Biomarkers in Atherosclerotic Lesions

Myeloperoxidase was first found to be expressed in human atherosclerotic lesions in 1994 [50]. Subsequently, the presence of HOCl-modified proteins (including 3-chlorotyrosine) as well as 5-chlorouracil in human atherosclerotic lesions was demonstrated [20, 51, 52]. Moreover, HOCl oxidizes high-density lipoprotein (HDL) in the human artery wall and impairs ATP-binding cassette A1 (ABCA1)-dependent cholesterol transport [42].

5.2.2. Modifications of Lipoproteins

HOCl causes modifications of lipoproteins, including both LDL and HDL particles. HOCl-modified LDL stimulates leukocytes to produce more ROS and to adhere to endothelial cells [53]. Other effects resulting from HOCl-modified LDL include: (1) augmented uptake of the modified LDL by macrophages via CD36- and scavenger receptor B1 (SR-B1)-dependent mechanisms [54]; (2) inhibition of endothelial nitric oxide synthase (eNOS) in endothelial cells [55]; and (3) stimulation of platelet aggregation [56]. Collectively, these effects of HOCl-modified

LDL may contribute to the development of atherosclerotic plaques and thrombus formation. In this context, passive immunization with specific antibodies against HOCl-oxidized LDL reduces plaque volume in LDL receptor-deficient mice [57], which further highlights the causal involvement of HOCl-induced LDL modifications in atherosclerosis.

As noted earlier, HOCl causes oxidation of HDL and compromises ABCA1-mediated reverse cholesterol transport [42, 58]. One of the major protein targets of HOCl in HDL is apolipoprotein A-I (ApoA-I). HOCl-induced modifications of ApoA-I generate dysfunctional HDL [59, 60]. As indicated above, SR-B1 receptor mediates the hepatic uptake of HDL and plays a critical role in HDL-mediated reverse cholesterol transport. A recent study shows that modification of the lysine residues of albumin by HOCl promotes the irreversible binding of albumin to SR-B1, resulting in permanent receptor blockage [61].

5.2.3. Modulation of Endothelial Nitric Oxide Synthase

eNOS and eNOS-derived nitric oxide play important physiological roles in cardiovascular homeostasis. As aforementioned, HOCl-oxidized LDL inhibits eNOS in endothelial cells, resulting in decreased production of vasoprotective nitric oxide [55]. Notably, HOCl is found to also cause uncoupling of eNOS [62]. Moreover, modifications of L-arginine by HOCl also contribute to the decreased production of endothelial nitric oxide [63, 64].

As discussed in Section 2.2 above, VPO1, like MPO, catalyzes the formation of HOCl from chloride and H_2O_2. VPO1-derived HOCl has been shown to increase the production of asymmetric dimethylarginine (ADMA), an endogenous inhibitor of NOS. It is suggested that angiotensin II-mediated upregulation of VPO1 may decrease endothelial nitric oxide production via HOCl-induced production of ADMA, thereby leading to hypertension [65]. In this context, decreased formation of nitric oxide from eNOS is an important mechanism of hypertension [66, 67].

5.2.4. Prothrombotic Activities

In addition to its involvement in promoting platelet aggregation and activation [56, 68], HOCl also affects a number of other pathways involved in the regulation of hemostasis. For example, HOCl induces endothelial apoptosis and tissue factor expression, promoting thrombogenesis [69]. Similarly, HOSCN

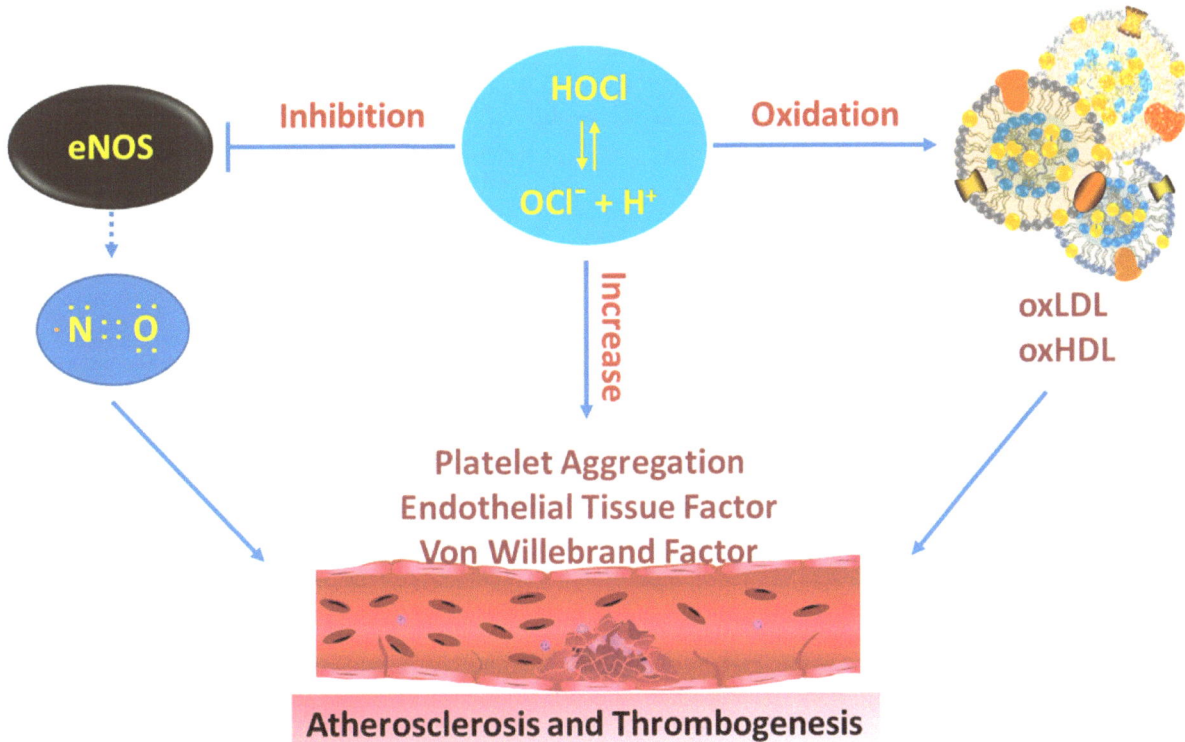

FIGURE 13.3. Potential mechanisms of hypochlorous acid (HOCl)-induced atherosclerosis and thrombogenesis. As illustrated, HOCl causes modifications of lipoproteins, including both low-density lipoprotein (LDL) and high-density lipoprotein (HDL). Oxidized LDL (oxLDL) elicits a number of adverse effects including enhanced uptake by macrophages. On the other hand, oxidized HDL (oxHDL) may impair the reverse cholesterol transport. HOCl inhibits vascular endothelial nitric oxide synthase (eNOS) and reduces the formation of vasoprotective nitric oxide. Furthermore, HOCl causes platelet aggregation and activation, induces endothelial tissue factor, and increases the levels of von Willebrand factor. These effects on hemostasis along with oxidation of lipoproteins and decreased bioavailability of vascular protective nitric oxide contribute to atherosclerotic cardiovascular injury associated with HOCl overproduction.

is also a potent inducer of endothelial cell tissue factor via nuclear factor kappaB (NF-κB)-mediated signaling mechanism [70].

von Willebrand factor (VWF) is required for platelet adhesion to sites of vessel injury, a process vital for both hemostasis and thrombosis. Elevated levels of VWF are associated with an increased risk of atherosclerotic cardiovascular disorders [71, 72]. Oxidative modifications of VWF by HOCl inhibit its cleavage by ADAMTS13 (also known as von Willebrand factor-cleaving protease, a zinc-containing metalloprotease) [73, 74]. Phagocyte (neutrophil)-generated HOCl is also found to directly inactivate ADAMTS13 [75]. Together, the above effects may lead to increased levels of VWF in the blood and thereby augmented thrombogenesis.

6. SUMMARY OF CHAPTER KEY POINTS

- HOCl and its salts (hypochlorites) have been used as disinfectants for more than a century. However, detailed biological studies on HOCl were not witnessed until after the demonstration of the production of this acid in biological systems in the 1970s and early 1980s.

- Two major pathways have been identified to contribute to the formation of HOCl in biological systems. They are the MPO-H_2O_2-chloride and the vascular peroxidase 1 (VPO1)-H_2O_2-chloride pathways, with the former being more extensively characterized in biological systems.

- HOCl is a weak acid with a pKa of ~7.5. As such, in physiologically relevant milieu, HOCl and its deprotonated form OCl⁻ are approximately at equal concentrations. HOCl possesses a high redox potential which makes it a potent oxidizing species towards cellular constituents, including lipids, proteins, and nucleic acids.

- Reaction of HOCl with the double-bond of the unsaturated fatty acid side-chains of lipids in cell membranes or lipoproteins results in the formation of chlorohydrins.
- HOCl oxidizes the sulfur-containing amino acid residues of proteins. Chlorination of tyrosine residue by HOCl leads to the formation of 3-chlorotyrosine, a biomarker for biological HOCl production. Reaction of HOCl with amine groups of amino acid side-chains of proteins and the α-amino groups of free amino acids yields chloramines, which are also reactive to biomolecules.
- Reaction of HOCl with DNA causes base modifications, leading to the formation of 5-Cl-dC and 8-Cl-dG, among others. Chlorination of DNA bases by HOCl may cause gene mutations, contributing to tumorigenesis associated with inflammation.
- HOCl also reacts with other ROS, such as superoxide, H_2O_2, and lipid hydroperoxides to form secondary reactive radical species, including singlet oxygen and hydroxyl radical.
- The half-life of HOCl in biological systems depends on the availability and levels of surrounding antioxidant molecules. GSH is a major cellular defense in the detoxification of HOCl.
- Formation of HOCl by phagocytic cells (mainly neutrophils) during respiratory burst plays an integral part in the innate immune defense system and participates in killing the invading pathogens. On the other hand, several mechanisms operate in bacteria to protect them from HOCl-induced killing.
- Under certain conditions such as chronic inflammation, overproduction of HOCl may cause damage to host cell and tissue injury, contributing to various disease processes, especially atherosclerotic cardiovascular injury.

7. SELF-ASSESSMENT QUESTIONS

7.1. HOCl is a weak acid (HOCl ↔ OCl⁻ + H⁺). At a physiological pH, the ratio of HOCl to OCl⁻ is approximately which of the following?

A. 0.25
B. 0.5
C. 1.0
D. 1.5

E. 2.0

7.2. In addition to MPO, which of the following mammalian enzymes may also be responsible for the peroxidation of chloride to form HOCl in the presence of hydrogen peroxide?

A. Endothelial nitric oxide synthase
B. Inducible nitric oxide synthase
C. Superoxide dismutase
D. Vascular peroxidase 1
E. Xanthine oxidoreductase

7.3. Currently, there is no known enzyme capable of directly catalyzing the detoxification of HOCl in mammalian systems. However, a mammalian enzyme has been recently shown to catalyze the metabolism of HOSCN. What is this enzyme?

A. Catalase
B. Glutathione peroxidase
C. Inducible nitric oxide synthase
D. Peroxiredoxin
E. Thioredoxin reductase

7.4. Which of the following molecules has been shown to react with HOCl to reduce HOCl-induced cytotoxicity?

A. Hydrogen peroxide
B. Nitric oxide
C. Nitrite
D. Peroxynitrite
E. Singlet oxygen

7.5. The *E. Coli* bacteria also express an enzyme system known as MsrPQ, which is responsible for repairing proteins containing methionine sulfoxide in the bacterial cell envelope. A recent study shows that MsrPQ uses electrons from which of the following sources in the bacterial cell?

A. Adenosine triphosphate
B. Glutathione disulfide
C. Hydrogen peroxide
D. Respiratory chain
E. Water

ANSWERS AND EXPLANATIONS

7.1. The answer is C. HOCl is a weak acid with a pKa of ~7.5. As such, in physiologically relevant milieu, HOCl and its deprotonated form OCl⁻ are approximately at equal concentrations.

7.2. The answer is D. Although the exact physiological function of VPO1 remains to be defined, studies suggest that VPO1, like MPO, can catalyze the peroxidation of chloride to form HOCl in the presence of H_2O_2 derived from NADPH oxidases (NOXs). VPO1-derived HOCl may be particularly relevant in vascular injury.

7.3. The answer is E. Mammalian thioredoxin reductase is shown to be able to catalyze the metabolism of HOSCN and protect against HOSCN-induced toxicity to cells.

7.4. The answer is C. Nitrite, a product that accumulates at sites of chronic inflammation, is found to react with HOCl to form nitryl chloride (NO_2Cl), which is less toxic to the cells. Nitrite may also decrease the formation of HOCl by inhibiting MPO. In cell cultures, nitrite protects against HOCl-induced cytotoxicity.

7.5. The answer is D. In *E. coli*, MsrPQ uses electrons from the respiratory chain to catalyze the reduction of oxidized methionine, thereby repairing proteins containing methionine sulfoxide in the bacterial cell envelope.

REFERENCES

1. Smith JL, Drennan AM, Rettie T, Campbell W. Experimental observations on the antiseptic action of hypochlorous acid and its application to wound treatment. *Br Med J* 1915; 2(2847):129–36.
2. Fraser J. The value of hypochlorous acid in the treatment of cases of gas gangrene. *Br Med J* 1915; 2(2858):525–9.
3. Sakarya S, Gunay N, Karakulak M, Ozturk B, Ertugrul B. Hypochlorous acid: an ideal wound care agent with powerful microbicidal, antibiofilm, and wound healing potency. *Wounds* 2014; 26(12):342–50.
4. Crew JR, Thibodeaux KT, Speyrer MS, Gauto AR, Shiau T, Pang L, Bley K, Debabov D. Flow-through instillation of hypochlorous acid in the treatment of necrotizing fasciitis. *Wounds* 2016; 28(2):40–7.
5. Cho HJ, Min HJ, Chung HJ, Park DY, Seong SY, Yoon JH, Lee JG, Kim CH. Improved outcomes after low-concentration hypochlorous acid nasal irrigation in pediatric chronic sinusitis. *Laryngoscope* 2016; 126(4):791–5.
6. Harrison JE, Schultz J. Studies on the chlorinating activity of myeloperoxidase. *J Biol Chem* 1976; 251(5):1371–4.
7. Babior BM, Kipnes RS, Curnutte JT. Biological defense mechanisms: the production by leukocytes of superoxide, a potential bactericidal agent. *J Clin Invest* 1973; 52(3):741–4.
8. Slivka A, LoBuglio AF, Weiss SJ. A potential role for hypochlorous acid in granulocyte-mediated tumor cell cytotoxicity. *Blood* 1980; 55(2):347–50.
9. Albrich JM, McCarthy CA, Hurst JK. Biological reactivity of hypochlorous acid: implications for microbicidal mechanisms of leukocyte myeloperoxidase. *Proc Natl Acad Sci USA* 1981; 78(1):210–4.
10. Weiss SJ, Slivka A. Monocyte and granulocyte-mediated tumor cell destruction: a role for the hydrogen peroxide-myeloperoxidase-chloride system. *J Clin Invest* 1982; 69(2):255–62.
11. Weiss SJ, Klein R, Slivka A, Wei M. Chlorination of taurine by human neutrophils: evidence for hypochlorous acid generation. *J Clin Invest* 1982; 70(3):598–607.
12. Lampert MB, Weiss SJ. The chlorinating potential of the human monocyte. *Blood* 1983; 62(3):645–51.
13. Winterbourn CC, Kettle AJ, Hampton MB. Reactive oxygen species and neutrophil function. *Annu Rev Biochem* 2016; 85:765–92.
14. Dunn WB, Hardin JH, Spicer SS. Ultrastructural localization of myeloperoxidase in human neutrophil and rabbit heterophil and eosinophil leukocytes. *Blood* 1968; 32(6):935–44.
15. Wang Z, DiDonato JA, Buffa J, Comhair SA, Aronica MA, Dweik RA, Lee NA, Lee JJ, Thomassen MJ, Kavuru M, Erzurum SC, Hazen SL. Eosinophil peroxidase catalyzed protein carbamylation participates in asthma. *J Biol Chem* 2016; 291(42):22118–35.
16. Cheng G, Salerno JC, Cao Z, Pagano PJ, Lambeth JD. Identification and characterization of VPO1, a new animal heme-containing peroxidase. *Free Radic Biol Med* 2008; 45(12):1682–94.
17. Shi R, Hu C, Yuan Q, Yang T, Peng J, Li Y, Bai Y, Cao Z, Cheng G, Zhang G. Involvement of vascular peroxidase 1 in angiotensin II-induced vascular smooth muscle cell proliferation. *Cardiovasc Res* 2011; 91(1):27–36.

18. Winterbourn CC, van den Berg JJ, Roitman E, Kuypers FA. Chlorohydrin formation from unsaturated fatty acids reacted with hypochlorous acid. *Arch Biochem Biophys* 1992; 296(2):547–55.

19. Hazell LJ, van den Berg JJ, Stocker R. Oxidation of low-density lipoprotein by hypochlorite causes aggregation that is mediated by modification of lysine residues rather than lipid oxidation. *Biochem J* 1994; 302 (Pt 1):297–304.

20. Hazen SL, Heinecke JW. 3-Chlorotyrosine, a specific marker of myeloperoxidase-catalyzed oxidation, is markedly elevated in low density lipoprotein isolated from human atherosclerotic intima. *J Clin Invest* 1997; 99(9):2075–81.

21. Fu S, Wang H, Davies M, Dean R. Reactions of hypochlorous acid with tyrosine and peptidyl-tyrosyl residues give dichlorinated and aldehydic products in addition to 3-chlorotyrosine. *J Biol Chem* 2000; 275(15):10851–8.

22. Hazen SL, d'Avignon A, Anderson MM, Hsu FF, Heinecke JW. Human neutrophils employ the myeloperoxidase-hydrogen peroxide-chloride system to oxidize alpha-amino acids to a family of reactive aldehydes: mechanistic studies identifying labile intermediates along the reaction pathway. *J Biol Chem* 1998; 273(9):4997–5005.

23. Englert RP, Shacter E. Distinct modes of cell death induced by different reactive oxygen species: amino acyl chloramines mediate hypochlorous acid-induced apoptosis. *J Biol Chem* 2002; 277(23):20518–26.

24. Suzuki T, Masuda M, Friesen MD, Fenet B, Ohshima H. Novel products generated from 2'-deoxyguanosine by hypochlorous acid or a myeloperoxidase-H_2O_2-Cl- system: identification of diimino-imidazole and amino-imidazolone nucleosides. *Nucleic Acids Res* 2002; 30(11):2555–64.

25. Fedeles BI, Freudenthal BD, Yau E, Singh V, Chang SC, Li D, Delaney JC, Wilson SH, Essigmann JM. Intrinsic mutagenic properties of 5-chlorocytosine: a mechanistic connection between chronic inflammation and cancer. *Proc Natl Acad Sci USA* 2015; 112(33):E4571–80.

26. Miyamoto S, Martinez GR, Rettori D, Augusto O, Medeiros MH, Di Mascio P. Linoleic acid hydroperoxide reacts with hypochlorous acid, generating peroxyl radical intermediates and singlet molecular oxygen. *Proc Natl Acad Sci USA* 2006; 103(2):293–8.

27. Peskin AV, Winterbourn CC. Kinetics of the reactions of hypochlorous acid and amino acid chloramines with thiols, methionine, and ascorbate. *Free Radic Biol Med* 2001; 30(5):572–9.

28. Vissers MC, Winterbourn CC. Oxidation of intracellular glutathione after exposure of human red blood cells to hypochlorous acid. *Biochem J* 1995; 307 (Pt 1):57–62.

29. Pullar JM, Vissers MC, Winterbourn CC. Glutathione oxidation by hypochlorous acid in endothelial cells produces glutathione sulfonamide as a major product but not glutathione disulfide. *J Biol Chem* 2001; 276(25):22120–5.

30. Whiteman M, Hooper DC, Scott GS, Koprowski H, Halliwell B. Inhibition of hypochlorous acid-induced cellular toxicity by nitrite. *Proc Natl Acad Sci USA* 2002; 99(19):12061–6.

31. van Dalen CJ, Winterbourn CC, Senthilmohan R, Kettle AJ. Nitrite as a substrate and inhibitor of myeloperoxidase: implications for nitration and hypochlorous acid production at sites of inflammation. *J Biol Chem* 2000; 275(16):11638–44.

32. Chapman AL, Mocatta TJ, Shiva S, Seidel A, Chen B, Khalilova I, Paumann-Page ME, Jameson GN, Winterbourn CC, Kettle AJ. Ceruloplasmin is an endogenous inhibitor of myeloperoxidase. *J Biol Chem* 2013; 288(9):6465–77.

33. Chandler JD, Nichols DP, Nick JA, Hondal RJ, Day BJ. Selective metabolism of hypothiocyanous acid by mammalian thioredoxin reductase promotes lung innate immunity and antioxidant defense. *J Biol Chem* 2013; 288(25):18421–8.

34. Pi J, Zhang Q, Woods CG, Wong V, Collins S, Andersen ME. Activation of Nrf2-mediated oxidative stress response in macrophages by hypochlorous acid. *Toxicol Appl Pharmacol* 2008; 226(3):236–43.

35. Winter J, Ilbert M, Graf PC, Ozcelik D, Jakob U. Bleach activates a redox-regulated chaperone by oxidative protein unfolding. *Cell* 2008; 135(4):691–701.

36. Gennaris A, Ezraty B, Henry C, Agrebi R, Vergnes A, Oheix E, Bos J, Leverrier P, Espinosa L, Szewczyk J, Vertommen D, Iranzo O, et al. Repairing oxidized proteins in the bacterial envelope using respiratory chain electrons. *Nature* 2015; 528(7582):409–12.

37. Lee WL, Gold B, Darby C, Brot N, Jiang X, de Carvalho LP, Wellner D, St John G, Jacobs WR,

Jr., Nathan C. *Mycobacterium tuberculosis* expresses methionine sulphoxide reductases A and B that protect from killing by nitrite and hypochlorite. *Mol Microbiol* 2009; 71(3):583–93.

38. Parker BW, Schwessinger EA, Jakob U, Gray MJ. The RclR protein is a reactive chlorine-specific transcription factor in *Escherichia coli*. *J Biol Chem* 2013; 288(45):32574–84.

39. Drazic A, Gebendorfer KM, Mak S, Steiner A, Krause M, Bepperling A, Winter J. Tetramers are the activation-competent species of the HOCl-specific transcription factor HypT. *J Biol Chem* 2014; 289(2):977–86.

40. Gray MJ, Wholey WY, Parker BW, Kim M, Jakob U. NemR is a bleach-sensing transcription factor. *J Biol Chem* 2013; 288(19):13789–98.

41. Reynolds WF, Chang E, Douer D, Ball ED, Kanda V. An allelic association implicates myeloperoxidase in the etiology of acute promyelocytic leukemia. *Blood* 1997; 90(7):2730–7.

42. Bergt C, Pennathur S, Fu X, Byun J, O'Brien K, McDonald TO, Singh P, Anantharamaiah GM, Chait A, Brunzell J, Geary RL, Oram JF, et al. The myeloperoxidase product hypochlorous acid oxidizes HDL in the human artery wall and impairs ABCA1-dependent cholesterol transport. *Proc Natl Acad Sci USA* 2004; 101(35):13032–7.

43. Ford DA. Lipid oxidation by hypochlorous acid: chlorinated lipids in atherosclerosis and myocardial ischemia. *Clin Lipidol* 2010; 5(6):835–52.

44. Zhang C, Yang J, Jennings LK. Leukocyte-derived myeloperoxidase amplifies high-glucose--induced endothelial dysfunction through interaction with high-glucose-stimulated, vascular non-leukocyte-derived reactive oxygen species. *Diabetes* 2004; 53(11):2950–9.

45. Kalogiannis M, Delikatny EJ, Jeitner TM. Serotonin as a putative scavenger of hypohalous acid in the brain. *Biochim Biophys Acta* 2016; 1862(4):651–61.

46. Kettle AJ, Chan T, Osberg I, Senthilmohan R, Chapman AL, Mocatta TJ, Wagener JS. Myeloperoxidase and protein oxidation in the airways of young children with cystic fibrosis. *Am J Respir Crit Care Med* 2004; 170(12):1317–23.

47. Crouch EC, Hirche TO, Shao B, Boxio R, Wartelle J, Benabid R, McDonald B, Heinecke J, Matalon S, Belaaouaj A. Myeloperoxidase-dependent inactivation of surfactant protein D in vitro and in vivo. *J Biol Chem* 2010;

285(22):16757–70.

48. Jeitner TM, Kalogiannis M, Krasnikov BF, Gomlin I, Peltier MR, Moran GR. Linking inflammation and Parkinson disease: hypochlorous acid generates parkinsonian poisons. *Toxicol Sci* 2016; 151(2):388–402.

49. Ray RS, Katyal A. Myeloperoxidase: bridging the gap in neurodegeneration. *Neurosci Biobehav Rev* 2016; 68:611–20.

50. Daugherty A, Dunn JL, Rateri DL, Heinecke JW. Myeloperoxidase, a catalyst for lipoprotein oxidation, is expressed in human atherosclerotic lesions. *J Clin Invest* 1994; 94(1):437–44.

51. Hazell LJ, Arnold L, Flowers D, Waeg G, Malle E, Stocker R. Presence of hypochlorite-modified proteins in human atherosclerotic lesions. *J Clin Invest* 1996; 97(6):1535–44.

52. Takeshita J, Byun J, Nhan TQ, Pritchard DK, Pennathur S, Schwartz SM, Chait A, Heinecke JW. Myeloperoxidase generates 5-chlorouracil in human atherosclerotic tissue: a potential pathway for somatic mutagenesis by macrophages. *J Biol Chem* 2006; 281(6):3096–104.

53. Kopprasch S, Leonhardt W, Pietzsch J, Kuhne H. Hypochlorite-modified low-density lipoprotein stimulates human polymorphonuclear leukocytes for enhanced production of reactive oxygen metabolites, enzyme secretion, and adhesion to endothelial cells. *Atherosclerosis* 1998; 136(2):315–24.

54. Marsche G, Zimmermann R, Horiuchi S, Tandon NN, Sattler W, Malle E. Class B scavenger receptors CD36 and SR-BI are receptors for hypochlorite-modified low density lipoprotein. *J Biol Chem* 2003; 278(48):47562–70.

55. Nuszkowski A, Grabner R, Marsche G, Unbehaun A, Malle E, Heller R. Hypochlorite-modified low density lipoprotein inhibits nitric oxide synthesis in endothelial cells via an intracellular dislocalization of endothelial nitric-oxide synthase. *J Biol Chem* 2001; 276(17):14212–21.

56. Coleman LG, Jr., Polanowska-Grabowska RK, Marcinkiewicz M, Gear AR. LDL oxidized by hypochlorous acid causes irreversible platelet aggregation when combined with low levels of ADP, thrombin, epinephrine, or macrophage-derived chemokine (CCL22). *Blood* 2004; 104(2):380–9.

57. van Leeuwen M, Kemna MJ, de Winther MP, Boon L, Duijvestijn AM, Henatsch D, Bos NA, Gijbels MJ, Tervaert JW. Passive immunization

with hypochlorite-oxLDL specific antibodies reduces plaque volume in LDL receptor-deficient mice. *PLoS One* 2013; 8(7):e68039.

58. Marsche G, Hammer A, Oskolkova O, Kozarsky KF, Sattler W, Malle E. Hypochlorite-modified high density lipoprotein, a high affinity ligand to scavenger receptor class B, type I, impairs high density lipoprotein-dependent selective lipid uptake and reverse cholesterol transport. *J Biol Chem* 2002; 277(35):32172–9.

59. Bergt C, Fu X, Huq NP, Kao J, Heinecke JW. Lysine residues direct the chlorination of tyrosines in YXXK motifs of apolipoprotein A-I when hypochlorous acid oxidizes high density lipoprotein. *J Biol Chem* 2004; 279(9):7856–66.

60. Hadfield KA, Pattison DI, Brown BE, Hou L, Rye KA, Davies MJ, Hawkins CL. Myeloperoxidase-derived oxidants modify apolipoprotein A-I and generate dysfunctional high-density lipoproteins: comparison of hypothiocyanous acid (HOSCN) with hypochlorous acid (HOCl). *Biochem J* 2013; 449(2):531–42.

61. Binder V, Ljubojevic S, Haybaeck J, Holzer M, El-Gamal D, Schicho R, Pieske B, Heinemann A, Marsche G. The myeloperoxidase product hypochlorous acid generates irreversible high-density lipoprotein receptor inhibitors. *Arterioscler Thromb Vasc Biol* 2013; 33(5):1020–7.

62. Xu J, Xie Z, Reece R, Pimental D, Zou MH. Uncoupling of endothelial nitric oxidase synthase by hypochlorous acid: role of NAD(P)H oxidase-derived superoxide and peroxynitrite. *Arterioscler Thromb Vasc Biol* 2006; 26(12):2688–95.

63. Zhang C, Patel R, Eiserich JP, Zhou F, Kelpke S, Ma W, Parks DA, Darley-Usmar V, White CR. Endothelial dysfunction is induced by proinflammatory oxidant hypochlorous acid. *Am J Physiol Heart Circ Physiol* 2001; 281(4):H1469–75.

64. Zhang C, Reiter C, Eiserich JP, Boersma B, Parks DA, Beckman JS, Barnes S, Kirk M, Baldus S, Darley-Usmar VM, White CR. L-Arginine chlorination products inhibit endothelial nitric oxide production. *J Biol Chem* 2001; 276(29):27159–65.

65. Peng H, Chen L, Huang X, Yang T, Yu Z, Cheng G, Zhang G, Shi R. Vascular peroxidase 1 up regulation by angiotensin II attenuates nitric oxide production through increasing asymmetrical dimethylarginine in HUVECs. *J Am Soc Hypertens* 2016; 10(9):741–51 e3.

66. Huang PL, Huang Z, Mashimo H, Bloch KD, Moskowitz MA, Bevan JA, Fishman MC. Hypertension in mice lacking the gene for endothelial nitric oxide synthase. *Nature* 1995; 377(6546):239–42.

67. Yuan Q, Yang J, Santulli G, Reiken SR, Wronska A, Kim MM, Osborne BW, Lacampagne A, Yin Y, Marks AR. Maintenance of normal blood pressure is dependent on IP3R1-mediated regulation of eNOS. *Proc Natl Acad Sci USA* 2016; 113(30):8532–7.

68. Assinger A, Koller F, Schmid W, Zellner M, Babeluk R, Koller E, Volf I. Specific binding of hypochlorite-oxidized HDL to platelet CD36 triggers proinflammatory and procoagulant effects. *Atherosclerosis* 2010; 212(1):153–60.

69. Sugiyama S, Kugiyama K, Aikawa M, Nakamura S, Ogawa H, Libby P. Hypochlorous acid, a macrophage product, induces endothelial apoptosis and tissue factor expression: involvement of myeloperoxidase-mediated oxidant in plaque erosion and thrombogenesis. *Arterioscler Thromb Vasc Biol* 2004; 24(7):1309–14.

70. Wang JG, Mahmud SA, Thompson JA, Geng JG, Key NS, Slungaard A. The principal eosinophil peroxidase product, HOSCN, is a uniquely potent phagocyte oxidant inducer of endothelial cell tissue factor activity: a potential mechanism for thrombosis in eosinophilic inflammatory states. *Blood* 2006; 107(2):558–65.

71. Spiel AO, Gilbert JC, Jilma B. von Willebrand factor in cardiovascular disease: focus on acute coronary syndromes. *Circulation* 2008; 117(11):1449–59.

72. Frankel DS, Meigs JB, Massaro JM, Wilson PW, O'Donnell CJ, D'Agostino RB, Tofler GH. Von Willebrand factor, type 2 diabetes mellitus, and risk of cardiovascular disease: the framingham offspring study. *Circulation* 2008; 118(24):2533–9.

73. Fu X, Chen J, Gallagher R, Zheng Y, Chung DW, Lopez JA. Shear stress-induced unfolding of VWF accelerates oxidation of key methionine residues in the A1A2A3 region. *Blood* 2011; 118(19):5283–91.

74. Chen J, Fu X, Wang Y, Ling M, McMullen B, Kulman J, Chung DW, Lopez JA. Oxidative modification of von Willebrand factor by neutrophil oxidants inhibits its cleavage by ADAMTS13. *Blood* 2010; 115(3):706–12.

75. Wang Y, Chen J, Ling M, Lopez JA, Chung DW,

Fu X. Hypochlorous acid generated by neutrophils inactivates ADAMTS13: an oxidative mechanism for regulating ADAMTS13 proteolytic activity during inflammation. *J Biol Chem* 2015; 290(3):1422–31.

Chapter 14

Singlet Oxygen in Biology and Medicine

ABSTRACT | The term singlet oxygen in biology and medicine, if not specified, typically refers to the $^1\Delta_g$ form, which is not a free radical. In biological systems, production of singlet oxygen results from photosensitivity reaction, phagocytic cell respiration burst, and lipid peroxidation. Singlet oxygen, as a potent reactive oxygen species (ROS), displays considerable reactivity towards cellular constituents, including lipids, proteins, and nucleic acids. Attack of these biomolecules by singlet oxygen causes lipid peroxidation, protein oxidation, and DNA base modifications, respectively. As an ROS synthesized endogenously in biological systems, singlet oxygen is a useful molecule responsible, at least partly, for host defense against invading pathogens. It is also the chief reactive species mediating photodynamic therapy-induced cancer cell killing. However, overproduction of singlet oxygen may cause injury to normal cells and tissues, contributing to certain pathophysiological processes.

KEYWORDS | Carotenoids; Furan-containing fatty acid; Haber–Weiss reaction; Immunity; Lipid peroxidation; Orange carotenoid protein; Ozone; Photodynamic therapy; Photosensitivity reaction; Porphyrias; Reactive oxygen species; Respiratory burst; Singlet oxygen resistant 1; Singlet oxygen

CITATION | Hopkins RZ and Li YR. Essentials of Free Radical Biology and Medicine. Cell Med Press, Raleigh, NC, USA. 2017. http://dx.doi.org/10.20455/efrbm.2017.14

ABBREVIATIONS | OCP, orange carotenoid protein; 8-OH-dG, 8-hydroxy-2′-deoxyguanosine; PDT, photodynamic therapy; PS, photosensitizer; ROS, reactive oxygen species; sor1, singlet oxygen resistant 1

CHAPTER AT A GLANCE

1. OVERVIEW

Singlet oxygen was first discovered in 1931 by W.H.J. Childe and R.Z. Mecke (see ref in [1]), and this reactive oxygen species (ROS) has received considerable attention in biology and medicine over the past several decades. As introduced in Chapter 2, singlet oxygen is an electronically excited form of molecular oxygen. There are two types of singlet oxygen, namely, $(^1\Delta_g)^1O_2$ and $(^1\Sigma_g^+)^1O_2$. The $^1\Sigma_g^+$ form is a free radical of higher energy that undergoes rapid decay rather than chemical reactions. This form of singlet oxygen is thus regarded to be too short-lived to be of any significance in biological systems. Therefore, in free radical biology and medicine, the term singlet oxygen, if not specified, typically refers to the $^1\Delta_g$ form, which is not a free radical. This chapter first considers the biological sources of singlet oxygen and then describes the basic chemical and biochemical properties of this ROS as well as its cell and tissue defenses. Finally, the chapter discusses the involvement of singlet oxygen in biology and medicine, outlining primarily its role in host defense, cancer photodynamic therapy, and disease process.

2. SOURCES

Singlet oxygen is formed via different pathways or chemical mechanisms in biological systems, including both animals and plants. The major sources of biological relevance include photosensitivity reaction, phagocytic cell respiratory burst, and lipid peroxidation (**Figure 14.1**).

2.1. Photosensitivity Reaction

In a photosensitivity reaction, an endogenous photosensitizer molecule (PS) (e.g., a porphyrin, flavin, or quinone molecule) is converted to an excited state (PS*) upon illumination by light. The excitation energy is then transferred to molecular oxygen (O_2), converting it to singlet oxygen, while the photosensitizer molecule returns to the ground state (Reactions 1 and 2). Photosensitivity reaction is a major source of singlet oxygen generation in plants [2]. It is also the chemical basis of cancer photodynamic therapy, in which an exogenous photosensitizer is typically employed [3] (see Section 5.2).

$$PS + light \rightarrow PS* \quad (1)$$

$$PS* + O_2 \rightarrow PS + {}^1O_2 \quad (2)$$

2.2. Phagocytic Cell Respiratory Burst

During the respiratory burst, the activated NADPH oxidase (also known as NOX2) of the phagocytic cells (mainly neutrophils) reduces molecular oxygen to superoxide, which then undergoes dismutation to form hydrogen peroxide. The phagocytic myeloperoxidase (MPO) catalyzes the reaction between hydrogen peroxide and chloride (Cl^-) to form hypochlorous acid (HOCl) (see Chapter 13). Hypochlorous acid in turn reacts with hydrogen peroxide to yield singlet oxygen (Reaction 3). Singlet oxygen formation may account for a significant portion (~20%) of the oxygen consumed during phagocytic cell respiratory burst and occur both intracellularly and extracellularly [4–6].

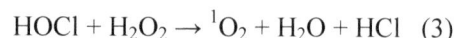

$$HOCl + H_2O_2 \rightarrow {}^1O_2 + H_2O + HCl \quad (3)$$

2.3. Lipid Peroxidation

On the one hand, ROS cause peroxidation of cell membrane lipids. On the other hand, lipid peroxidation generates ROS, including singlet oxygen. In this regard, peroxyl radicals (LOO·) formed during lipid peroxidation react with each other to yield singlet oxygen along with the formation of alcohol (LOH) and ketone (LO). This reaction proceeds via a linear tetraoxide intermediate (LOOOOL) (Reaction 4) [7].

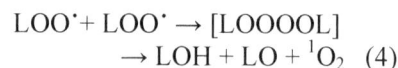

$$LOO· + LOO· \rightarrow [LOOOOL]$$
$$\rightarrow LOH + LO + {}^1O_2 \quad (4)$$

2.4. Other Sources

Singlet oxygen may also be formed via other sources of biological relevance. These include: (1) the Haber–Weiss reaction between superoxide and hydrogen peroxide ($O_2^{·-} + H_2O_2 \rightarrow {}^1O_2 + OH· + OH^-$) [8, 9]; (2) the reaction of ozone with biomolecules (e.g., cysteine, methionine, reduced form of glutathione, albumin, uric acid, and ascorbic acid) [10]; (3) the reaction between peroxynitrite and lipid hydroperoxides [11]; and (4) metabolic activation of certain drugs (e.g., bleomycin) [12].

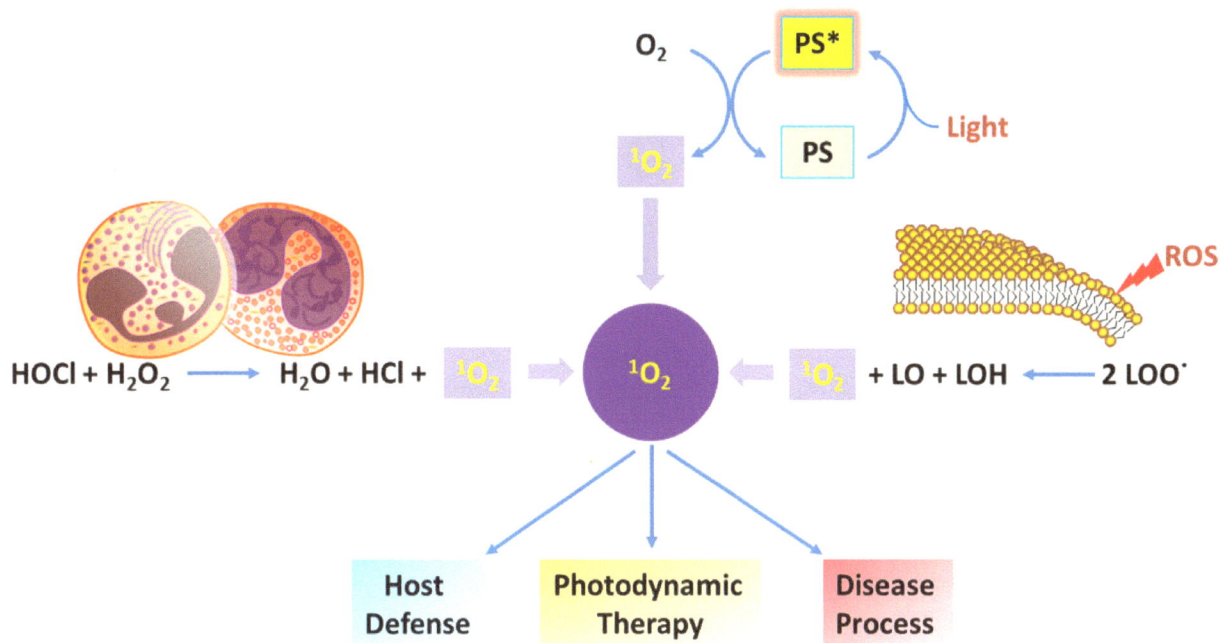

FIGURE 14.1. Singlet oxygen ($^1O_2$) production in biological systems and its involvement in biology and medicine. As illustrated, biological singlet oxygen is produced by three major sources, including photosensitivity reaction, phagocytic cell respiratory burst, and lipid peroxidation. In a photosensitivity reaction, a photosensitizer molecule (PS) is converted to an excited state (PS*) upon illumination by light. The excitation energy is then transferred to O_2, converting it to singlet oxygen, while the photosensitizer molecule returns to the ground state. In phagocytic cells, hypochlorous acid (HOCl) and H_2O_2 are produced during respiratory burst, and the reaction between them forms singlet oxygen. During lipid peroxidation, the reaction between two lipid peroxyl radicals (LOO·) results in the formation of singlet oxygen, lipid alcohol (LOH), and ketone (LO). As also depicted, phagocytic cell-derived singlet oxygen participates in the killing of invading pathogens. Singlet oxygen is the major reactive species responsible for photodynamic therapy-induced cancer cell killing.

3. CHEMISTRY AND BIOCHEMISTRY

3.1. General Chemical Properties

Singlet oxygen has an energy level of 22–23 kcal/mol above the ground state. The spontaneous decay of singlet oxygen to the ground state gives rise to photoemission, generating two types of chemiluminescence: (1) monomol emission ($^1O_2 \rightarrow O_2 + h\nu$; λ = 1268 nm) and (2) dimol emission ($^1O_2 \rightarrow O_2 + h\nu$; λ = 634 and 703 nm). This characteristic chemiluminescence is employed for the detection of singlet oxygen in biological systems [9, 13, 14].

Singlet oxygen is a strong oxidant that displays considerable reactivity towards cellular constituents, including lipids, proteins, and nucleic acids. There are two modes of reactivity by singlet oxygen: (1)

direct chemical reaction and (2) physical quenching. Physical quenching results in energy transfer and de-excitation of the singlet state, but it causes no chemical changes in the energy acceptor. Direct chemical reaction is the major mode of reactivity by singlet oxygen in biological systems.

3.2. Reaction with Cellular Constituents

Attack of lipid molecules in biomembranes or lipoproteins by singlet oxygen triggers lipid peroxidation, resulting in the formation of lipid peroxidation products, including reactive aldehydes. As noted earlier, lipid peroxidation also gives rise to singlet oxygen.

Singlet oxygen reacts with amino acid residues (e.g., tryptophan, tyrosine, histidine, methionine, and cysteine) of proteins. The reaction of singlet oxygen with proteins can result in multiple effects including oxidation of side-chains, backbone fragmentation, dimerization or aggregation, unfolding or conformational changes, enzyme inactivation, and alterations in cellular handling and turnover.

Reaction of singlet oxygen with DNA leads to base modifications, including the formation of 8-hydroxy-2′-deoxyguanosine (8-OH-dG) [15, 16]. Singlet oxygen can also cause DNA strand breaks. These genetic effects may collectively cause mutagenesis in organisms [17].

3.3. Half-Life, Diffusion, and Membrane Permeability

Singlet oxygen is short-lived species in biological systems. In this context, the lifetime of singlet oxygen in deuterated water is more than 10 times longer than that in water [18]. Singlet oxygen is membrane permeable and may diffuse across both plasma membrane and intracellular membranes. This property is in line with the potential of singlet oxygen to act as a biological signaling molecule [19, 20].

4. CELL AND TISSUE DEFENSES

4.1. Small Molecules in Mammalian Systems

Singlet oxygen reacts with most cellular biomolecules, including the non-enzymatic antioxidants, which include the reduced form of glutathione (GSH), vitamin E, vitamin C, nicotinamide adenine dinucleotide (NADH), nicotinamide adenine dinucleotide phosphate (NADPH), and carotenoids. Thus, reaction with these low-molecular-weight molecules protects the macromolecules (e.g., DNA, proteins, and lipids) from being damaged by singlet oxygen. Although carotenoids, as a chemical class, are considered potent scavengers of singlet oxygen, a recent study shows that β-carotene does not quench singlet oxygen in mammalian cells [21].

4.2. Specific Proteins in Plants and Microorganisms

Currently, there is no known enzyme capable of directly catalyzing the detoxification of singlet oxygen in mammalian systems. In plant cells and microorganisms, specific protein molecules involved in the detoxification of singlet oxygen have been identified. For example, in *Chlamydomonas reinhardtii*, a transcription factor, known as singlet oxygen resistant 1

(sor1), is inducible by singlet oxygen. Activation of sor1 increases the expression of detoxification genes, which serves as part of the singlet oxygen-induced acclimation process in the plant cells [22].

Cyanobacteria have developed a photoprotective mechanism that decreases the energy arriving at the photosynthetic reaction centers under high-light conditions. The photoactive orange carotenoid protein (OCP) is crucial in this mechanism as both a light sensor and an energy quencher. OCP is also shown to be a potent singlet oxygen quencher [23].

4.3. Specific Lipids in Microorganisms

Microorganisms may also synthesize specific lipid molecules to scavenge singlet oxygen. For example, the 19 carbon furan-containing fatty acid, 10,13-epoxy-11-methyl-octadecadienoate (9-(3-methyl-5-pentylfuran-2-yl)nonanoic acid) (19Fu-FA), in phospholipids from *Rhodobacter sphaeroides* may act as a membrane-bound scavenger of singlet oxygen [24]. As singlet oxygen is naturally produced by *R. sphaeroides* photosynthetic apparatus, 19Fu-FA may serve as an endogenous defense against singlet oxygen toxicity to the bacteria.

5. BIOLOGY AND MEDICINE

As an ROS synthesized endogenously in biological systems, singlet oxygen is a useful molecule responsible, at least partly, for host defense against pathogens. Due to its destructive power towards cellular constituents, singlet oxygen can be generated locally for killing cancer cells, a practice known as cancer photodynamic therapy. Owing to the same damaging property, uncontrolled production of singlet oxygen may cause injury to normal cells and tissues, contributing to disease process (**Figure 14.1**).

5.1. Immunity

Approximately, 20% of the oxygen utilized during phagocytic respiratory burst is converted to singlet oxygen [4]. This suggests that singlet oxygen production may play an important part in the host defense against invading pathogens. Indeed, singlet oxygen either derived from phagocytic cells or produced by photosensitivity reactions kills bacteria [25–27]. Singlet oxygen also inactivates various types of viruses [28–30]. It is noteworthy that some novel antiviral drugs may act via a singlet oxygen-mediated mechanism [31].

5.2. Cancer Photodynamic Therapy

Photodynamic therapy (PDT) uses photosensitizers and visible light in combination with molecular oxygen to produce ROS that kill the cancer cells. Singlet oxygen is recognized as the chief tumoricidal ROS produced by most PDT modalities, including recently developed innovative photosensitizers or associated platforms [32–35]. In addition to PDT, singlet oxygen formed via non-photosensitizing reactions in combination with conventional anticancer drugs has been employed for cancer therapy to overcome drug resistance [36].

5.3. Disease Process

Although controlled production of singlet oxygen plays a beneficial role in host defense against pathogens as well as cancer therapy, overproduction of this ROS and the subsequent oxidation of the critical biomolecules including lipids, proteins, and nucleic acids can lead to cell and tissue injury and potentially contribute to certain disease processes, such as adverse effects associated with photodynamic therapy and hereditary porphyrias. Hereditary porphyrias are a group of eight metabolic disorders of the heme biosynthesis pathway that are characterized by acute neurovisceral symptoms, skin lesions, or both. Cutaneous porphyrias present with either acute painful photosensitivity or skin fragility and blisters [37]. Although the detailed pathophysiological mechanisms of cutaneous porphyrias remain to be defined, singlet oxygen derived from the deposit of porphyrins upon exposure of the skin to sunlight is recognized as an important mechanism [38, 39].

6. SUMMARY OF CHAPTER KEY POINTS

- In free radical biology and medicine, the term singlet oxygen, if not specified, typically refers to the $^1\Delta_g$ state of singlet oxygen, which is a non-radical ROS.
- The major sources of biological singlet oxygen include photosensitivity reaction, phagocytic cell respiratory burst, and lipid peroxidation.
- Singlet oxygen has an energy level of 22–23 kcal/mol above the ground state. It is a strong oxidant that displays considerable reactivity towards cellular constituents, including lipids, proteins, and nucleic acids. It causes 8-OH-dG formation.
- Due to quenching by water in biological milieu, the biological half-life of singlet oxygen is in the range of a few microseconds. In mammalian systems, many small molecules of antioxidants including GSH, vitamin C, vitamin E, and carotenoids are capable of effectively quenching singlet oxygen, thereby protecting critical cellular targets from being damaged by this ROS.
- Specific proteins and lipids have been identified in certain plants and microorganisms to specifically and potently scavenge singlet oxygen.
- About 20% of the oxygen utilized during phagocytic cell respiratory burst is converted to singlet oxygen, which appears to play an important role in host defenses against invading pathogens.
- Singlet oxygen is the major ROS produced by most PDT modalities and is responsible for the cancer cell killing efficacy of PDT.
- Overproduction of singlet oxygen leads to cell and tissue injury and potentially contributes to certain disease processes, such as adverse effects associated with PDT and hereditary porphyrias.

7. SELF-ASSESSMENT QUESTIONS

7.1. Which of the following reactive species is not a free radical?

A. Delta state of singlet oxygen
B. Nitric oxide
C. Nitrogen dioxide
D. Sigma state of singlet oxygen
E. Superoxide anion

7.2. The spontaneous decay of $(^1\Delta_g)^1O_2$ to the ground state results in photo emission, giving rise to chemiluminescence. Which of the following is the maximal wavelength (λ) of the monomor emission of singlet oxygen?

A. 240 nm
B. 340 nm
C. 634 nm
D. 703 nm
E. 1268 nm

7.3. Which of the following species is known to be both an initiator and a product of lipid peroxidation?

A. Hydrogen peroxide
B. Nitric oxide
C. Nitrogen dioxide
D. Singlet oxygen
E. Superoxide

7.4. It has been shown that about 20% of the oxygen utilized during neutrophil respiratory burst is converted to singlet oxygen. Which of the following species is most likely involved in the reaction to give rise to singlet oxygen in the neutrophils?

A. Hydroxyl radical
B. Hypochlorous acid
C. Nitric oxide
D. Nitrogen dioxide
E. Ozone

7.5. Photodynamic therapy (PDT) is an effective approach to the management of certain types of cancer. Which of the following species is most likely to be responsible for PDT-induced cancer cell killing?

A. Carbon monoxide
B. Nitric oxide
C. Ozone
D. Singlet oxygen
E. Superoxide

ANSWERS AND EXPLANATIONS

7.1. The answer is A. There are two states of singlet oxygen, namely, $(^1\Delta_g)^1O_2$ and $(^1\Sigma_g^+)^1O_2$. The $^1\Sigma_g^+$ state is a free radical because it contains two unpaired electrons. In contrast, the $^1\Delta_g$ form is not a free radical as all electrons are paired. Nitric oxide, nitrogen dioxide, and superoxide anion are all free radicals as each of them contains an unpaired electron.

7.2. The answer is E. The spontaneous decay of singlet oxygen to the ground state gives rise to photoemission, generating two types of chemiluminescence, namely, monomol emission ($^1O_2 \rightarrow O_2 + h\nu$; $\lambda = 1268$ nm) and (2) dimol emission ($^1O_2 \rightarrow O_2 + h\nu$; $\lambda = 634$ and 703 nm). This characteristic chemiluminescence is commonly employed for the detection of singlet oxygen in biological systems.

7.3. The answer is D. Among the reactive species, only singlet oxygen can both directly trigger lipid peroxidation and be formed during lipid peroxidation (see Reaction 4 in Section 2.2).

7.4. The answer is B. During neutrophil respiratory burst, activation of NOX2 produces superoxide, which then undergoes dismutation to form hydrogen peroxide. The phagocytic myeloperoxidase catalyzes the reaction between hydrogen peroxide and chloride to form hypochlorous acid. Hypochlorous acid in turn reacts with hydrogen peroxide to yield singlet oxygen.

7.5. The answer is D. PDT uses photosensitizers and visible light in combination with molecular oxygen to produce ROS that kill the cancer cells. Singlet oxygen is recognized as the chief tumoricidal ROS produced by most PDT modalities.

REFERENCES

1. Hurst JR, Schuster GB. Nonradiative relaxation of singlet oxygen in solution. *J Am Chem Soc* 1983; 105(18):5756–60.
2. Triantaphylides C, Havaux M. Singlet oxygen in plants: production, detoxification and signaling. *Trends Plant Sci* 2009; 14(4):219–28.
3. Cengel KA, Simone CB, 2nd, Glatstein E. PDT: what's past is prologue. *Cancer Res* 2016; 76(9):2497–9.
4. Steinbeck MJ, Khan AU, Karnovsky MJ. Intracellular singlet oxygen generation by phagocytosing neutrophils in response to particles coated with a chemical trap. *J Biol Chem* 1992; 267(19):13425–33.
5. Steinbeck MJ, Khan AU, Karnovsky MJ. Extracellular production of singlet oxygen by stimulated macrophages quantified using 9,10-diphenylanthracene and perylene in a polystyrene film. *J Biol Chem* 1993; 268(21):15649–54.
6. Kanofsky JR, Hoogland H, Wever R, Weiss SJ. Singlet oxygen production by human eosinophils. *J Biol Chem* 1988; 263(20):9692–6.
7. Kanofsky JR. Singlet oxygen production from the reactions of alkylperoxy radicals: evidence from 1268-nm chemiluminescence. *J Org Chem* 1986; 51(17):3386–8.
8. Kellogg EW, 3rd, Fridovich I. Superoxide, hydrogen peroxide, and singlet oxygen in lipid peroxidation by a xanthine oxidase system. *J Biol Chem* 1975; 250(22):8812–7.
9. Khan AU, Kasha M. Singlet molecular oxygen in the Haber–Weiss reaction. *Proc Natl Acad Sci USA* 1994; 91(26):12365–7.
10. Kanofsky JR, Sima P. Singlet oxygen production from the reactions of ozone with biological molecules. *J Biol Chem* 1991; 266(14):9039–42.
11. Miyamoto S, Martinez GR, Martins AP, Medeiros MH, Di Mascio P. Direct evidence of

singlet molecular oxygen [$O_2(^1\Delta_g)$] production in the reaction of linoleic acid hydroperoxide with peroxynitrite. *J Am Chem Soc* 2003; 125(15):4510–7.

12. Kanofsky JR. Singlet oxygen production by bleomycin: a comparison with heme-containing compounds. *J Biol Chem* 1986; 261(29):13546–50.

13. Chou P-T, Chen Y-C, Wei C-Y, Lee M-Z. Evidence on the O_2 ($^1\Delta_g$) dimol-sensitized luminescence in solution. *J Am Chem Soc* 1998; 120(19):4883–4.

14. Khan AU, Kasha M. Direct spectroscopic observation of singlet oxygen emission at 1268 nm excited by sensitizing dyes of biological interest in liquid solution. *Proc Natl Acad Sci USA* 1979; 76(12):6047–9.

15. Ravanat JL, Di Mascio P, Martinez GR, Medeiros MH. Singlet oxygen induces oxidation of cellular DNA. *J Biol Chem* 2001; 276(8):40601–4.

16. Dumont E, Gruber R, Bignon E, Morell C, Moreau Y, Monari A, Ravanat JL. Probing the reactivity of singlet oxygen with purines. *Nucleic Acids Res* 2016; 44(1):56–62.

17. Noma K, Jin Y. Optogenetic mutagenesis in *Caenorhabditis elegans*. *Nat Commun* 2015; 6:8868.

18. Schweitzer C, Schmidt R. Physical mechanisms of generation and deactivation of singlet oxygen. *Chem Rev* 2003; 103(5):1685–757.

19. Basu-Modak S, Tyrrell RM. Singlet oxygen: a primary effector in the ultraviolet A/near-visible light induction of the human heme oxygenase gene. *Cancer Res* 1993; 53(19):4505–10.

20. Kim C, Meskauskiene R, Apel K, Laloi C. No single way to understand singlet oxygen signalling in plants. *EMBO Rep* 2008; 9(5):435–9.

21. Bosio GN, Breitenbach T, Parisi J, Reigosa M, Blaikie FH, Pedersen BW, Silva EF, Martire DO, Ogilby PR. Antioxidant beta-carotene does not quench singlet oxygen in mammalian cells. *J Am Chem Soc* 2013; 135(1):272–9.

22. Fischer BB, Ledford HK, Wakao S, Huang SG, Casero D, Pellegrini M, Merchant SS, Koller A, Eggen RI, Niyogi KK. SINGLET OXYGEN RESISTANT 1 links reactive electrophile signaling to singlet oxygen acclimation in *Chlamydomonas reinhardtii*. *Proc Natl Acad Sci USA* 2012; 109(20):E1302–11.

23. Sedoud A, Lopez-Igual R, Ur Rehman A, Wilson A, Perreau F, Boulay C, Vass I, Krieger-Liszkay A, Kirilovsky D. The cyanobacterial photoactive orange carotenoid protein is an excellent singlet oxygen quencher. *Plant Cell* 2014; 26(4):1781–91.

24. Lemke RA, Peterson AC, Ziegelhoffer EC, Westphall MS, Tjellstrom H, Coon JJ, Donohue TJ. Synthesis and scavenging role of furan fatty acids. *Proc Natl Acad Sci USA* 2014; 111(33):E3450–7.

25. Tatsuzawa H, Maruyama T, Hori K, Sano Y, Nakano M. Singlet oxygen (($^1\Delta_g$)O_2) as the principal oxidant in myeloperoxidase-mediated bacterial killing in neutrophil phagosome. *Biochem Biophys Res Commun* 1999; 262(3):647–50.

26. Tatsuzawa H, Maruyama T, Misawa N, Fujimori K, Nakano M. Quenching of singlet oxygen by carotenoids produced in *Escherichia coli*: attenuation of singlet oxygen-mediated bacterial killing by carotenoids. *FEBS Lett* 2000; 484(3):280–4.

27. Maisch T, Baier J, Franz B, Maier M, Landthaler M, Szeimies RM, Baumler W. The role of singlet oxygen and oxygen concentration in photodynamic inactivation of bacteria. *Proc Natl Acad Sci USA* 2007; 104(17):7223–8.

28. Muller-Breitkreutz K, Mohr H, Briviba K, Sies H. Inactivation of viruses by chemically and photochemically generated singlet molecular oxygen. *J Photochem Photobiol B* 1995; 30(1):63–70.

29. Kasermann F, Kempf C. Inactivation of enveloped viruses by singlet oxygen thermally generated from a polymeric naphthalene derivative. *Antiviral Res* 1998; 38(1):55–62.

30. Hollmann A, Castanho MA, Lee B, Santos NC. Singlet oxygen effects on lipid membranes: implications for the mechanism of action of broad-spectrum viral fusion inhibitors. *Biochem J* 2014; 459(1):161–70.

31. Hollmann A, Goncalves S, Augusto MT, Castanho MA, Lee B, Santos NC. Effects of singlet oxygen generated by a broad-spectrum viral fusion inhibitor on membrane nanoarchitecture. *Nanomedicine* 2015; 11(5):1163–7.

32. He J, Wang Y, Missinato MA, Onuoha E, Perkins LA, Watkins SC, St Croix CM, Tsang M, Bruchez MP. A genetically targetable near-infrared photosensitizer. *Nat Methods* 2016; 13(3):263–8.

33. Pinto A, Mace Y, Drouet F, Bony E, Boidot R, Draoui N, Lobysheva I, Corbet C, Polet F,

Martherus R, Deraedt Q, Rodriguez J, et al. A new ER-specific photosensitizer unravels $^1O_2$-driven protein oxidation and inhibition of deubiquitinases as a generic mechanism for cancer PDT. *Oncogene* 2016; 35(30):3976–85.

34. Cheng Y, Cheng H, Jiang C, Qiu X, Wang K, Huan W, Yuan A, Wu J, Hu Y. Perfluorocarbon nanoparticles enhance reactive oxygen levels and tumour growth inhibition in photodynamic therapy. *Nat Commun* 2015; 6:8785.

35. Ge J, Lan M, Zhou B, Liu W, Guo L, Wang H, Jia Q, Niu G, Huang X, Zhou H, Meng X, Wang P, et al. A graphene quantum dot photodynamic therapy agent with high singlet oxygen generation. *Nat Commun* 2014; 5:4596.

36. Lebedeva IV, Washington I, Sarkar D, Clark JA,

Fine RL, Dent P, Curiel DT, Turro NJ, Fisher PB. Strategy for reversing resistance to a single anticancer agent in human prostate and pancreatic carcinomas. *Proc Natl Acad Sci USA* 2007; 104(9):3484–9.

37. Puy H, Gouya L, Deybach JC. Porphyrias. *Lancet* 2010; 375(9718):924–37.

38. Franck B, Dust M, Stange A, Hoppe PP. Role of singlet oxygen in porphyria diseases. *Naturwissenschaften* 1982; 69(8):401–2.

39. Babes A, Sauer SK, Moparthi L, Kichko TI, Neacsu C, Namer B, Filipovic M, Zygmunt PM, Reeh PW, Fischer MJ. Photosensitization in porphyrias and photodynamic therapy involves TRPA1 and TRPV1. *J Neurosci* 2016; 36(19):5264–78.

Chapter 15

Other Relevant Chemical Species in Biology and Medicine

ABSTRACT | This chapter considers several other relevant chemical species in free radical biology and medicine, including alkoxyl and peroxyl radicals, ozone, carbon dioxide, carbon monoxide, hydrogen sulfide, molecular hydrogen, and transition metal ions. Alkoxyl radical and peroxyl radical are formed during lipid peroxidation and responsible for the propagation of lipid peroxidation. As potent oxidizing species, both alkoxyl and peroxyl radicals cause damage to cellular macromolecules, leading to cell and tissue injury. Ozone is an environmental pollutant, and exposure to high levels of environmental ozone is associated with an increased risk of diverse diseases. Ozone may also be produced in biological systems (e.g., neutrophils) via an antibody- or amino acid-catalyzed water oxidation pathway. The endogenously formed ozone may contribute to certain disease processes, such as atherosclerosis. On the other hand, controlled production of biological ozone may be part of the innate immunity against invading pathogens. Carbon dioxide is present in high concentrations in the body. While it is not an oxidant, carbon dioxide potentiates peroxynitrite- and hydrogen peroxide-induced toxicity, likely via the formation of secondary radical species, such as carbonate radical. Both carbon monoxide and hydrogen sulfide are air pollutants and among the significant causes of poisoning-related death. They are also produced endogenously via enzymatic reactions catalyzed by heme oxygenase and cystathionine β-synthase (or cystathionine γ-lyase), respectively. Both carbon monoxide and hydrogen sulfide are endogenously formed signaling molecules playing important roles in diverse physiological processes. While hydrogen atom is a reactive radical species, molecular hydrogen is found to act as a potential antioxidant and protect against oxidative tissue injury and disease pathophysiology. Transition metal ions, including iron and copper ions are essential elements of cell physiology. They also contribute to free radical generation and oxidative stress, especially when the free ion form is present.

KEYWORDS | Alkoxyl radical; Carbon dioxide; Carbon monoxide; Hydrogen sulfide; Molecular hydrogen; Ozone; Peroxyl radical; Transition metals

CITATION | Hopkins RZ and Li YR. *Essentials of Free Radical Biology and Medicine. Cell Med Press, Raleigh, NC, USA. 2017. http://dx.doi.org/10.20455/efrbm.2017.15*

ABBREVIATIONS | ATP, adenosine triphosphate; CBS, cystathionine β-synthase; CSE, cystathionine γ-lyase; GSH, reduced form of glutathione; 8-OH-dG, 8-hydroxy-2′-deoxyguanosine; ROS, reactive oxygen species; SOD, superoxide dismutase

CHAPTER AT A GLANCE

1. OVERVIEW

The preceding chapters have covered the most commonly encountered reactive oxygen species (ROS) with regard to their sources, basic chemical and biochemical properties, and cell and tissue defenses, as well as their potential involvement in physiology and disease process. This chapter provides a brief overview on less commonly encountered ROS, such as alkoxyl radical, peroxyl radical, and ozone, as well as several other relevant chemical species, including carbon dioxide, carbon monoxide, hydrogen sulfide, molecular hydrogen, and transition metal ions. The chapter focuses on discussing some major aspects of these species, such as their biological sources and possible roles in physiology and disease process.

2. ALKOXYL RADICAL AND PEROXYL RADICAL

2.1. Sources

Alkoxyl radical ($LO^{\cdot}$) and peroxyl radical ($LOO^{\cdot}$) are formed during lipid peroxidation. Hydroxyl radical ($OH^{\cdot}$) abstracts a hydrogen atom from a lipid molecule (LH), leading to the formation of a carbon-centered radical ($L^{\cdot}$). In the presence of molecular oxygen, the carbon-centered radical is converted to a peroxyl radical (Reactions 1 and 2).

$$OH^{\cdot} + LH \rightarrow L^{\cdot} + H_2O \quad (1)$$

$$L^{\cdot} + O_2 \rightarrow LOO^{\cdot} \quad (2)$$

Both alkoxyl and peroxyl radicals can abstract hydrogen atom from an adjacent lipid molecule, resulting in the propagation of lipid peroxidation. After abstracting a hydrogen atom, peroxyl radical is reduced to lipid hydroperoxide (LOOH). Decomposition of lipid hydroperoxide in the presence of metal ions, such as iron ion leads to the formation of alkoxyl radical or peroxyl radical dependent on the form of the iron ions (Reactions 3 and 4).

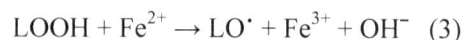

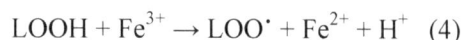

$$LOOH + Fe^{2+} \rightarrow LO^{\cdot} + Fe^{3+} + OH^- \quad (3)$$

$$LOOH + Fe^{3+} \rightarrow LOO^{\cdot} + Fe^{2+} + H^+ \quad (4)$$

Another source of peroxyl radical formation is the biotransformation of certain xenobiotics. For example, biotransformation of carbon tetrachloride (CCl_4) by liver cytochrome P450 2E1 produces trichloromethyl radical ($CCl_3^{\cdot}$), a carbon-centered radical, which then reacts with molecular oxygen to give rise to trichloromethylperoxyl radical ($CCl_3OO^{\cdot}$) (Reactions 5 and 6) [1]. The trichloromethylperoxyl radical triggers lipid peroxidation and is likely a major reactive metabolite responsible for carbon tetrachloride-induced liver injury [2].

$$CCl_4 \rightarrow CCl_3^{\cdot} \quad (5)$$

$$CCl_3^{\cdot} + O_2 \rightarrow CCl_3OO^{\cdot} \quad (6)$$

$$^1O_2 + H_2O \rightarrow H_2O_3 \quad (7)$$

$$H_2O_3 + {}^1O_2 \rightarrow O_3 + H_2O_2 \quad (8)$$

2.2. Biological Effects

Both alkoxyl and peroxyl radicals are strong oxidants with highly positive reduction potentials, being +1600 and +1000 mV, respectively (see Table 5.1 of Chapter 5). The higher reduction potential makes alkoxyl radical a generally more potent oxidant than the peroxyl radical. The protonated form of superoxide ($HO_2^{\cdot}$) is the simplest peroxyl radical.

Both alkoxyl and peroxyl radicals can abstract a hydrogen atom from a lipid molecule, triggering lipid peroxidation in biomembranes or lipoproteins. As such, the alkoxyl and peroxyl radicals formed during lipid peroxidation are responsible for the propagation of the lipid peroxidation chain-reactions. Alkoxyl and peroxyl radicals are also able to oxidize proteins, leading to protein dysfunction and enzyme inactivation. Oxidation of DNA by these free radicals causes oxidative base modifications including formation of 8-hydroxy-2′-deoxyguanosine (8-OH-dG), a widely used biomarker for oxidative DNA damage [3, 4]. As described in Chapter 14, peroxyl radicals react with each other yielding singlet oxygen, a potent ROS capable of damaging biomolecules.

Alkoxyl and peroxyl radicals react readily with cellular non-protein antioxidants, such as vitamin E, vitamin C, and reduced form of glutathione (GSH). These antioxidants act to protect more vital biomolecules from damage by alkoxyl and peroxyl radicals.

3. OZONE

3.1. Sources

Ozone (O_3) is a gas in the stratosphere (commonly known as stratospheric ozone) that protects animals on Earth from solar irradiation (**Figure 15.1**). O_3 is also an air pollutant near Earth's surface (commonly known as tropospheric O_3), where it is formed by photochemical reactions involving nitrogen oxides, volatile organic compounds, and carbon monoxide. Notably, O_3 may be produced in biological systems (e.g., by neutrophils) via an antibody- or amino acid-catalyzed water oxidation pathway [5–8]. The proposed reactions are depicted in **Figure 15.1** and also given below (Reactions 7 and 8). The reactant singlet oxygen ($^1O_2$) is derived from neutrophils (see Figure 14.1 of Chapter 14).

3.2. Biological Effects

O_3 is not a free radical, but has potent oxidizing capacity. It reacts with diverse biomolecules, including lipids, proteins, and nucleic acids, leading to cell and tissue injury. Exposure to environmental O_3 is associated with an increased risk of many human diseases, including asthma, chronic pulmonary obstructive disease (COPD), and atherosclerotic cardiovascular diseases, among many others [9–11]. O_3 is also reported to be present in the atherosclerotic arteries of humans [12], which is in line with its role in atherosclerotic cardiovascular disorders. Despite its causal role in disease process, controlled production of biological O_3 may be part of the host defense against invading pathogens [6–8] (**Figure 15.1**).

4. CARBON DIOXIDE

4.1. Sources

Carbon dioxide (CO_2) is a colorless and odorless gas that is vital to life of both plant and animal kingdoms on Earth. CO_2 is produced by all aerobic organisms, and along with its hydrated derivative bicarbonate (HCO_3^-), is present in high concentrations in the body.

4.2. Biological Effects

CO_2 is neither a free radical nor reactive to biomolecules. However, it is involved in free radical reactions. For example, the reaction between CO_2 and peroxynitrite ($ONOO^-$) leads to the formation of carbonate radical ($CO_3^{\cdot -}$) and nitrogen dioxide (NO_2): $CO_2 + ONOO^- \rightarrow [ONOOCO_2^-] \rightarrow CO_3^{\cdot -} + NO_2$. Both carbonate radical and nitrogen dioxide are highly reactive free radical species capable of damaging biomolecules. Formation of these free radical species is responsible, at least partly, for peroxynitrite-induced damage to target molecules, such as manganese superoxide dismutase (MnSOD) [13].

CO_2 potentiates hydrogen peroxide-induced oxidative damage to cellular targets, including CuZnSOD and protein tyrosine phosphatase [14, 15]. At the cellular level CO_2 also leads to increases in the death rates due to hydrogen peroxide stress in *Escherichia coli* in a concentration-dependent manner. This exac-

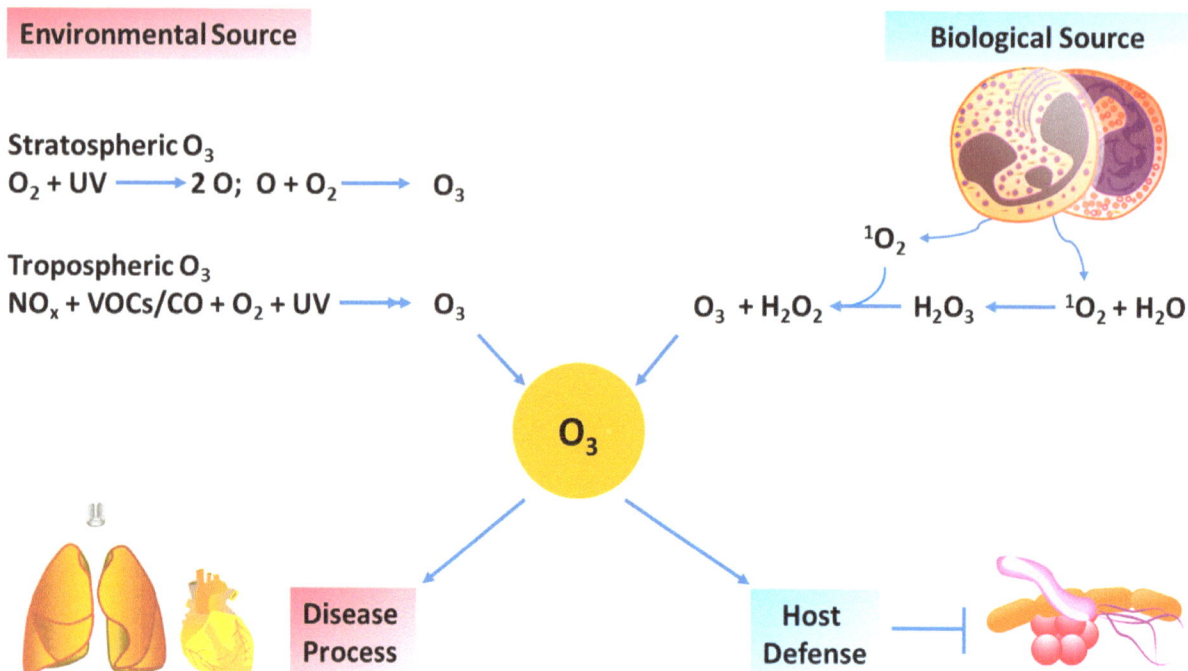

FIGURE 15.1. Sources of ozone (O_3) and its involvement in disease process as well as host defense. As illustrated, stratospheric O_3 is formed naturally by chemical reactions involving solar ultraviolet (UV) light. Solar UV light breaks apart an oxygen molecule (O_2) to form two separate oxygen atoms (O). The oxygen atom then reacts with O_2 to form O_3. Stratospheric O_3 protects life on Earth from solar irradiation-induced damage. The O_3 near Earth's surface, known as tropospheric O_3, is formed via chemical reactions involving solar UV light, naturally occurring gases, and pollutants, such as nitrogen oxides (NO_x), volatile organic compounds (VOCs), and carbon monoxide (CO). Exposure to high levels of tropospheric O_3 is associated with an increased risk of diverse disease conditions, such as pulmonary disorders and cardiovascular diseases. As also depicted, O_3 may be formed in biological systems, such as by neutrophils. Antibodies and certain amino acids may catalyze the reaction between singlet oxygen (derived from neutrophils or other biological processes) and water to eventually form O_3. The endogenously formed O_3 may also be involved in disease pathophysiology (not depicted). Notably, antibody-catalyzed formation of O_3 has been suggested to be an important pathway of the host defense against invading pathogens.

erbation is correlated with an increase in hydrogen peroxide-induced mutagenesis and formation of 8-OH-dG [16].

5. CARBON MONOXIDE

5.1. Environmental Sources and Poisoning

Carbon monoxide (CO) is an air pollutant and one of the significant causes of poisoning-related death [17, 18]. CO is neither a free radical nor an oxidant. However, exposure to high levels of environmental CO results in decreased oxygen-carrying capacity of

hemoglobin owing to its much higher binding affinity to hemoglobin than oxygen. High levels of CO also cause significant inhibition of mitochondrial respiration and decreased production of adenosine triphosphate (ATP) as a result of its high affinity binding to and inhibition of mitochondrial cytochrome c oxidase (complex IV) (**Figure 15.2**).

5.2. Endogenous Sources and Signaling

CO is also produced endogenously in mammals including humans via the action of heme oxygenase. This enzyme catalyzes the conversion of heme to biliverdin with the formation of CO and release of

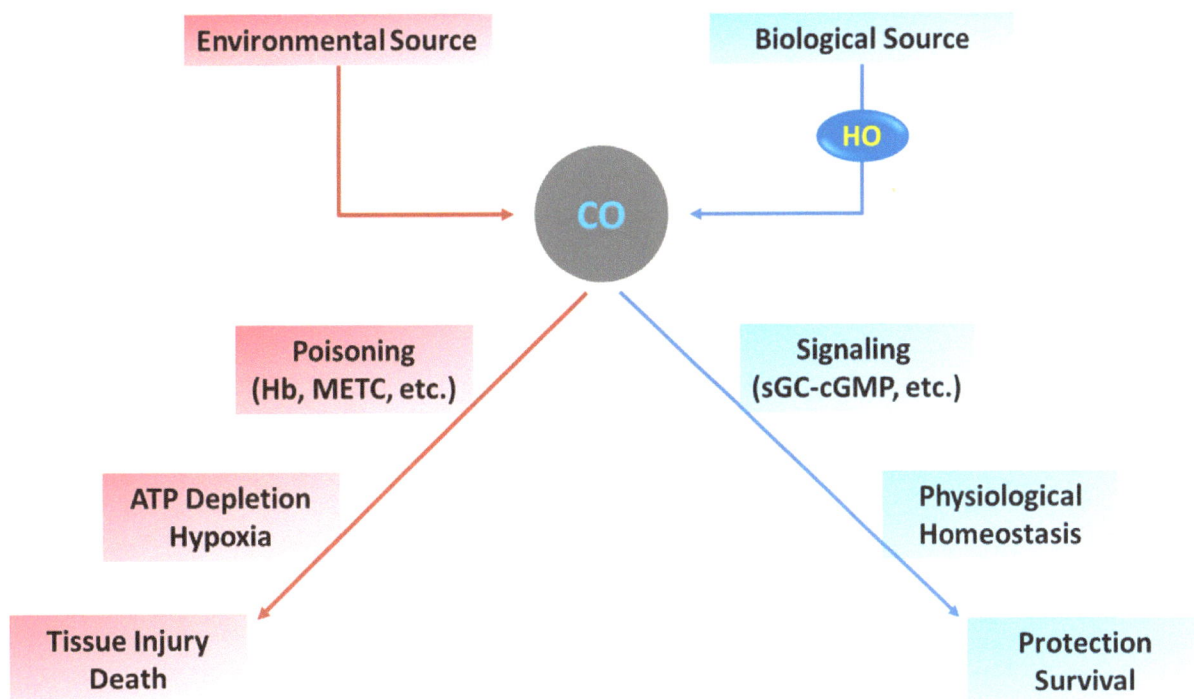

FIGURE 15.2. Environmental carbon monoxide (CO)-induced poisoning and endogenous CO-mediated cell signaling. Exposure to high levels of environmental CO causes significant inhibition of hemoglobin-mediated oxygen transport as well as suppression of mitochondrial respiration (via inhibiting the electron transport chain [METC] complex IV, also known as cytochrome c oxidase). These collectively cause depletion of adenosine triphosphate (ATP) and hypoxia, leading to tissue injury and death. On the other hand, CO formed endogenously via heme oxygenase (HO) may act as a signaling molecule via activating the soluble guanylate cyclase (sGC) and cyclic guanosine monophosphate (cGMP) pathway, and probably other mechanisms. As a signaling molecule, CO plays an important role in maintaining normal physiological homeostasis, thereby affording tissue protection and promoting host survival.

iron (see Appendix B). As indicated above, a significant chemical property of CO is its ability to react with metalloproteins, including hemoglobin, cytochrome c oxidase, cytochrome P450 enzymes, and soluble guanylate cyclase. The endogenously formed CO acts as a signaling molecule [19] and is involved in a number of physiological processes, including regulation of vascular tone, inflammatory processes, mitochondrial function, and the circadian clock, among others [20–22] (**Figure 15.2**).

5.3. As a Disease Protector

In line with its role in physiological homeostasis, CO either formed endogenously or given as a therapeutic modality has been shown to protect against the pathogenesis of many human disorders. These include cardiovascular diseases [23–25], neurological injury [26–28], and inflammatory/immunological disorders [29–32], among others.

5.4. As a Player in Host Defense

Studies also show an important role for CO in host defense against invading bacteria, and CO-releasing compounds may be used as an effective therapy of bacterial infections, especially for those that are resistant to conventional antibiotic treatment [33–36]. How CO boosts innate immunity to enhance bacterial clearance remains to be elucidated. A recent study suggested that macrophage-generated CO promoted ATP production and release by bacteria, which then activated the Nacht, LRR, and PYD domains-containing protein 3 (NALP3)/interleukin-1β inflammasome, thereby intensifying bacterial phagocytosis by macrophages [35].

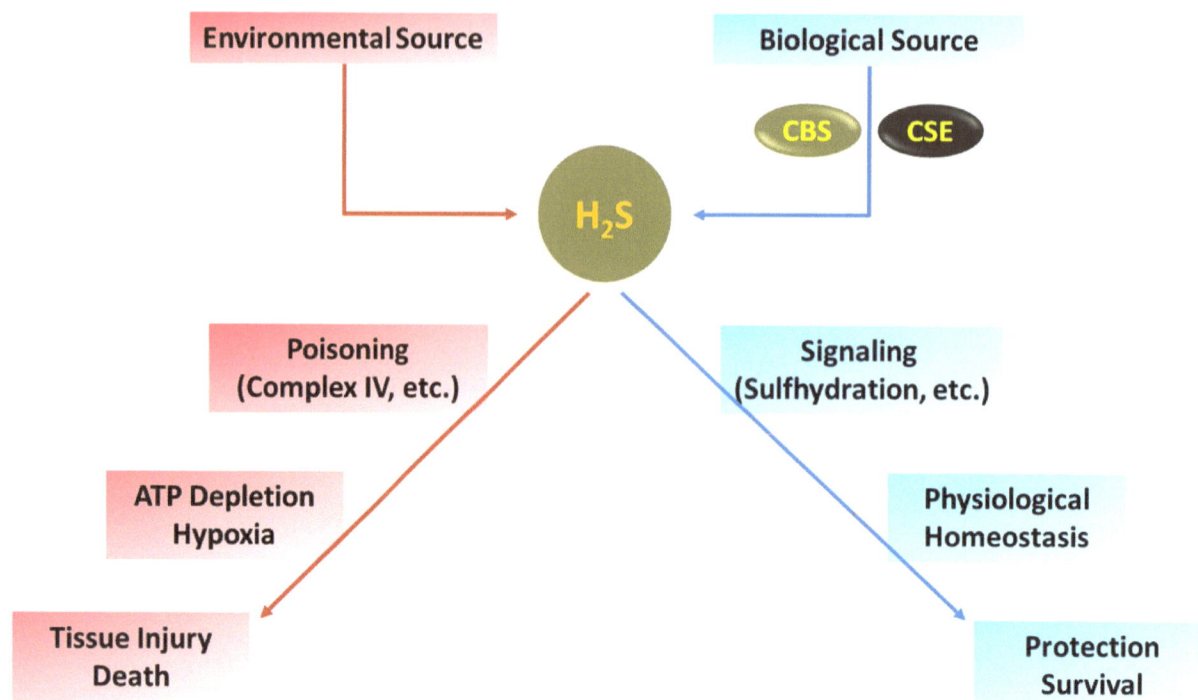

FIGURE 15.3. Environmental hydrogen sulfide (H$_2$S)-induced poisoning and endogenous H$_2$S-mediated cell signaling. Exposure to high levels of environmental H$_2$S causes significant suppression of mitochondrial respiration (via inhibiting the electron transport chain complex IV). This causes depletion of adenosine triphosphate (ATP) and hypoxia, leading to tissue injury and death. On the other hand, H$_2$S formed endogenously via cystathionine β-synthase (CBS) or cystathionine γ-lyase (CSE) may act as a signaling molecule via mechanisms involving sulfhydration of protein cysteine residues, among others. As a signaling molecule, H$_2$S plays an important role in maintaining normal physiological homeostasis, thereby affording tissue protection and promoting host survival.

6. HYDROGEN SULFIDE

6.1. Environmental Sources and Poisoning

Hydrogen disulfide (H$_2$S) is an air pollutant with a characteristic smell of rotten eggs. It is neither a free radical nor a potent oxidant, but exposure to high levels of environmental H$_2$S can cause significant toxicity to all organs, particularly the central nervous system and respiratory system in humans. While its mechanisms of toxicity remain partially understood, high levels of H$_2$S can suppress mitochondrial respiration by inhibiting mitochondrial electron transport chain complex IV (also known as cytochrome c oxidase). In this context, high levels of H$_2$S, like carbon monoxide and cyanide, cause ATP depletion and hypoxia, thereby leading to cell injury and death [37] (**Figure 15.3**).

6.2. Endogenous Sources and Signaling

Like carbon monoxide, H$_2$S is also formed endogenously in mammals including humans, and can be detected in significant amounts in biological samples [38–40]. For example, in the mammalian brain tissue, the levels of H$_2$S can be as high as 50–160 μM, and in the blood its concentrations may range from 10 to 100 μM. H$_2$S is produced endogenously via enzymatic activity of cystathionine β-synthase (CBS) or cystathionine γ-lyase (CSE), nonenzymatic pathways (such as reduction of thiol-containing molecules), and is also released from intracellular sulfur stores (sulfane sulfur) [41]. Both CBS and CSE use L-cysteine as a substrate and depend on pyridoxal-5'-phosphate, and are the major enzymatic machineries for endogenous production of H$_2$S in the mammalian systems.

Similar to nitric oxide and carbon monoxide, H_2S has the ability to interact with metalloproteins. It also reacts with various free radicals, leading to the formation of less reactive products. In addition, H_2S is able to upregulate antioxidant enzymes in cells and tissues via the activation of the nuclear factor E2-related factor 2 (Nrf2) signaling [42–44]. As such, endogenously formed H_2S is viewed as an antioxidant. Studies over the past few years have established H_2S as an endogenously formed signaling molecule involved in the maintenance of physiological homeostasis, including vasodilation and blood pressure regulation [45, 46], angiogenesis [47], stem cell function [48], anti-inflammation and cytoprotection [49], mitochondrial energy production [50], immunity [51], and possibly longevity [52–54], among others. The molecular mechanisms underlying H_2S-mediated physiological functions remain to be defined. One potential pathway involves posttranslational modification of protein cysteine residues through a process known as sulfhydration (protein–SH + H_2S → protein–SSH) [55–57] (**Figure 15.3**).

6.3. As a Disease Protector

Given its important role in physiological homeostasis, it is not surprising that dysregulation of endogenous H_2S production contributes to the pathogenesis of a number of diseases, especially cardiovascular disorders [39]. Likewise, drugs are currently being developed to modulate H_2S levels to achieve therapeutic efficacy for diverse disease conditions [58].

7. MOLECULAR HYDROGEN

7.1. Sources

Molecular hydrogen (H_2) is a colorless, odorless, and highly combustible gas present in the air in small quantities, accounting for only ~0.00005% of air. In humans, H_2 is mainly produced in the gut via bacteria-mediated fermentation of dietary components, and can be excreted via the lungs [59, 60].

7.2. Biological Effects

While hydrogen atom (H) is a reactive radical species, molecular hydrogen (H_2) is found to act as a potential antioxidant. H_2 reduces hydroxyl radical and peroxynitrite, and protects cultured neurons from ischemia-reperfusion injury. Inhalation of H_2 gas is also shown to protect against brain ischemia-reperfusion injury in rats [61]. In experimental animals, consumption of H_2-rich water was shown to (1) prevent atherosclerosis in apolipoprotein E-knockout mice [62]; (2) prevent chronic allograft nephropathy in rats [63]; (3) prevent progression of nonalcoholic steatohepatitis and accompanying hepatocarcinogenesis in mice [64]; and (4) improve the neurological outcome in a rat model of cardiac arrest [65]. It was suggested that H_2 might regulate cytoprotective gene expression, stimulate energy metabolism, and function as an anti-inflammatory, anti-allergic, and anti-apoptotic molecule [66–68].

8. TRANSITION METAL IONS

8.1. As Double-Edged Swords

Transition metal ions, including iron and copper ions are essential elements in animals, including humans. On the one hand, they play important roles in various physiological processes. On the other hand, these metal ions, particularly iron and copper ions also contribute to free radical damage in biological systems. The detrimental effects of transition metal ions are believed to be associated with their unique chemical properties as outlined below (**Figure 15.4**).

(1) The redox chemistry of the transition metal ions makes them being involved in the conversion of less reactive ROS to more reactive ROS. For example, reaction of ferrous (Fe^{2+}) or cuprous (Cu^{1+}) ion with hydrogen peroxide produces hydroxyl radical, an extremely potent ROS capable of damaging the entire spectrum of biomolecules. The above reactions involving iron and copper are commonly referred to as the Fenton reaction and Fenton-type reaction, respectively (also see Section 3.3 of Chapter 8).

(2) Transition metal ions catalyze the autoxidation of cellular biomolecules, such as vitamin C, L-cysteine, NADH, NADPH, and catecholamines to produce ROS and related reactive species [69–71]. Interaction of certain xenobiotics/drugs, such as doxorubicin with transition metal ions also results in the formation of reactive species contributing to cell and tissue injury [72].

8.2. Binding and Mobilization

It should be noted that in order for transition metal ions to participate in the above reactions, the metal

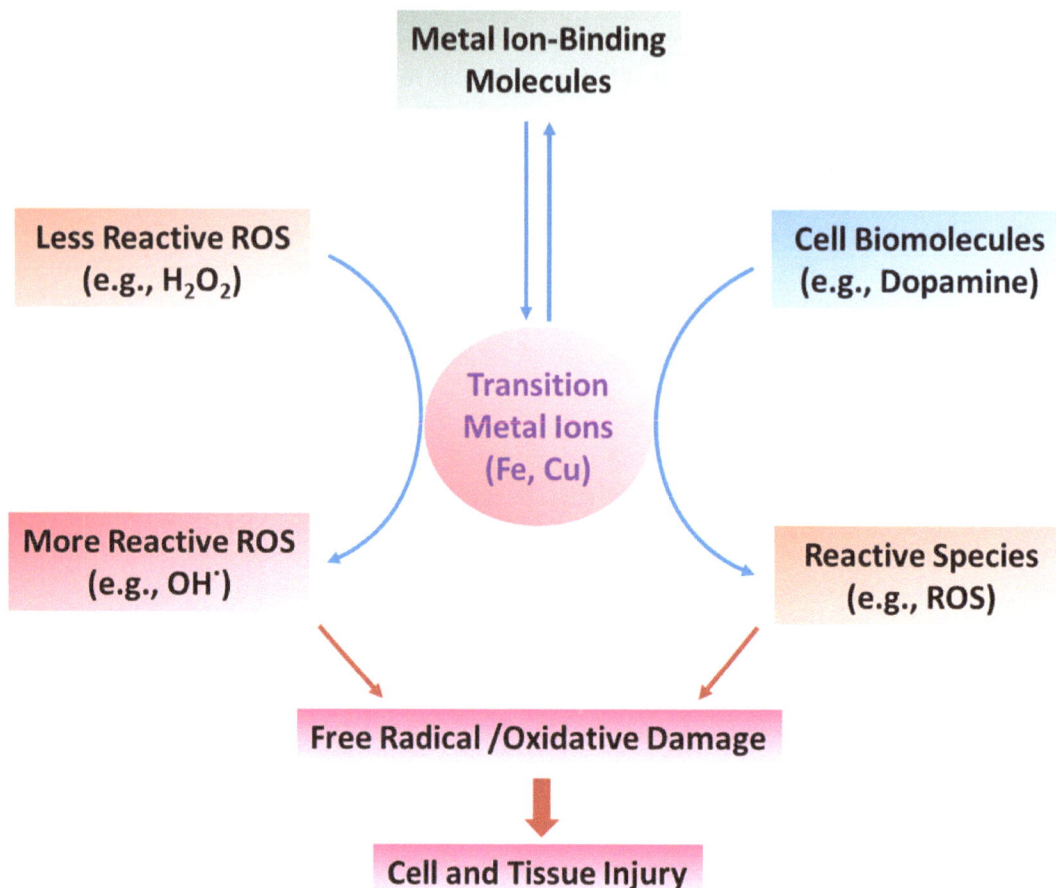

FIGURE 15.4. Transition metal ions in free radical damage. On the one hand, transition metal ions, including iron and copper ions are essential for normal physiology. On the other hand, the redox chemistry of these metal ions especially iron and copper ions enables them to participate in the redox reactions that either convert less toxic reactive oxygen species (ROS) to more toxic ones, or catalyze the autoxidation of cellular biomolecules to form toxic free radicals/ROS. These may collectively contribute to oxidative tissue injury. To minimize iron or copper ion-mediated oxidative injury, cells possess diverse molecules to bind to these metal ions so that the free ion form can be kept at very low levels under physiological conditions.

ions typically need to be in the free form. In cells and tissues, various proteins and non-protein biomolecules can bind to these metal ions so that free metal ion concentrations are kept extremely low in vivo [73, 74]. These metal ion-binding proteins or non-protein biomolecules are critical for both intracellular dynamics of metal distribution and preventing them from mediating free radical generation and tissue damage [73, 74] (**Figure 15.4**).

However, under certain pathophysiological conditions, such as myocardial ischemia, copper and iron ions may be mobilized and released from the binding proteins to participate in the redox reactions, thereby

generating ROS to cause tissue injury [75]. As stated in Chapter 8 (Section 3.1 and Figure 8.3), superoxide causes iron release from certain iron-sulfur cluster-containing enzymes, such as mitochondrial aconitase and electron transport chain enzyme complexes.

Although protein-bound copper or iron ions are generally considered redox-inactive, they may still participate in redox reactions, generating ROS under certain conditions. For example, it was reported that copper ions bound to β-amyloid fibrils in Alzheimer's disease could still be redox-active and thereby degrade hydrogen peroxide, forming hydroxyl radicals [76, 77].

9. SUMMARY OF CHAPTER KEY POINTS

- Alkoxyl radical and peroxyl radical are formed from lipid peroxidation. Peroxyl radical may also be formed during the biotransformation of certain xenobiotics.
- Both alkoxyl and peroxyl radicals are strong oxidants and attack lipids, proteins, and nucleic acids, causing oxidative damage.
- O_3 is present in the environment and may also be produced endogenously in biological systems (e.g., by neutrophils) via antibody- or amino acid-catalyzed water oxidation.
- While environmental O_3 is associated with an increased risk of diverse diseases, neutrophil-derived O_3 may play a role in host defense against invading pathogens.
- CO_2 along with bicarbonate is present in high concentrations in the body. Although it is not an oxidant, CO_2 can augment the toxicity of peroxynitrite and hydrogen peroxide, possibly via the formation of secondary free radicals.
- CO is an air pollutant and a significant cause of poisoning-related death. CO is also produced endogenously in mammals via the action of heme oxygenase.
- The endogenously formed CO acts as a signaling molecule and is involved in diverse physiological processes.
- CO either formed endogenously or given as a therapeutic modality has been shown to protect against the pathogenesis of many human disorders.
- H_2S is an air pollutant that can cause significant toxicity to all organs. Like CO, endogenously formed H_2S is a signaling molecule, playing important physiological roles.
- While hydrogen atom is a reactive radical species, H_2 is found to act as a potential antioxidant. H_2 protects against a number of pathophysiological processes.
- Transition metal ions, including iron and copper ions are double-edged swords. On the one hand they are essential in normal physiology. On the other hand, via redox chemistry, transition metal ions may cause free radical formation and oxidative damage.

10. SELF-ASSESSMENT QUESTIONS

10.1. Which of the following ROS is most likely to be produced from the reaction of lipid hydroperoxide with ferric ion?

A. Alkoxyl radical
B. Hydrogen peroxide
C. Lipid peroxyl radical
D. Singlet oxygen
E. Superoxide

10.2. It has been demonstrated that ozone may be formed endogenously by neutrophils. Which of the following species is most likely to be involved in the reactions giving rise to ozone?

A. Hydrogen peroxide
B. Hypochlorous acid
C. Nitric oxide
D. Peroxynitrite
E. Singlet oxygen

10.3. Which of the following chemical species has been shown to potentiate both peroxynitrite- and hydrogen peroxide-mediated oxidative damage to molecular targets?

A. Carbon dioxide
B. Carbon monoxide
C. Hydrogen gas
D. Molecular oxygen
E. Nitrogen gas

10.4. Which of the following gases is a "smelly" signaling molecule playing important physiological roles in mammalian systems?

A. Carbon dioxide
B. Carbon monoxide
C. Hydrogen gas
D. Hydrogen sulfide
E. Nitric oxide

10.5. Which of the following has been shown to be an antioxidant gas that protects against experimental cerebral ischemia-reperfusion injury?

A. Carbon dioxide
B. Hydrogen gas
C. Methane
D. Nitrogen dioxide
E. Nitrogen gas

ANSWERS AND EXPLANATIONS

10.1. The answer is C. Decomposition of lipid hydroperoxide in the presence of ferric iron ion leads to the formation of peroxyl radical. This reaction is depicted as: $LOOH + Fe^{3+} \rightarrow LOO^{\cdot} + Fe^{2+} + H^+$.

10.2. The answer is E. Antibody-catalyzed reaction of singlet oxygen with water has been suggested to give rise to ozone.

10.3. The answer is A. CO_2 has been shown to potentiate peroxynitrite- and hydrogen peroxide-induced oxidative damage to target molecules, such as MnSOD and CuZnSOD.

10.4. The answer is D. H_2S smells like rotten eggs and the endogenously formed H_2S acts as a signaling molecule involved in the maintenance of physiological homeostasis.

10.5. The answer is B. H_2 is an antioxidant gas, and inhalation of H_2 gas is shown to protect against brain ischemia-reperfusion injury in rats.

REFERENCES

1. Connor HD, Thurman RG, Galizi MD, Mason RP. The formation of a novel free radical metabolite from CCl_4 in the perfused rat liver and in vivo. *J Biol Chem* 1986; 261(10):4542–8.
2. Kono N, Inoue T, Yoshida Y, Sato H, Matsusue T, Itabe H, Niki E, Aoki J, Arai H. Protection against oxidative stress-induced hepatic injury by intracellular type II platelet-activating factor acetylhydrolase by metabolism of oxidized phospholipids in vivo. *J Biol Chem* 2008; 283(3):1628–36.
3. Adam W, Kurz A, Saha-Moller CR. Peroxidase-catalyzed oxidative damage of DNA and 2'-deoxyguanosine by model compounds of lipid hydroperoxides: involvement of peroxyl radicals. *Chem Res Toxicol* 2000; 13(12):1199–207.
4. Lim P, Wuenschell GE, Holland V, Lee DH, Pfeifer GP, Rodriguez H, Termini J. Peroxyl radical mediated oxidative DNA base damage: implications for lipid peroxidation induced mutagenesis. *Biochemistry* 2004; 43(49):15339–48.
5. Wentworth P, Jr., Jones LH, Wentworth AD, Zhu X, Larsen NA, Wilson IA, Xu X, Goddard WA, 3rd, Janda KD, Eschenmoser A, Lerner RA. Antibody catalysis of the oxidation of water. *Science* 2001; 293(5536):1806–11.
6. Wentworth P, Jr., McDunn JE, Wentworth AD, Takeuchi C, Nieva J, Jones T, Bautista C, Ruedi JM, Gutierrez A, Janda KD, Babior BM, Eschenmoser A, et al. Evidence for antibody-catalyzed ozone formation in bacterial killing and inflammation. *Science* 2002; 298(5601):2195–9.
7. Babior BM, Takeuchi C, Ruedi J, Gutierrez A, Wentworth P, Jr. Investigating antibody-catalyzed ozone generation by human neutrophils. *Proc Natl Acad Sci USA* 2003; 100(6):3031–4.
8. Yamashita K, Miyoshi T, Arai T, Endo N, Itoh H, Makino K, Mizugishi K, Uchiyama T, Sasada M. Ozone production by amino acids contributes to killing of bacteria. *Proc Natl Acad Sci USA* 2008; 105(44):16912–7.
9. Islam T, McConnell R, Gauderman WJ, Avol E, Peters JM, Gilliland FD. Ozone, oxidant defense genes, and risk of asthma during adolescence. *Am J Respir Crit Care Med* 2008; 177(4):388–95.
10. Zanobetti A, Schwartz J. Ozone and survival in four cohorts with potentially predisposing diseases. *Am J Respir Crit Care Med* 2011; 184(7):836–41.
11. Ruidavets JB, Cournot M, Cassadou S, Giroux M, Meybeck M, Ferrieres J. Ozone air pollution is associated with acute myocardial infarction. *Circulation* 2005; 111(5):563–9.
12. Wentworth P, Jr., Nieva J, Takeuchi C, Galve R, Wentworth AD, Dilley RB, DeLaria GA, Saven A, Babior BM, Janda KD, Eschenmoser A, Lerner RA. Evidence for ozone formation in human atherosclerotic arteries. *Science* 2003; 302(5647):1053–6.
13. Surmeli NB, Litterman NK, Miller AF, Groves JT. Peroxynitrite mediates active site tyrosine nitration in manganese superoxide dismutase. Evidence of a role for the carbonate radical anion. *J Am Chem Soc* 2010; 132(48):17174–85.
14. Liochev SI, Fridovich I. CO_2, not HCO_3^-, facilitates oxidations by Cu,Zn superoxide dismutase plus H_2O_2. *Proc Natl Acad Sci USA* 2004; 101(3):743–4.
15. Zhou H, Singh H, Parsons ZD, Lewis SM, Bhattacharya S, Seiner DR, LaButti JN, Reilly TJ, Tanner JJ, Gates KS. The biological buffer bicarbonate/CO_2 potentiates H_2O_2-mediated inactivation of protein tyrosine phosphatases. *J Am Chem Soc* 2011; 133(40):15803–5.
16. Ezraty B, Chabalier M, Ducret A, Maisonneuve E, Dukan S. CO_2 exacerbates oxygen toxicity. *EMBO Rep* 2011; 12(4):321–6.
17. Rose JJ, Wang L, Xu Q, McTiernan CF, Shiva S,

Tejero J, Gladwin MT. Carbon monoxide poisoning: pathogenesis, management and future directions of therapy. *Am J Respir Crit Care Med* 2016.

18. Weaver LK. Clinical practice. Carbon monoxide poisoning. *N Engl J Med* 2009; 360(12):1217–25.

19. Verma A, Hirsch DJ, Glatt CE, Ronnett GV, Snyder SH. Carbon monoxide: a putative neural messenger. *Science* 1993; 259(5093):381–4.

20. Mustafa AK, Gadalla MM, Snyder SH. Signaling by gasotransmitters. *Sci Signal* 2009; 2(68):re2.

21. Szabo C. Gaseotransmitters: new frontiers for translational science. *Sci Transl Med* 2010; 2(59):59ps4.

22. Klemz R, Reischl S, Wallach T, Witte N, Jurchott K, Klemz S, Lang V, Lorenzen S, Knauer M, Heidenreich S, Xu M, Ripperger JA, et al. Reciprocal regulation of carbon monoxide metabolism and the circadian clock. *Nat Struct Mol Biol* 2017; 24(1):15–22.

23. Otterbein LE, Zuckerbraun BS, Haga M, Liu F, Song R, Usheva A, Stachulak C, Bodyak N, Smith RN, Csizmadia E, Tyagi S, Akamatsu Y, et al. Carbon monoxide suppresses arteriosclerotic lesions associated with chronic graft rejection and with balloon injury. *Nat Med* 2003; 9(2):183–90.

24. True AL, Olive M, Boehm M, San H, Westrick RJ, Raghavachari N, Xu X, Lynn EG, Sack MN, Munson PJ, Gladwin MT, Nabel EG. Heme oxygenase-1 deficiency accelerates formation of arterial thrombosis through oxidative damage to the endothelium, which is rescued by inhaled carbon monoxide. *Circ Res* 2007; 101(9):893–901.

25. Otterbein LE, Foresti R, Motterlini R. Heme oxygenase-1 and carbon monoxide in the heart: the balancing act between danger signaling and pro-survival. *Circ Res* 2016; 118(12):1940–59.

26. Morikawa T, Kajimura M, Nakamura T, Hishiki T, Nakanishi T, Yukutake Y, Nagahata Y, Ishikawa M, Hattori K, Takenouchi T, Takahashi T, Ishii I, et al. Hypoxic regulation of the cerebral microcirculation is mediated by a carbon monoxide-sensitive hydrogen sulfide pathway. *Proc Natl Acad Sci USA* 2012; 109(4):1293–8.

27. Schallner N, Pandit R, LeBlanc R, 3rd, Thomas AJ, Ogilvy CS, Zuckerbraun BS, Gallo D, Otterbein LE, Hanafy KA. Microglia regulate blood clearance in subarachnoid hemorrhage by heme oxygenase-1. *J Clin Invest* 2015;

125(7):2609–25.

28. Choi YK, Maki T, Mandeville ET, Koh SH, Hayakawa K, Arai K, Kim YM, Whalen MJ, Xing C, Wang X, Kim KW, Lo EH. Dual effects of carbon monoxide on pericytes and neurogenesis in traumatic brain injury. *Nat Med* 2016; 22(11):1335–41.

29. Lee TS, Chau LY. Heme oxygenase-1 mediates the anti-inflammatory effect of interleukin-10 in mice. *Nat Med* 2002; 8(3):240–6.

30. Wang H, Lee SS, Gao W, Czismadia E, McDaid J, Ollinger R, Soares MP, Yamashita K, Bach FH. Donor treatment with carbon monoxide can yield islet allograft survival and tolerance. *Diabetes* 2005; 54(5):1400–6.

31. Hegazi RA, Rao KN, Mayle A, Sepulveda AR, Otterbein LE, Plevy SE. Carbon monoxide ameliorates chronic murine colitis through a heme oxygenase 1-dependent pathway. *J Exp Med* 2005; 202(12):1703–13.

32. Xue J, Habtezion A. Carbon monoxide-based therapy ameliorates acute pancreatitis via TLR4 inhibition. *J Clin Invest* 2014; 124(1):437–47.

33. Chung SW, Liu X, Macias AA, Baron RM, Perrella MA. Heme oxygenase-1-derived carbon monoxide enhances the host defense response to microbial sepsis in mice. *J Clin Invest* 2008; 118(1):239–47.

34. Onyiah JC, Sheikh SZ, Maharshak N, Steinbach EC, Russo SM, Kobayashi T, Mackey LC, Hansen JJ, Moeser AJ, Rawls JF, Borst LB, Otterbein LE, et al. Carbon monoxide and heme oxygenase-1 prevent intestinal inflammation in mice by promoting bacterial clearance. *Gastroenterology* 2013; 144(4):789–98.

35. Wegiel B, Larsen R, Gallo D, Chin BY, Harris C, Mannam P, Kaczmarek E, Lee PJ, Zuckerbraun BS, Flavell R, Soares MP, Otterbein LE. Macrophages sense and kill bacteria through carbon monoxide-dependent inflammasome activation. *J Clin Invest* 2014; 124(11):4926–40.

36. Wareham LK, Poole RK, Tinajero-Trejo M. CO-releasing metal carbonyl compounds as antimicrobial agents in the post-antibiotic era. *J Biol Chem* 2015; 290(31):18999–9007.

37. Reiffenstein RJ, Hulbert WC, Roth SH. Toxicology of hydrogen sulfide. *Annu Rev Pharmacol Toxicol* 1992; 32:109–34.

38. Szabo C. Hydrogen sulphide and its therapeutic potential. *Nat Rev Drug Discov* 2007; 6(11):917–35.

39. Polhemus DJ, Lefer DJ. Emergence of hydrogen sulfide as an endogenous gaseous signaling

molecule in cardiovascular disease. *Circ Res* 2014; 114(4):730–7.

40. Farrugia G, Szurszewski JH. Carbon monoxide, hydrogen sulfide, and nitric oxide as signaling molecules in the gastrointestinal tract. *Gastroenterology* 2014; 147(2):303–13.

41. Li L, Rose P, Moore PK. Hydrogen sulfide and cell signaling. *Annu Rev Pharmacol Toxicol* 2011; 51:169–87.

42. Calvert JW, Jha S, Gundewar S, Elrod JW, Ramachandran A, Pattillo CB, Kevil CG, Lefer DJ. Hydrogen sulfide mediates cardioprotection through Nrf2 signaling. *Circ Res* 2009; 105(4):365–74.

43. Calvert JW, Elston M, Nicholson CK, Gundewar S, Jha S, Elrod JW, Ramachandran A, Lefer DJ. Genetic and pharmacologic hydrogen sulfide therapy attenuates ischemia-induced heart failure in mice. *Circulation* 2010; 122(1):11–9.

44. Xie L, Gu Y, Wen M, Zhao S, Wang W, Ma Y, Meng G, Han Y, Wang Y, Liu G, Moore PK, Wang X, et al. Hydrogen sulfide induces Keap1 S-sulfhydration and suppresses diabetes-accelerated atherosclerosis via Nrf2 activation. *Diabetes* 2016; 65(10):3171–84.

45. Yang G, Wu L, Jiang B, Yang W, Qi J, Cao K, Meng Q, Mustafa AK, Mu W, Zhang S, Snyder SH, Wang R. H_2S as a physiologic vasorelaxant: hypertension in mice with deletion of cystathionine gamma-lyase. *Science* 2008; 322(5901):587–90.

46. Peng YJ, Nanduri J, Raghuraman G, Souvannakitti D, Gadalla MM, Kumar GK, Snyder SH, Prabhakar NR. H_2S mediates O_2 sensing in the carotid body. *Proc Natl Acad Sci USA* 2010; 107(23):10719–24.

47. Papapetropoulos A, Pyriochou A, Altaany Z, Yang G, Marazioti A, Zhou Z, Jeschke MG, Branski LK, Herndon DN, Wang R, Szabo C. Hydrogen sulfide is an endogenous stimulator of angiogenesis. *Proc Natl Acad Sci USA* 2009; 106(51):21972–7.

48. Liu Y, Yang R, Liu X, Zhou Y, Qu C, Kikuiri T, Wang S, Zandi E, Du J, Ambudkar IS, Shi S. Hydrogen sulfide maintains mesenchymal stem cell function and bone homeostasis via regulation of Ca^{2+} channel sulfhydration. *Cell Stem Cell* 2014; 15(1):66–78.

49. King AL, Polhemus DJ, Bhushan S, Otsuka H, Kondo K, Nicholson CK, Bradley JM, Islam KN, Calvert JW, Tao YX, Dugas TR, Kelley EE, et al. Hydrogen sulfide cytoprotective signaling is endothelial nitric oxide synthase-nitric oxide

dependent. *Proc Natl Acad Sci USA* 2014; 111(8):3182–7.

50. Fu M, Zhang W, Wu L, Yang G, Li H, Wang R. Hydrogen sulfide (H_2S) metabolism in mitochondria and its regulatory role in energy production. *Proc Natl Acad Sci USA* 2012; 109(8):2943–8.

51. Yang R, Qu C, Zhou Y, Konkel JE, Shi S, Liu Y, Chen C, Liu S, Liu D, Chen Y, Zandi E, Chen W, et al. Hydrogen sulfide promotes Tet1- and Tet2-mediated Foxp3 Demethylation to drive regulatory T cell differentiation and maintain immune homeostasis. *Immunity* 2015; 43(2):251–63.

52. Miller DL, Roth MB. Hydrogen sulfide increases thermotolerance and lifespan in Caenorhabditis elegans. *Proc Natl Acad Sci USA* 2007; 104(51):20618–22.

53. Hine C, Harputlugil E, Zhang Y, Ruckenstuhl C, Lee BC, Brace L, Longchamp A, Trevino-Villarreal JH, Mejia P, Ozaki CK, Wang R, Gladyshev VN, et al. Endogenous hydrogen sulfide production is essential for dietary restriction benefits. *Cell* 2015; 160(1–2):132–44.

54. Wei Y, Kenyon C. Roles for ROS and hydrogen sulfide in the longevity response to germline loss in *Caenorhabditis elegans*. *Proc Natl Acad Sci USA* 2016; 113(20):E2832–41.

55. Paul BD, Snyder SH. H_2S signalling through protein sulfhydration and beyond. *Nat Rev Mol Cell Biol* 2012; 13(8):499–507.

56. Nishida M, Sawa T, Kitajima N, Ono K, Inoue H, Ihara H, Motohashi H, Yamamoto M, Suematsu M, Kurose H, van der Vliet A, Freeman BA, et al. Hydrogen sulfide anion regulates redox signaling via electrophile sulfhydration. *Nat Chem Biol* 2012; 8(8):714–24.

57. Vandiver MS, Paul BD, Xu R, Karuppagounder S, Rao F, Snowman AM, Ko HS, Lee YI, Dawson VL, Dawson TM, Sen N, Snyder SH. Sulfhydration mediates neuroprotective actions of parkin. *Nat Commun* 2013; 4:1626.

58. Wallace JL, Wang R. Hydrogen sulfide-based therapeutics: exploiting a unique but ubiquitous gasotransmitter. *Nat Rev Drug Discov* 2015; 14(5):329–45.

59. Levitt MD. Production and excretion of hydrogen gas in man. *N Engl J Med* 1969; 281(3):122–7.

60. Levitt MD, Hirsh P, Fetzer CA, Sheahan M, Levine AS. H_2 excretion after ingestion of complex carbohydrates. *Gastroenterology* 1987; 92(2):383–9.

61. Ohsawa I, Ishikawa M, Takahashi K, Watanabe M, Nishimaki K, Yamagata K, Katsura K, Katayama Y, Asoh S, Ohta S. Hydrogen acts as a therapeutic antioxidant by selectively reducing cytotoxic oxygen radicals. *Nat Med* 2007; 13(6):688–94.

62. Ohsawa I, Nishimaki K, Yamagata K, Ishikawa M, Ohta S. Consumption of hydrogen water prevents atherosclerosis in apolipoprotein E knockout mice. *Biochem Biophys Res Commun* 2008; 377(4):1195–8.

63. Cardinal JS, Zhan J, Wang Y, Sugimoto R, Tsung A, McCurry KR, Billiar TR, Nakao A. Oral hydrogen water prevents chronic allograft nephropathy in rats. *Kidney Int* 2010; 77(2):101–9.

64. Kawai D, Takaki A, Nakatsuka A, Wada J, Tamaki N, Yasunaka T, Koike K, Tsuzaki R, Matsumoto K, Miyake Y, Shiraha H, Morita M, et al. Hydrogen-rich water prevents progression of nonalcoholic steatohepatitis and accompanying hepatocarcinogenesis in mice. *Hepatology* 2012; 56(3):912–21.

65. Hayashida K, Sano M, Kamimura N, Yokota T, Suzuki M, Ohta S, Fukuda K, Hori S. Hydrogen inhalation during normoxic resuscitation improves neurological outcome in a rat model of cardiac arrest independently of targeted temperature management. *Circulation* 2014; 130(24):2173–80.

66. Ohta S. Molecular hydrogen is a novel antioxidant to efficiently reduce oxidative stress with potential for the improvement of mitochondrial diseases. *Biochim Biophys Acta* 2012; 1820(5):586–94.

67. Ohta S. Molecular hydrogen as a novel antioxidant: overview of the advantages of hydrogen for medical applications. *Methods Enzymol* 2015; 555:289–317.

68. Iuchi K, Imoto A, Kamimura N, Nishimaki K, Ichimiya H, Yokota T, Ohta S. Molecular hydrogen regulates gene expression by modifying the free radical chain reaction-dependent generation of oxidized phospholipid mediators. *Sci Rep* 2016; 6:18971.

69. Wang Y, Van Ness B. Site-specific cleavage of supercoiled DNA by ascorbate/Cu(II). *Nucleic Acids Res* 1989; 17(17):6915–26.

70. Oikawa S, Kawanishi S. Site-specific DNA damage induced by NADH in the presence of copper(II): role of active oxygen species. *Biochemistry* 1996; 35(14):4584–90.

71. Hare DJ, Double KL. Iron and dopamine: a toxic couple. *Brain* 2016; 139(Pt 4):1026–35.

72. Ichikawa Y, Ghanefar M, Bayeva M, Wu R, Khechaduri A, Naga Prasad SV, Mutharasan RK, Naik TJ, Ardehali H. Cardiotoxicity of doxorubicin is mediated through mitochondrial iron accumulation. *J Clin Invest* 2014; 124(2):617–30.

73. Banci L, Bertini I, Ciofi-Baffoni S, Kozyreva T, Zovo K, Palumaa P. Affinity gradients drive copper to cellular destinations. *Nature* 2010; 465(7298):645–8.

74. Xu W, Barrientos T, Andrews NC. Iron and copper in mitochondrial diseases. *Cell Metab* 2013; 17(3):319–28.

75. Chevion M, Jiang Y, Har-El R, Berenshtein E, Uretzky G, Kitrossky N. Copper and iron are mobilized following myocardial ischemia: possible predictive criteria for tissue injury. *Proc Natl Acad Sci USA* 1993; 90(3):1102–6.

76. Mayes J, Tinker-Mill C, Kolosov O, Zhang H, Tabner BJ, Allsop D. beta-amyloid fibrils in Alzheimer disease are not inert when bound to copper ions but can degrade hydrogen peroxide and generate reactive oxygen species. *J Biol Chem* 2014; 289(17):12052–62.

77. Parthasarathy S, Yoo B, McElheny D, Tay W, Ishii Y. Capturing a reactive state of amyloid aggregates: NMR-based characterization of copper-bound Alzheimer disease amyloid beta-fibrils in a redox cycle. *J Biol Chem* 2014; 289(14):9998–10010.

Common Chemical Formulas and Abbreviations in Free Radical Biology and Medicine

CITATION | *Hopkins RZ and Li YR. Essentials of Free Radical Biology and Medicine. Cell Med Press, Raleigh, NC, USA. 2017. http://dx.doi.org/10.20455/efrbm.2017.appendixA*

CONTENTS AT A GLANCE

1. OVERVIEW

In free radical biology and medicine, chemical formulas, symbols, and/or abbreviations are commonly used to denote reactive species, antioxidants, and related entities. In this context, and to facilitate the reader's understanding of the contents of the book, this appendix lists some of the commonly used formulas or abbreviations for chemical entities in free radical biology and medicine. These include widely accepted formulas or abbreviations for: (1) free radicals and related reactive species (FRRS) as well as other relevant chemical species; (2) antioxidants and related entities; and (3) enzymes involved in the production of FRRS.

2. FRRS AND OTHER RELEVANT CHEMICAL SPECIES

$(^1\Delta_g)^1O_2$: Delta state singlet oxygen
$(^1\Sigma_g^+)^1O_2$: Sigma state singlet oxygen
$^1O_2$: Singlet oxygen
$Asc^{\cdot-}$: Ascorbate radical
$CCl_3^{\cdot}$: Trichloromethyl radical
$CCl_3OO^{\cdot}$: Trichloromethylperoxyl radical
CO: Carbon monoxide
CO_2: Carbon dioxide
$CO_3^{\cdot-}$: Carbonate radical
Cu^{1+}: Cuprous ion
Cu^{2+}: Cupric ion
Fe^{2+}: Ferrous ion
Fe^{3+}: Ferric ion
GS^-: Glutathione anion or glutathione thiolate anion
$GS^{\cdot}$: Glutathione radical
GSNO: S-Nitrosoglutathione
$GSSG^{\cdot-}$: Glutathione disulfide radical or glutathione disulfide radical anion
H (or $H^{\cdot}$): Hydrogen atom
H^+: Hydrogen ion
H_2: Molecular hydrogen or hydrogen gas
H_2O_2: Hydrogen peroxide
H_2S: Hydrogen sulfide
H_2O_3: Hydrogen trioxide
HCO_3^-: Bicarbonae or bicarbonate ion
HCO_4^-: Peroxymonocarbonate
HNO_2: Nitrous acid
$HO_2^{\cdot}$: Hydroperoxyl radical or perhydroxyl radical
HOBr: Hypobromous acid
HOCl: Hypochlorous acid
HOSCN: Hypothiocyanous acid
$L^{\cdot}$: Carbon-centered radical
$LO^{\cdot}$: Lipid alkoxyl radical
LOH: Lipid alcohol
LONO: Lipid alkyl nitrite
$LONO_2$: Lipid alkyl nitrate

LOO$^{\bullet}$: Lipid peroxyl radical
LOOH: Lipid hydroperoxide
LOONO: Lipid peroxynitrite
LOOOOL: Lipid tetraoxide
Metal–NO: Nitrosyl group
N_2O_3: Dinitrogen trioxide
NO$^-$: Nitroxyl anion
NO (or NO$^{\bullet}$): Nitric oxide or nitrogen monoxide
NO$^+$: Nitroxyl cation
NO_2 (or $NO_2{}^{\bullet}$): Nitrogen dioxide or nitric oxide radical
$NO_2{}^-$: Nitrite
–NO_2: Nitro group
$NO_3{}^-$: Nitrate
NO_x: Nitrogen oxides
$O(^1D_2)$: Excited oxygen atom
O_2 (or $^3O_2$): Ground state (triplet) molecular dioxygen
$O_2{}^{\bullet -}$ (or $O_2{}^-$): Superoxide, superoxide anion, or superoxide anion radical
O_3: Ozone
OCl$^-$: Hypochlorite or hypochlorite ion
OH$^-$: Hydroxide ion or hydroxide
OH$^{\bullet}$(or $^{\bullet}$OH): Hydroxyl radical
ONOO$^-$: Peroxynitrite anion or peroxynitrite
ONOOCO$_2{}^-$: Nitrosoperoxycarbonate
ONOOH: Peroxynitrous acid
R–NO: Nitroso group
RNS: Reactive nitrogen species
RO$^{\bullet}$: Alkoxyl radical
ROO$^{\bullet}$: Peroxyl radical
ROS: Reactive oxygen species
–SH: Sulfhydryl group or thiol group
–SO_2H: Sulfinic acid
–SO_3H: Sulfonic acid
–SOH: Sulfenic acid
SQ$^{\bullet -}$: Semiquinone, semiquinone radical, or semiquinone anion radical
–SSH: S-Sulfhydration group or persulfide

3. ANTIOXIDANTS AND RELATED ENTITIES

ARE: Antioxidant response element
CuZnSOD (or CuZn-SOD or SOD1): Copper, zinc superoxide dismutase
ECSOD (or EC-SOD or SOD3): Extracellular superoxide dismutase
FeSOD (or Fe-SOD): Iron superoxide dismutase
γGCL (or γGCS): γ-Glutamylcysteine ligase or γ-glutamylcysteine synthetase
G6PD: Glucose-6-phosphate dehydrogenase
GPx: Glutathione peroxidase

GR (or GSR): Glutathione reductase or glutathione disulfide reductase
Grx: Glutaredoxin
GSH: Reduced form of glutathione or reduced glutathione
GSSG: Glutathione disulfide or oxidized form of glutathione
GST: Glutathione S-transferase or glutathione transferase
HO-1: Heme oxygenase-1
HO-2: Heme oxygenase -2
Keap1: Kelch-like ECH-associated protein 1
MnSOD (or Mn-SOD or SOD2): Manganese superoxide dismutase
Msr: Methionine sulfoxide reductase
NAD$^+$: Nicotinamide adenine dinucleotide (oxidized form)
NADH: Nicotinamide adenine dinucleotide (reduced form)
NADP$^+$: Nicotinamide adenine dinucleotide phosphate (oxidized form)
NADPH: Nicotinamide adenine dinucleotide phosphate (reduced form)
NiSOD (or Ni-SOD): Nickel superoxide dismutase
NQO1: NAD(P)H:quinone oxidoreductase 1
Nrf2: Nuclear factor erythroid 2-related factor 2 or nuclear factor E2-related factor 2
PON: Paraoxonase
Prx (or TPx): Peroxiredoxin or thioredoxin peroxidase
SOD: Superoxide dismutase
Srx: Sulfiredoxin
TGR: Thioredoxin glutathione reductase
Trx: Thioredoxin
TrxR: Thioredoxin reductase

4. ENZYMES INVOLVED IN THE PRODUCTION OF FRRS AND OTHER RELEVANT CHEMICAL SPECIES

CBS: Cystathionine β-synthase
CSE: Cystathionine γ-lyase
CYP: Cytochrome P450
DUOX: Dual oxidase
eNOS (or NOS3): Endothelial nitric oxide synthase
EPO: Eosinophil peroxidase
ERO1: Endoplasmic reticulum oxidoreductin 1
iNOS (or NOS2): Inducible nitric oxide synthase
LPO: Lipoxygenase
MAO: Monoamine oxidase
mARC: Mitochondrial amidoxime reducing component

METC: Mitochondrial electron transport chain
MPO: Myeloperoxidase
nNOS (or NOS1): Neuronal nitric oxide synthase
NOS: Nitric oxide synthase
NOX: NADPH oxidase

VPO: Vascular peroxidase
VPO1: Vascular peroxidase-1
XDH: Xanthine dehydrogenase
XO: Xanthine oxidase
XOR: Xanthine oxidoreductase

Common Cellular Antioxidants and Related Entities in Free Radical Biology and Medicine

CITATION | *Hopkins RZ and Li YR. Essentials of Free Radical Biology and Medicine. Cell Med Press, Raleigh, NC, USA. 2017. http://dx.doi.org/10.20455/efrbm.2017.appendixB*

CONTENTS AT A GLANCE

1. OVERVIEW

As indicated by the title, this book is intended to provide a concise coverage of the key principles and concepts regarding free radicals and related reactive species (FRRS). However, even a concise coverage of the essentials of FRRS would have to include discussion of antioxidants. Indeed, FRRS and antioxidants are two essential components of free radical biology and medicine. Accordingly, this appendix

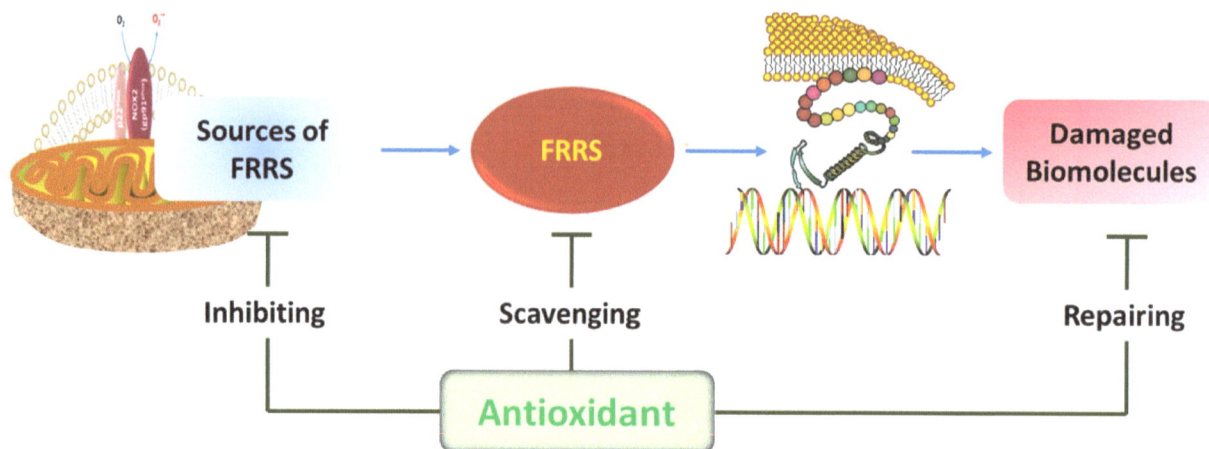

FIGURE B.1. The three modes of action of antioxidants in biology and medicine. As illustrated, an antioxidant may protect against oxidative injury by inhibiting the formation of free radicals and related reactive species (FRRS), directly scavenging FRRS, and/or repairing the oxidatively damaged cellular targets. It should be noted that a particular antioxidant molecule may possess more than one mode in protecting against FRRS-induced molecular damage. Although lipids, proteins, and nucleic acids are the major cellular targets depicted in the scheme, FRRS, dependent on their chemical properties, may also cause damage to other cellular molecules, such as carbohydrates and the nucleotide pool.

provides an overview of common cellular antioxidants and related entities that are involved in the metabolism of FRRS, focusing primarily on their basic biochemistry and major biological functions. The appendix begins with a brief introduction to the definition and classification of antioxidants. It then considers common antioxidants which are categorized into: (1) superoxide dismutase and catalase; (2) glutathione system; (3) thioredoxin system; and (4) other antioxidant enzymes.

2. DEFINING AND CLASSIFYING ANTIOXIDANTS

2.1. Defining Antioxidants

The word antioxidant is probably one of the most widely encountered terms among biomedical scientists and health professionals, as well as the general public in today's societies. However, the term is loosely defined in both the literature and the public media. In fact, there is no universally accepted definition for antioxidant. Nevertheless, the term has been defined in various ways for different purposes. In biology and medicine, antioxidant may be defined as any substance that, when present at a level of bio-

logical, physiological, or pharmacological relevance, can prevent, reduce, or repair the FRRS-induced damage of a target biomolecule. According to this definition, there are three potential modes of action by which antioxidants protect biomolecules from FRRS-induced damage (**Figure B.1**).

2.1.1. Inhibition of FRRS Formation

As described in Chapter 6, FRRS are produced by a number of cellular sources, including the mitochondrial electron transport chain, NADPH oxidases (also known as NOX enzymes), cytochrome P450 enzyme system, and xanthine oxidase (XO), among many others. Antioxidants may act on these cellular sources, inhibiting or preventing the production of FRRS. For example, apocynin inhibits NOX enzymatic activity, thereby reducing NOX-derived reactive oxygen species (ROS) and the subsequent oxidative tissue injury [1–3]. Another example is the XO specific inhibitor, allopurinol. Inhibition of XO by allopurinol attenuates ROS production and oxidative tissue injury in diverse disease models [4–6]. Hence, both apocynin and allopurinol can be regarded as antioxidant compounds that act via inhibiting the ROS production from their respective cellular sources.

TABLE B.1. Classification of antioxidants in biology and medicine

Criterion	Category	Example
Source	Endogenous antioxidants	Superoxide dismutase, catalase
	Exogenous antioxidants	Vitamin C, resveratrol
Location	Intracellular antioxidants	Cu,Zn superoxide dismutase, glutathione peroxidase-1
	Extracellular antioxidants	Extracellular superoxide dismutase, glutathione peroxidase-3
Enzymatic activity	Enzymatic antioxidants	Superoxide dismutase, catalase
	Non-enzymatic antioxidants	Vitamin C, reduced form of glutathione
Protein nature	Protein antioxidants	Superoxide dismutase, ferritin
	Non-protein antioxidants	Vitamin C, reduced form of glutathione
Direct effect on FRRS	Direct antioxidants	Superoxide dismutase, catalase
	Indirect antioxidants	Apocynin, sulforaphane
Dependence on Nrf2/ARE	Nrf2/ARE-dependent antioxidants	Glutathione reductase, heme oxygenase-1
	Nrf2/ARE-independent antioxidants	Glutathione peroxidase-1, manganese superoxide dismutase

Note: It should be noted that the different ways of classification are not mutually exclusive. For example, Cu,Zn superoxide dismutase can be classified as an endogenous, intracellular, enzymatic, protein, or direct antioxidant dependent on the classification scheme used.

Certain endogenous molecules may also act to reduce ROS formation from cellular sources. For instance, a recently characterized protein, known as negative regulator of ROS (NRROS), is able to suppress cellular ROS formation. NRROS is localized to the endoplasmic reticulum (ER), where it directly interacts with nascent NOX2 monomer, one of the membrane-bound subunits of the NADPH oxidase complex, and facilitates the degradation of NOX2 through the ER-associated degradation pathway [7]. Thus, NRROS may be viewed as an endogenous antioxidant molecule that acts to suppress ROS production by NOX2. Investigations of the existence of endogenous inhibitors of ROS may provide important insights into the development of novel drug molecules to selectively target cellular sources of ROS formation for the treatment of ROS-associated disease processes.

2.1.2. Scavenging of FRRS Already Formed

Many endogenous and exogenous antioxidants can directly scavenge or detoxify FRRS. Scavenging of FRRS can occur through enzyme-catalyzed reactions. For example, superoxide dismutase catalyzes the dismutation of superoxide to form hydrogen perox-

ide and molecular oxygen, and catalase catalyzes the decomposition of hydrogen peroxide to form water and molecular oxygen (see Section 3 below). Non-enzymatic antioxidants typically scavenge FRRS through direct chemical reactions. Such non-enzymatic reactions, often time, can lead to the formation of secondary free radical species from the non-enzymatic antioxidants. For example, the antioxidant α-tocopherol scavenges lipid peroxyl radical by reducing the lipid peroxyl radical to lipid hydroperoxide (see Figure 5.3 of Chapter 5). In the reaction, α-tocopherol is oxidized to α-tocopherol radical. The α-tocopherol radical is, however, much less reactive than the lipid peroxyl radical and unable to abstract a hydrogen atom from an adjacent polyunsaturated fatty acid, thereby leading to the inhibition of lipid peroxyl radical-mediated propagation of lipid peroxidation chain reaction (see Figure 7.2 of Chapter 7).

2.1.3. Repairing of FRRS-Induced Damage

FRRS can cause damage or modifications to cellular biomolecules, including proteins, lipids, and nucleic acids. Mammalian cells are equipped with various mechanisms to remove or repair the FRRS-damaged or modified biomolecules. For example, FRRS oxidize methionine residues in proteins, yielding methionine sulfoxide. The enzyme methionine sulfoxide reductase (Msr) reduces the methionine sulfoxide in proteins back to the normal methionine (see Section 6 below). This is an important repairing mechanism for oxidative protein damage in mammals. Mammalian cells also contain enzymes for repairing oxidative damage of lipids and nucleic acids [8–10].

2.2. Classifying Antioxidants

In biology and medicine, antioxidants are classified based on various criteria, including source, location, enzymatic activity, protein nature, action on FRRS, and molecular regulation. **Table B.1** lists the major categories of biological antioxidants and the classification criteria.

2.2.1. Endogenous and Exogenous Antioxidants

Based on the source, antioxidants are classified into endogenous and exogenous antioxidants. Endogenous antioxidants refer to those that are synthesized in mammalian cells. Examples include superoxide dismutase (SOD), catalase, and the reduced form of glutathione (GSH), to name a few. On the other hand, those derived from dietary sources or synthesized in laboratories are called exogenous antioxidants. Plant-derived polyphenols (e.g., resveratrol) and various synthetic antioxidant mimetics (e.g., the peroxynitrite scavenger FeTMPyP) are examples of exogenous antioxidants.

2.2.2. Intracellular and Extracellular Antioxidants

Based on the cellular location, antioxidants are classified into intracellular and extracellular antioxidants. Intracellular antioxidants are those present inside cells, such as manganese SOD (MnSOD), catalase, and glutathione reductase. Extracellular antioxidants exist in the extracellular environment, including the plasma. Extracellular superoxide dismutase (ECSOD) and plasma glutathione peroxidase (GPx) (also known as GPx3) are typical examples of extracellular antioxidant enzymes. Many antioxidants, such as GSH, vitamin C, and thioredoxin, are located both intracellularly and extracellularly.

2.2.3. Enzymatic and Non-Enzymatic Antioxidants

Based on the enzyme activity, antioxidants are classified into enzymatic and non-enzymatic antioxidants. Some antioxidants, such as SOD, GPx, and catalase are enzymes that catalyze the dismutation or degradation of ROS. Some other antioxidants, such as the transition metal ion-sequestering proteins (e.g., metallothionein and ferritin) are non-enzymes.

2.2.4. Protein and Non-Protein Antioxidants

Based on the protein nature, antioxidants are classified into protein and non-protein antioxidants. All enzymatic antioxidants are protein antioxidants. The non-protein antioxidants include the GSH, vitamin C, and vitamin E. Many synthetic antioxidant enzyme mimetics (e.g., the SOD mimetic MnTMPyP) are non-protein antioxidants.

2.2.5. Direct and Indirect Antioxidants

Based on the direct scavenging effects on FRRS, antioxidants are classified into direct and indirect antioxidants. Direct antioxidants refer to those that directly scavenge or metabolize FRRS either enzymatically or non-enzymatically. For example, SOD, GPx, catalase, vitamin C, and vitamin E act as direct antioxidants. One the other hand, indirect antioxidants refer to those that do not directly act on FRRS. Indirect antioxidants may inhibit the enzymes or cellular pathways that give rise to FRRS. For example, the inhibitors of NOXs (e.g., apocynin) are considered as indirect antioxidants because they indirectly reduce the levels of ROS by inhibiting the ROS-generating NOX enzymes. The uncoupling protein-2 (UCP-2) is also viewed as an indirect antioxidant because of its ability to reduce the ROS formation by the mitochondrial electron transport chain [11]. The enzymes involved in repairing the damage caused by FRRS, such as methionine sulfoxide reductase may also be classified as indirect antioxidants.

Many endogenous antioxidant enzymes are inducible by exogenous compounds, such as sulforaphane, an isothiocyanate compound found in cruciferous vegetables. Although sulforaphane cannot directly scavenge FRRS, it protects against oxidative damage by upregulating endogenous antioxidant defenses via a nuclear factor E2-related factor 2 (Nrf2)-dependent mechanism [12–15].

2.2.6. Nrf2/ARE-Dependent and -Independent Antioxidants

The transcription factor Nrf2 is recognized as a major regulator of antioxidant genes. Nrf2 binds to the cis-element, known as antioxidant response element (ARE) in the promoter region of antioxidant genes,

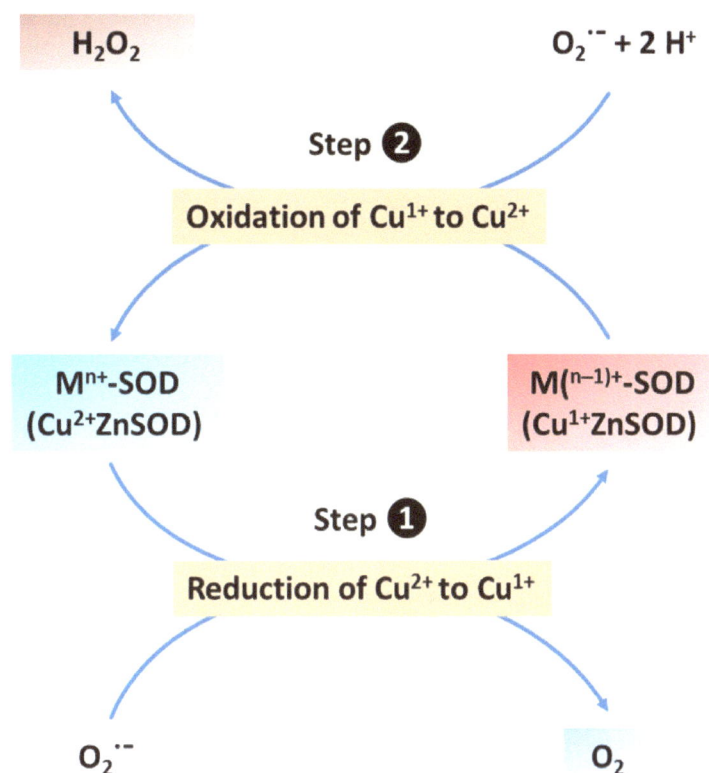

FIGURE B.2. Mechanism of superoxide dismutase (SOD)-catalyzed dismutation of superoxide ($O_2^{\cdot-}$) to form hydrogen peroxide (H_2O_2) and molecular oxygen. As illustrated, the overall mechanism by which SOD functions is called "ping-pong" mechanism as it involves the sequential reduction and oxidation of the metal center (M), with the concomitant oxidation and reduction of superoxide.

causing increased transcriptional expression [16–18]. Indeed, the expression of many antioxidant genes is upregulated following Nrf2-ARE activation. These include ferritin, γ-glutamylcysteine ligase, glutathione peroxidase-2, glutathione reductase, heme oxygenase-1, NAD(P)H:quinone oxidoreductase 1, and thioredoxin, among many others. Hence, treatment with Nrf2 activators, such as sulforaphane mentioned earlier, can result in the increased expression of many antioxidant genes and the consequent increased levels of the antioxidant enzymes or proteins.

Although Nrf2-ARE is a major regulator of antioxidant genes, many other antioxidant genes, due to lack of ARE in their promoter region, are not directly subject to Nrf2-ARE-mediated transcriptional activation. These antioxidants include catalase, GPx1, MnSOD, and Msr, to name a few. However, these antioxidant genes may be responsive to the changes of the cellular redox environment induced by Nrf2 activation.

3. SUPEROXIDE DISMUTASE AND CATALASE

SOD and catalase are frequently discussed together because they are the enzymes involved in the eventual conversion of superoxide to water. SOD converts superoxide to hydrogen peroxide, which is in turn decomposed to water by catalase.

3.1. Superoxide Dismutase

3.1.1. General Characteristics

The term superoxide dismutase (SOD) refers to a family of enzymes that catalyze the dismutation of superoxide to hydrogen peroxide and molecular oxygen. There are three isozymes of SOD in mammalian systems: (1) copper, zinc superoxide dismutase (CuZnSOD or SOD1); (2) manganese superoxide dismutase (MnSOD or SOD2); and (3) extracellular superoxide dismutase (ECSOD or SOD3). Prokaryotic cells also contain iron SOD (FeSOD) and nickel SOD (NiSOD). This appendix focuses on mammalian antioxidant enzymes and related entities.

CuZnSOD is a homodimer with a molecular mass of 32 kDa. Both MnSOD and ECSOD are homotetramers with a molecular mass of 86–88 and 135 kDa, respectively. ECSOD also contains copper and zinc. CuZnSOD is present in cytosol. It is also found in nuclei and mitochondrial intermembrane space. MnSOD exists in mitochondrial matrix. ECSOD is associated with plasma membrane or present in extracellular space. The human genes for CuZnSOD, MnSOD, and ECSOD are localized on chromosomes 21q22, 6q25, and 4q21, respectively.

3.1.2. Biochemistry

The three mammalian SOD isoforms catalyze dismutation of superoxide ($O_2^{\cdot-}$) to form hydrogen peroxide (H_2O_2) and molecular oxygen with a similar reaction rate constant of about $1.6 \times 10^9 \, M^{-1}s^{-1}$. The overall mechanism by which SOD functions has been called "ping-pong" mechanism as it involves the sequential reduction and oxidation of the metal center, with the concomitant oxidation and reduction of superoxide (**Figure B.2**).

3.1.3. Biological Functions

3.1.3.1. PRIMARY FUNCTIONS

The primary biological function of SOD is to dismutate superoxide and protect against superoxide-mediated toxicity. While homozygous deletion of CuZnSOD or ECSOD does not affect animal survival under normal conditions, homozygous knockout of MnSOD causes embryonic or early neonatal death in mice [19]. This suggests that MnSOD is essential for survival. Although CuZnSOD deletion does not affect survival, its deficiency impairs olfactory sexual signaling and alters bioenergetic function in mice [20]. On the other hand, a "gain-of-function" type of mutation of CuZnSOD is recognized as a cause of familial amyotrophic lateral sclerosis [21, 22]. The mutant CuZnSOD results in the formation of aggregates and neuron degeneration. The CuZnSOD aggregates may spread the disease in a prion-like fashion in the central nerve system [23].

Since the dismutation product of SOD is hydrogen peroxide, which is also an ROS of biological activity, SOD may exert detrimental effects under certain conditions. For example, MnSOD overexpression is found to play a role in promoting tumorigenesis [24, 25]. Several mechanisms have been suggested. First, MnSOD maintains highly functional mitochondria, by scavenging superoxide to support the high metabolic activity of the cancer cells. Second, MnSOD increases H_2O_2 production, which in turn stimulates cancer cell proliferation and metastasis. Indeed, MnSOD upregulation in cancer cells establishes a steady flow of H_2O_2 originating from mitochondria that sustains AMP-activated kinase (AMPK) activation and the metabolic shift to glycolysis [25].

3.1.3.2. NOVEL FUNCTIONS

In addition to its function in catalyzing the dismutation of superoxide to hydrogen peroxide, CuZnSOD may also possess other novel biological functions. For example, a recent study reports that CuZnSOD acts as a nuclear transcription factor to regulate oxidative stress resistance [26]. In response to elevated endogenous and exogenous reactive oxygen species, including H_2O_2, CuZnSOD rapidly relocates into the nucleus, and in the nucleus, CuZnSOD binds to promoters and regulates the expression of oxidative resistance and repair genes [26].

3.2. Catalase

3.2.1. General Characteristics

Mammalian catalase is a homotetrameric protein with a molecular mass of ~240 kDa. It is widely distributed throughout the body with high levels in the liver, kidney, and red blood cells. In cells, catalase is primarily localized in peroxisomes. Catalase is also found to be present in cardiac mitochondria [27]. In humans, the catalase gene is localized on chromosome 11p13.

3.2.2. Biochemistry

Catalase is best known for its high efficiency in catalyzing the decomposition of H_2O_2 to form water and molecular oxygen (Reaction 1). This is a dismutation reaction because one molecule of H_2O_2 is reduced to water and another molecule is oxidized to molecular oxygen.

$$2 \, H_2O_2 \rightarrow H_2O + O_2 \quad (1)$$

Catalase catalyzes the decomposition of H_2O_2 via a two-stage process. In the first step, one H_2O_2 molecule oxidizes the heme iron of the resting enzyme to

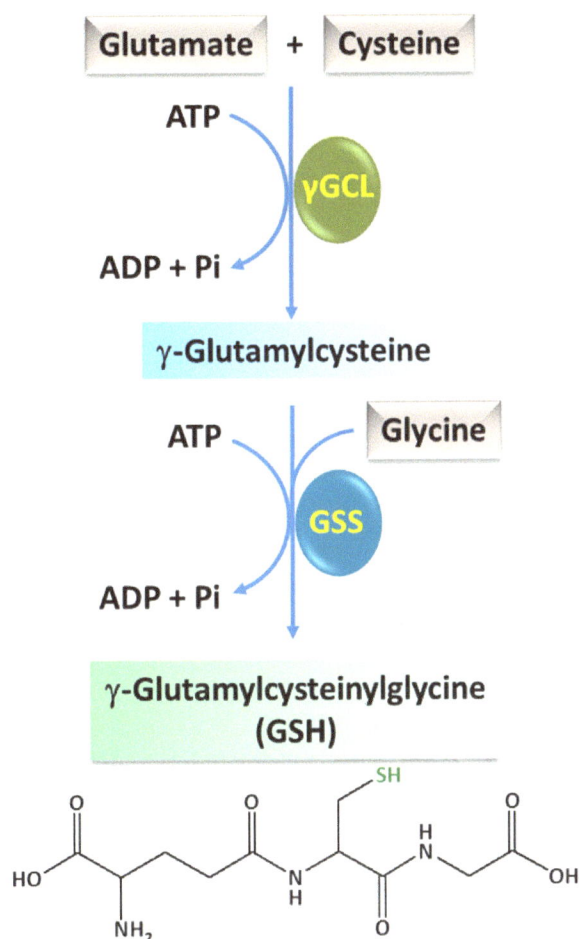

FIGURE B.3. Biosynthesis of the reduced form of glutathione (GSH). As illustrated, GSH is synthesized from three amino acids through two successive reactions catalyzed by γ-glutamylcysteine ligase (γGCL) and glutathione synthetase (GSS), respectively. Two molecules of adenosine triphosphate (ATP) are consumed for synthesizing each molecule of GSH. It is noteworthy that γGCL is the key enzyme of GSH biosynthesis. This enzyme is subject to Nrf2/ARE-mediated transcriptional regulation.

form an oxyferryl species with a π-cationic porphyrin radical, termed compound I (Reaction 2). The second H_2O_2 molecule is utilized as a reductant of compound I to regenerate the resting-stage enzyme along with the formation of water and molecular oxygen (Reaction 3, where Por denotes porphyrin).

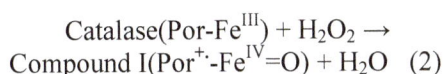

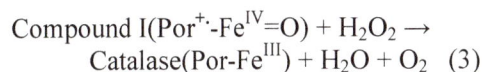

$$\text{Catalase(Por-Fe}^{III}) + H_2O_2 \rightarrow$$
$$\text{Compound I(Por}^{+\cdot}\text{-Fe}^{IV}\text{=O)} + H_2O \quad (2)$$

$$\text{Compound I(Por}^{+\cdot}\text{-Fe}^{IV}\text{=O)} + H_2O_2 \rightarrow$$
$$\text{Catalase(Por-Fe}^{III}) + H_2O + O_2 \quad (3)$$

$$\text{The sum: } 2\,H_2O_2 \rightarrow 2\,H_2O + O_2$$

Catalase also possesses peroxidase and oxidase activities toward a number of substrates, including alcohols, the tryptophan precursor indole, and the neurotransmitter precursor β-phenylethylamine [28]. Reaction 4 illustrates the peroxidase activity of catalase in converting alcohol (AH_2) to aldehyde (A).

$$H_2O_2 + AH_2 \rightarrow A + 2\,H_2O \quad (4)$$

3.2.3. Biological Functions

3.2.3.1. PRIMARY FUNCTION

The primary function of mammalian catalase is to catalyze the decomposition of H_2O_2 to form water and serves as one of the major defense mechanisms against H_2O_2-induced toxicity and disease process. For example, overexpression of catalase targeted to mitochondria significantly attenuates cardiac aging and extends the life span of mice by over 5 months [29, 30]. Targeted expression of catalase to mitochondria also prevents age-associated reductions in mitochondrial function and insulin resistance in mice [31]. In line with this, hereditary catalase deficiencies in humans are associated with an increased risk of diabetes [32].

3.2.3.2. OTHER FUNCTIONS

Catalase is one of the three enzymes involved in the metabolism of ethanol in the liver to acetaldehyde [33, 34]. The other two enzymes are alcohol dehydrogenase and cytochrome P450 2E1.

4. GLUTATHIONE SYSTEM

The glutathione system is a major cellular defense mechanism in the detoxification of FRRS. This system includes the reduced form of glutathione (GSH) and the enzymes (i.e., γ-glutatmylcysteine ligase and glutathione synthetase) involved in its biosynthesis, as well as the enzymes that use GSH as a cofactor/electron donor. The latter enzymes include glutathione peroxidase, glutathione S-transferase, and glutaredoxin. This antioxidant system also includes glutathione reductase, an enzyme that regenerates GSH from glutathione disulfide (GSSG).

4.1. Glutathione and Its Synthesizing Enzymes

4.1.1. General Characteristics

The term glutathione, if not specified, may refer to both the reduced form (GSH) and the oxidized form (GSSG) of glutathione. This section focuses on the reduced form, i.e., GSH and the enzymes involved in its biosynthesis.

GSH is a tripeptide (γ-glutamylcysteinylglycine) with a molecular mass of 307 (structure in **Figure B.3**). In mammalian cells, the cytosolic concentrations of GSH are in the range of 1–10 mM. GSH is also present in high concentrations in the mitochondria and nuclei. In contrast, the extracellular levels of GSH are much lower, and GSH levels in the plasma are usually in the range of lower micromolar concentrations. In mammalian cells, GSH biosynthesis involves two cytosolic enzymes, namely, γ-glutamylcysteine ligase (γGCL) and glutathione synthetase (GSS). γGCL consists of two subunits: the heavy catalytic subunit designated as GCLC with a molecular mass of ~73 kDa and the light modifier subunit designated as GCLM with a molecular mass of ~31 kDa. GCLC and GCLM are encoded by separate genes that are localized on chromosomes 6p12 and 1p22.1, respectively, in humans. Human GSS gene is localized on chromosome 20q11.2.

4.1.2. Biochemistry

GSH is synthesized from three amino acids via two successive enzymatic reactions in the cytoplasm (**Figure B.3**). The first step involves combination of L-cysteine and L-glutamate to produce γ-glutamylcysteine. This reaction is catalyzed by γGCL, also formerly known as γ-glutamylcysteine synthetase (γGCS). This reaction requires coupled ATP hydrolysis. The next step involves the enzyme GSS, which catalyzes the addition of glycine to the dipeptide to form γ-glutamylcysteinylglycine (GSH). This enzyme also requires coupled hydrolysis of adenosine triphosphate (ATP).

4.1.3. Biological Functions

4.1.3.1. Primary Functions

In mammalian systems, GSH is a major antioxidant involved in at least four types of biochemical reactions. They are: (1) reaction with ROS leading to their detoxification; (2) reaction with electrophiles; (3) regeneration of α-tocopherol (a form of vitamin E) and vitamin C; and (4) protein deglutathionylation catalyzed by glutaredoxin.

(1) Reaction with ROS: GSH is a major defense against ROS. GSH can directly react with ROS, leading to the detoxification of these reactive species. GSH is also used as a cofactor by glutathione peroxidase in the detoxification of H_2O_2 and other peroxides, as well as peroxynitrite. In addition, the reaction between GSH and nitric oxide (or nitric oxide-derived species) leads to the formation of S-nitrosoglutathione. In biological systems, S-nitrosoglutathione may act as a second messenger to transduce nitric oxide bioactivity [35, 36]

(2) Reaction with electrophilic compounds: Electrophiles (electron-deficient species), such as reactive aldehydes are derived from xenobiotic biotransformation as well as lipid peroxidation. GSH reacts with electrophiles, forming less reactive conjugates. Thus, conjugation with GSH represents an important mechanism for the detoxification of electrophilic species. The conjugation reactions with GSH may occur spontaneously, but are markedly accelerated by glutathione S-transferase. It is noteworthy that for certain xenobiotics, GSH conjugation may result in their bioactivation, thereby leading to increased toxicity [37].

(3) Regeneration of vitamin C: While GSH is the most abundant non-protein thiol antioxidant in mammalian cells, there are also many other cellular non-protein antioxidants, such as α-tocopherol and vitamin C (also known as ascorbic acid or ascorbate). α-Tocopherol reduces lipid peroxyl radical to form lipid hydroperoxide, and in the reaction α-tocopherol is oxidized to α-tocopherol radical. The α-tocopherol radical can be reduced back to α-tocopherol by ascorbate, which is oxidized to ascorbate radical and then to dehydroascorbate. Dehydroascorbate can then be restored to the reduced form by a GSH-dependent reaction catalyzed by dehydroascorbate reductase (**Figure B.4**). Because of this role GSH deficiency results in decreased tissue levels of vitamin C in animal models [38, 39].

(4) Protein deglutathionylation: Reversible protein S-glutathionylation (protein-SSG) is an important post-translational modification involved in redox signaling. Analogous to protein dephosphoryla-

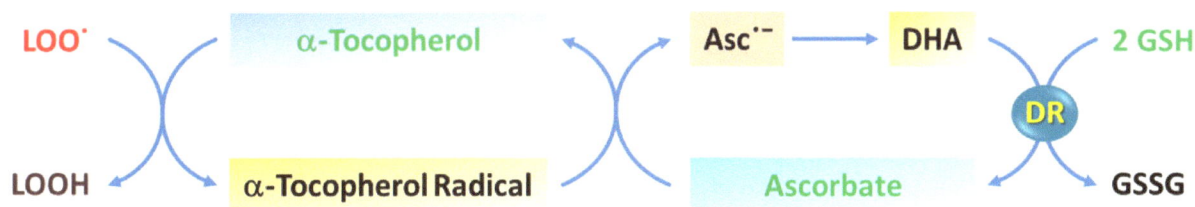

FIGURE B.4. Role of the reduced form of glutathione (GSH) in the regeneration of α-topopherol and ascorbate. As illustrated, α-tocopherol reduces lipid peroxyl radical (LOO˙) to lipid hydroperoxide (LOOH), and in the reaction, α-tocopherol is oxidized to α-tocopherol radical. The α-tocopherol radical can be reduced back to α-tocopherol by ascorbate, which is oxidized to ascorbate radical (Asc˙⁻) and then to dehydroascorbate (DHA). DHA can be reduced back to ascorbate by a GSH-dependent reaction catalyzed by DHA reductase (DR). During this reaction, GSH is oxidized to glutathione disulfide (GSSG).

tion catalyzed by phosphatases, glutaredoxin using GSH as a cofactor/electron donor catalyzes deglutathionylation of proteins. This participates in regulating diverse intracellular signaling pathways [40, 41].

4.1.3.2. ATYPICAL FUNCTIONS

In addition to the above well-established functions, GSH also possesses atypical biological activities, including both beneficial and detrimental effects. For example, GSH is the cofactor for glyoxalase 1, an enzyme involved in the detoxification of glycolysis-derived α-oxoaldehyde, methylglyoxal, and protection against hyperglycemia-induced oxidative stress [42–44]. On the contrary, as a GSH-dependent enzyme, glyoxalase 1 may be also involved in the development of anxiety. Local overexpression of glyoxalase 1 in the mouse brain results in increased anxiety-like behavior, while local inhibition of glyoxalase 1 expression by RNA interference decreases the anxiety-like behavior [45]. This is possibly due to the ability of glyoxalase 1 to decrease brain levels of methylglyoxal, a γ-aminobutyric acid (GABA) type A receptor agonist [46].

Intracellular GSH may play a role in promoting the virulence of pathogens in host cells. Infection by the human bacterial pathogen *Listeria monocytogenes* is mainly controlled by the positive regulatory factor A (PrfA), a member of the Crp/Fnr family of transcriptional activators. Activation of PrfA is dependent on host cell GSH, and the GSH-dependent PrfA activation is mediated by allosteric binding of GSH to PrfA [47]. By binding to PrfA in the cytosol of the host cell, GSH induces the correct fold of the HTH motifs,

thus priming the PrfA protein for DNA interaction and promoting the virulence [48].

Increased GSH content in cancer cells is a major mechanism underlying cancer cell resistance to chemotherapy [49, 50]. In this context, many classical anticancer drugs are electrophilic compounds that are detoxified by GSH conjugation in the cancer cells. In experimental models, GSH and thioredoxin synergize to drive cancer initiation, proliferation, and progression [51, 52].

4.2. Glutathione Peroxidase

4.2.1. General Characteristics

Glutathione peroxidase (GPx) is the general name for a family of multiple isozymes that catalyze the reduction of H_2O_2 or organic hydroperoxides to water or corresponding alcohols using GSH as an electron donor. In mammalian tissues, there are currently eight GPx isozymes, namely, GPx1, 2, 3, 4, 5, 6, 7, and 8. GPx1, 2, 3, and 4 are selenoproteins. GPx6 is also a selenoprotein in humans and pigs, but not in rats and mice. GPx5 is a non-selenoprotein. GPx7 and 8 are the newest members of the family and have been shown to be endoplasmic reticulum-resident protein disulfide isomerase peroxidases [53]. GPx7 is a novel putative non-selenocysteine-containing phospholipid hydroperoxide glutathione peroxidase (NPGPx) that lacks GPx enzymatic activity, but protects against oxidative stress-induced tissue injury via possibly serving as an oxidative stress sensor/transducer [54, 55]. Complete loss of NPGPx in animals causes systemic oxidative stress, increases carcinogenesis, and shortens life span [56]. The exact

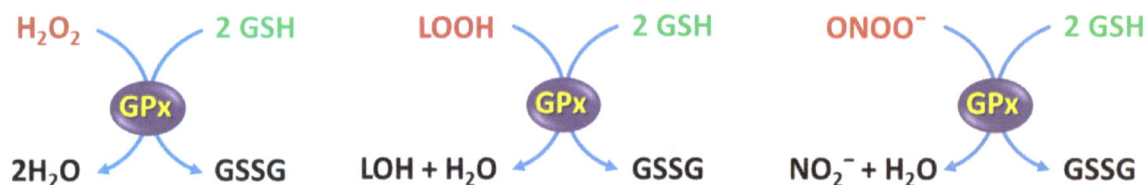

FIGURE B.5. Glutathione peroxidase (GPx)-catalyzed decomposition of hydrogen peroxide (H_2O_2), lipid hydroperoxide (LOOH), and peroxynitrite ($ONOO^-$). As illustrated, GPx catalyzes the decomposition of H_2O_2, LOOH, and $ONOO^-$ to form water, lipid alcohol (LOH), and nitrite (NO_2^-), respectively. During the reaction, the reduced form of glutathione (GSH) is oxidized to glutathione disulfide (GSSG).

biological activities of GPx7 and 8 remain elucidative. Henec, this section focuses on GPx1–6.

GPx1, 2, 3, and 6 are homotetrameric proteins with a subunit molecular mass of ~20–25 kDa, whereas GPx4 is a 20–22 kDa monomeric enzyme. GPx5 is a homodimeric enzyme with a subunit molecular mass of 24 kDa. The nomenclature and cellular and chromosomal localization of the various GPx isozymes are described below.

(1) GPx1: GPx1 is also known as classical or cytosolic GPx (cGPx). It is the first mammalian GPx identified and one of the most abundant and ubiquitously expressed selenoproteins. GPx1 is present in the cytosol, mitochondria, and nuclei. In humans, GPx1 gene is localized on chromosome 3p21.3.

(2) GPx2: GPx2 is also known as gastrointestinal GPx (GI-GPx). It is mainly expressed in the gastrointestinal tract. It is also found in the liver and lung. GPx2 is present in the cytosol and nuclei. In humans, GPx2 gene is localized on chromosome 14q24.1.

(3) GPx3: GPx3 is also known as plasma GPx (pGPx). It is a secreted form of enzyme found in the plasma. The kidney is the major source of GPx3. This enzyme is also expressed in many other tissues, including the lung and heart, and is present in the cytosol. In humans, GPx3 gene is localized on chromosome 5q23.

(4) GPx4: GPx4 is also known as phospholipid hydroperoxide GPx (PHGPx). It is ubiquitously expressed in a variety of tissues. GPx4 is also found to be a main structural component of the sperm mitochondrial capsule in mature spermatozoa, where it exists as an enzymatically-inactive, oxidatively cross-linked, insoluble protein [57]. Subcellular distribution of GPx4 includes the cytosol, nuclei, mitochondria, and membranes. Membrane-associated GPx4 plays an important role in repairing oxidative damage to membrane lipids. Recently, GPx4 is found to be an inhibitor of ferroptotic cell death [58]. Ferroptosis is a newly discovered type of cell death that differs from apoptosis, necrosis, and autophagy, and results from iron-dependent lipid peroxide accumulation triggered by insufficiency of GPx4 [59–61]. Inactivation of GPx4 causes ferroptosis and triggers lipid peroxidation-induced acute renal failure [62]. Conditional ablation of the ferroptosis inhibitor GPx4 in neurons results in rapid motor neuron degeneration and paralysis in mice [63]. In humans, GPx4 gene is localized on chromosome 19p13.3.

(5) GPx5: GPx5 is also known as epididymal GPx (eGPx). It is selectively expressed in the epididymis. The enzyme is secreted into the epididymal lumen. GPx5 is essential in maintaining sperm DNA integrity in mice [64]. In humans, GPx5 gene is localized on chromosome 6p22.1.

(6) GPx6: The expression of GPx6 is believed to be restricted to the developing embryo and in olfactory epithelium in adults. A recent study with a mouse model suggests GPx6 as a modulator of Huntington's disease. Overexpression of GPx6 can dramatically alleviate both behavioral and molecular phenotypes associated with Huntington's disease [65]. In humans, GPx6 gene is localized on chromosome 6p22.1.

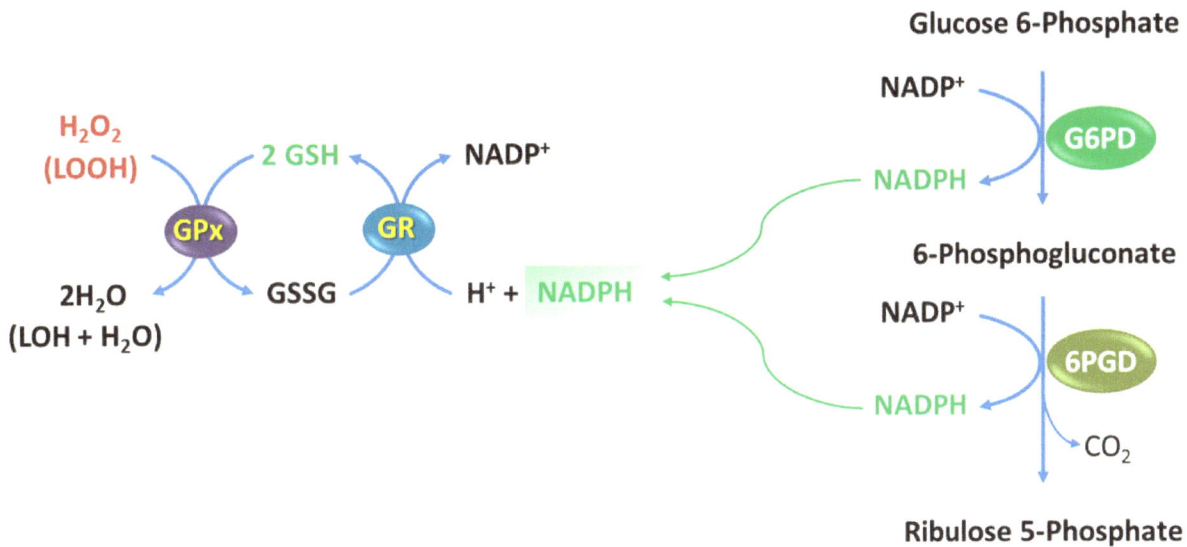

FIGURE B.6. Glutathione reductase (GR)-catalyzed reduction of glutathione disulfide (GSSG) to the reduced form of glutathione (GSH). As illustrated, glutathione peroxidase (GPx) catalyzes the decomposition of peroxides at the expense of GSH. GR then catalyzes the reduction of GSSG to GSH using NADPH as the electron donor. NADPH is primarily provided by the pentose phosphate pathway with glucose-6-phosphate dehydrogenase (G6PD) as the key enzyme. 6PGD, 6-phosphogluconate dehydrogenase; LOOH, lipid hydroperoxide; LOH, lipid alcohol.

4.2.2. Biochemistry

GPx1–6 isozymes are all able to catalyze the reduction of H_2O_2 or organic hydroperoxides (LOOH) to water or corresponding alcohols (LOH) using GSH as an electron donor (**Figure B.5**). GPx4 is also able to reduce phopholipid hydroperoxides in membranes, and as such is named phospholipid hydroperoxide GPx (PHGPx). Due to the low levels of GSH in extracellular fluid, GPx3 may also use extracellular thioredoxin and glutaredoxin as electron donors [66]. In addition to decomposing H_2O_2 and LOOH, GPx isozymes also reduce peroxynitrite in vitro [67].

4.2.3. Biological Functions

4.2.3.1. PRIMARY FUNCTIONS

The primary biological function of GPx1–6 isozymes is to decompose H_2O_2 and organic peroxides, thereby protecting against peroxide-induced oxidative stress and tissue injury. H_2O_2 and organic peroxides (such as lipid peroxides) are among the major ROS that contribute to oxidative tissue injury. As such, GPx1–6 enzymes are among the most important antioxidant defenses against oxidative stress-associated disease pathophysiology.

4.2.3.2. ATYPICAL FUNCTIONS

As a main structural component of the sperm mitochondrial capsule in mature spermatozoa, GPx4 is also involved in sperm maturation and male fertility, independent of its enzymatic activity [68, 69].

4.3. Glutathione Reductase

4.3.1. General Characteristics

Glutathione reductase (GR) is a homodimeric flavoprotein that catalyzes the formation of GSH from GSSG at the expense of the reduced form of nicotinamide adenine dinucleotide phosphate (NADPH). Mammalian GR is a homodimeric flavoprotein with a molecular mass of 104 kDa. It is ubiquitously expressed in various tissues. GR is present in both cytosol and mitochondria. These two isozymes of GR are biochemically indistinguishable, and are encoded by a single gene. In humans, GR gene is localized on chromosome 8p21.1.

TABLE B.2. Human and mouse cytosolic glutathione S-transferase genes

Class (Human)	Gene (Human)	Class (Mouse)	Gene (Mouse)
Alpha (A)	GSTA1 GSTA2 GSTA3 GSTA4 GSTA5	Alpha (A)	Gsta1 Gsta2 Gsta3 Gsta4 Gsta5
Mu (M)	GSTM1 GSTM2 GSTM3 GSTM4 GSTM5	Mu (M)	Gst1 Gst2 Gst3 Gst4 Gst5 Gst6 Gst7
Pi (P)	GSTP1	Pi (P)	Gstp1 Gstp2
Theta (T)	GSTT1 GSTT2	Theta (T)	Gstt1 Gstt2 Gstt3
Zeta (Z)	GSTZ1	Zeta (Z)	Gstz1
Omega (O)	GSTO1	Omega (O)	Gsto1 Gsto2
Sigma (S)	GSTS1	Sigma (S)	Gsts1

4.3.2. Biochemistry

GR catalyzes the reduction of GSSG to GSH with NADPH as the reducing cofactor. One molecule of NADPH is required for reducing each molecule of GSSG to form 2 molecules of GSH (**Figure B.6**).

As stated above, mammalian GR is a homodimer. The binding sites for NADPH and GSSG are at the opposite sides of each subunit of the dimer, and flavin adenine dinucleotide (FAD) is bound to the center of each subunit. NADPH reduces the FAD, which then passes its electrons onto a disulfide bridge in the active site of the enzyme. The two –SH groups formed via the above mechanism then interact with GSSG and reduce it to 2 molecules of GSH, and the enzyme disulfide is reformed [70, 71].

4.3.3. Biological Functions

As noted earlier, GSH is a major cellular antioxidant against oxidative stress. Upon reaction with ROS, GSH is oxidized to GSSG (also known as glutathione disulfide). In mammalian cells, the ratios of intracellular GSH to GSSG are high, usually in the range of 10:1 to 100:1. Maintenance of such high ratios of intracellular GSH to GSSG is critical for normal cellular activities, including redox signaling. GR reduces GSSG to GSH and is thus critical for maintaining the high ratios of intracellular GSH to GSSG [71]. While GR is the primary enzyme for reducing GSSG to GSH, thioredoxin 2 and glutaredoxin 2 may act as efficient backup systems to GR for cytosolic GSSG reduction [72].

4.4. Glutathione S-Transferase

4.4.1. General Characteristics

Glutathione S-transferase (GST), also called glutathione transferase, is a general name for a superfamily of enzymes that catalyze the conjugation of GSH to a wide variety of xenobiotics and play important roles in protecting mammalian cells and tissues from electrophilic and oxidative stress. Some GST isozymes also regulate cellular processes via non-GSH conjugation-dependent mechanisms. As listed below, this superfamily of enzymes consists of three main families, which are widely distributed in mammalian tissues. Among the three main families, cytosolic GSTs are the most extensively studied enzymes involved in the detoxification of electrophilic xenobiotics and ROS.

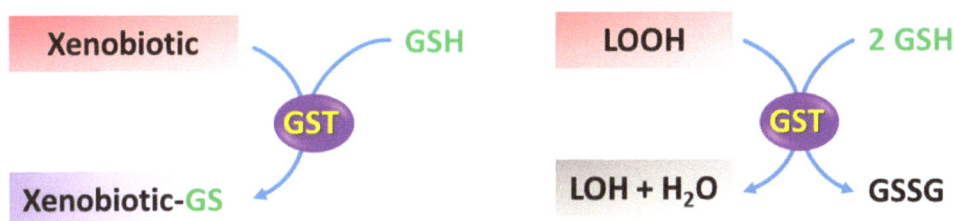

FIGURE B.7. Glutathione S-transferase (GST)-catalyzed xenobiotic conjugation reaction and decomposition of lipid peroxide (LOOH). As illustrated, GST-catalyzed conjugation reaction between an electrophilic xenobiotc compound and GSH typically forms a less reactive xenobiotic-GSH conjugate (Xenobiotic-GS). GST-catalyzed decomposition of LOOH results in the formation of the corresponding lipid alcohol (LOH). In this reaction, GSH is oxidized to glutathione disulfide (GSSG), and GST may be considered as a glutathione peroxidase-like enzyme.

(1) Cytosolic GSTs: Mammalian cytosolic GSTs are all dimeric with a molecular mass of ~50 kDa. They are classified into seven classes, namely, alpha (A), mu (M), pi (P), sigma (S), theta (T), omega (O), and zeta (Z). **Table B.2** lists the human and mouse cytosolic GST genes.

(2) Mitochondrial GSTs: Mammalian mitochondrial class kappa GST isozymes are dimeric. Mouse, rat and human possess only a single kappa GST (GSTK). This enzyme catalyzes GSH conjugation reactions with certain xenobiotics.

(3) Microsomal GSTs: Microsomal GSTs are also known as membrane-associated proteins in eicosanoid and glutathione metabolism (MAPEG). Most of the mammalian MAPEG enzymes are involved in the production of eicosanoids. Six human MAPEG isoenzymes have been identified. Some of the isoenzymes are involved in the detoxification of xenobiotics via catalyzing GSH conjugation.

4.4.2. Biochemistry

Cytosolic GSTs are among the most extensively studied enzymes involved in the detoxification of xenobiotics and ROS. As illustrated in **Figure B.7**, these enzymes catalyze the conjugation reactions of GSH with various electrophilic xenobiotics, including reactive aldehydes and quinone compounds, to form less reactive conjugates (xenobiotic-GS). Some GST isozymes also exhibit glutathione peroxidase

activity, catalyzing the reduction of organic hydroperoxide (LOOH) to form alcohol (LOH) and protect against oxidative stress injury [73–75].

4.4.3. Biological Functions

The biological activities of GST isozymes can be summarized into the following three categories: (1) protection against toxicity of electrophilic xenobiotics and ROS via enzymatic reactions; (2) protection against carcinogenesis; and (3) regulation of cell signaling.

4.4.3.1. PROTECTION AGAINST TOXICITY OF ELECTROPHILES AND ROS VIA ENZYMATIC REACTIONS

GSTs play a central role in phase 2 biotransformation, in which they catalyze the GSH conjugation reactions with various substrates containing electrophilic moieties. The resulting more water-soluble conjugates are excreted via the multidrug resistant protein efflux pumps or undergo further metabolism to mercapturic acids.

Substrates of GST isozymes include a wide range of endogenous metabolites, environmental xenobiotics, as well as alkylating and free radical-generating anticancer drugs. As noted above, some GST isozymes also function as glutathione peroxidases, catalyzing the reduction of organic peroxides, including those derived from lipid peroxidation. In this regard, certain GST isozymes are reported to protect against ROS-induced injury [73]. Thus, GSTs play an important role in the detoxification of both electrophilic species and ROS.

In line with the above notion, downregulation of adipose GSTA4 is shown to lead to increased protein carbonylation, oxidative stress, and mitochondrial dysfunction in mice [76]. Genetic deficiency of GSTP also increases myocardial sensitivity to ischemia-reperfusion injury in mice due to decreased detoxification of lipid peroxidation-derived reactive aldehydes [77]. In humans, downregulation of GSTP may also contribute to enhanced oxidative stress in asthma [78]. Less commonly studied GST isozymes, such as GSTS1 and GSTO1 have been shown to also protect against oxidative neurodegeneration in animal models of Parkinson's disease [79, 80]. It should be noted that although GST-catalyzed glutathione conjugation is generally regarded as a detoxification mechanism, GSH conjugation of certain xenobiotics, such as halogen-containing compounds may lead to their bioactivation, resulting in increased toxicity in biological systems [37].

4.4.3.2. PROTECTION AGAINST CARCINOGENESIS

Many carcinogens are electrophilic compounds and also substrates for GSTs. Thus, GST-catalyzed GSH conjugation of carcinogenic chemicals or their reactive metabolites represents an important detoxification mechanism for chemical carcinogens. Indeed, induction of GSTs by pharmacological agents is a major mechanism of chemoprotection against chemical carcinogenesis. On the contrary, deficiency of GST isozymes (e.g., GSTP) sensitizes animals to chemical-induced carcinogenesis [81, 82]. Moreover, in an initiated mouse model of colon cancer, deletion of GSTP results in increased inflammatory responses and marked enhancement of colon tumorigenesis as indicated by early tumor onset and decreased survival [83]. This suggests that GSTs may affect other cellular processes to protect against tumorigenesis. Indeed, as discussed below, GST isozymes, especially GSTP also regulate cell signaling to impact cancer development.

4.4.3.3. REGULATION OF CELL SIGNALING

In addition to catalyzing GSH conjugation reactions, GST isozymes, especially GSTP also possess other functions, regulating a number of cellular processes such as kinase cascades and S-glutathionylation that contribute to the intrinsic ability of mammalian cells to survive genotoxic, metabolic, and oxidative stress [84–86]. These atypical functions may contribute to the protective activities of GSTP in various disease conditions, especially cancer development. On the other hand, dysregulation of GSTP-mediated signaling may contribute to cancer development as well. For example, in brain cancer cells, phosphorylation of GSTP by epidermal growth factor receptor is found to promote formation of the GSTP1-c-Jun N-terminal kinase (JNK) complex and suppress JNK downstream signaling, leading to significant suppression of both spontaneous and drug-induced apoptosis in the tumor cells [87].

4.5. Glutaredoxin

4.5.1. General Characteristics

Glutaredoxin (Grx) refers to a family of GSH-dependent enzymes that catalyze the reduction of glutathionylated proteins. This reduction reaction is known as deglutathionylation. Protein glutathionylation refers to covalent attachment of glutathione to a protein cysteine residue via a disulfide bridge. Protein glutathionylation increases during oxidative stress. It represents a post-translational modification of proteins. Analogous to protein phosphorylation and dephosphorylation, protein glutathionylation and deglutathionylation may play an important role in cell signal transduction. Because of the reversible nature of protein glutathionylation, it is considered a transient protective mechanism for critical cysteine residues of proteins.

Grx isozymes are usually named by numbers in the order of their discovery in various species. In mammals, there are multiple Grx isozymes, namely, Grx1, 2, 3, and 5 with Grx1 and Grx2 being most extensively investigated. Grx4 is present in lower eukaryotes. Grx1 and 2 are dithiol Grxs as they contain the characteristic Cys-Pro-Tyr-Cys active site motif. On the other hand, Grx3 and 5 are monothiol Grxs, because they lack the C-terminal active site thiol in its Cys-Gly-Phe-Ser active site, but contain all structural and functional elements to bind and utilize GSH as the substrate. While Grx5 is a single domain monothiol Grx that consists of only one Grx domain, Grx3 is a multidomain monothiol Grx.

Grxs have a small molecular mass of ~10–12 kDa. Both Grx1 and Grx2 are widely distributed in mammalian tissues. Grx1 is mainly located in the cytosol. Grx2 is primarily localized in the mitochondria, and it can also be present in the nuclei. Grx3 is also known as protein kinase C interacting cousin of thioredoxin (PICOT), and is a cytosolic Grx. Grx5 is mainly present in the mitochondria. In humans, Grx1,

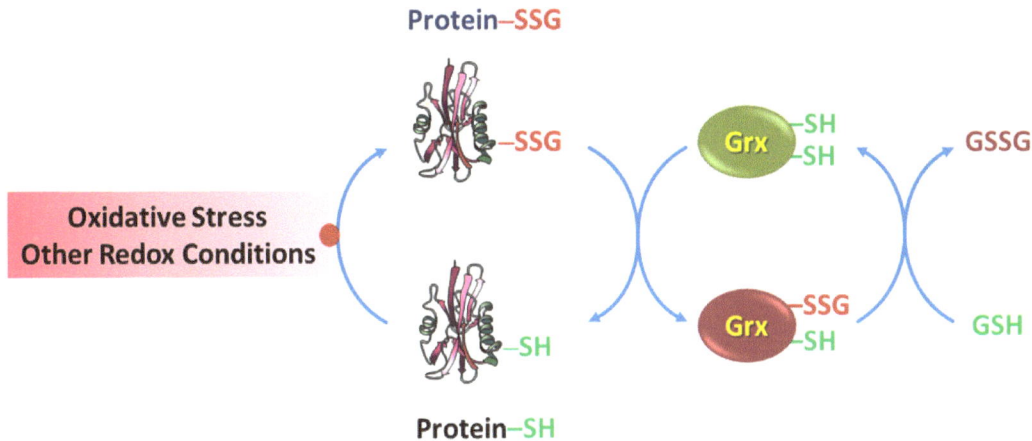

FIGURE B.8. Glutaredoxin (Grx)-catalyzed protein deglutathionylation. As illustrated, protein glutathionylation occurs under oxidative stress and other redox conditions. Grx catalyzes the reduction of the glutathionylated protein (protein–SSG) to the native protein–SH, and during the reaction Grx becomes glutathionylated. The glutathionylated Grx is then reduced back to Grx by the reduced form of glutathione (GSH), and during the reaction, GSH is converted to glutathione disulfide (GSSG).

Grx2, Grx3, and Grx5 are localized on chromosomes 5q15, 1q31.2, 10q26.3, and 14q32.13, respectively.

4.5.2. Biochemistry

Grxs contain active cysteine residues, and catalyze the reduction (deglutathionylation) of glutathionylated proteins. During the reaction the Grxs are oxidized with the formation of a disulfide bridge, which is then reduced back to the active cysteine groups by utilizing GSH (**Figure B.8**). Thus, Grxs are GSH-dependent oxidoreductases. Mitochondrial Grx2 is shown to also catalyze glutathionylation of mitochondrial membrane thiol proteins [88]. Moreover, Grxs possess dehydroascorbate reductase activity [89], suggesting a possible role in maintaining ascorbate homeostasis.

4.5.3. Biological Functions

4.5.3.1. PRIMARY BIOLOGICAL FUNCTIONS

The primary function of Grxs is to maintain cellular redox homeostasis and participate in cellular redox signaling. In this context, protein glutathonylation/deglutathionylation has been emerging as an important mechanism of cell redox regulation of a number of biological processes, including metabolic oxidative stress [90], cell growth and apoptosis [91,

92], inflammation [93, 94], and embryonic development [95, 96], among others.

4.5.3.2. NOVEL BIOLOGICAL FUNCTIONS

As they catalyze the reduction of disulfide formed in ribonucleotide reductase [97, 98], Grxs also play a role in regulating DNA synthesis. Moreover, Grxs participate in regulating iron homeostasis. For example, Grx5 is essential for iron-sulfur cluster biosynthesis and the maintenance of normal mitochondrial and cytosolic iron homeostasis [99]. Deficiency of Grx5 causes sideroblastic anemia [100, 101]. Grx3 is also able to transfer its [2Fe-2S] clusters to anamorsin, a physical and functional protein partner of Grx3 in the cytosol, whose [2Fe-2S] cluster-bound form is involved in the biogenesis of cytosolic and nuclear Fe-S proteins [41].

5. THIOREDOXIN SYSTEM

While the glutathione system is generally viewed as a classical cellular antioxidant defense mechanism, thioredoxin system represents relatively new machineries for defending against ROS and oxidative stress. The thioredoxin system currently includes four members. They are thioredoxin, peroxiredoxin, thioredoxin reductase, and sulfiredoxin.

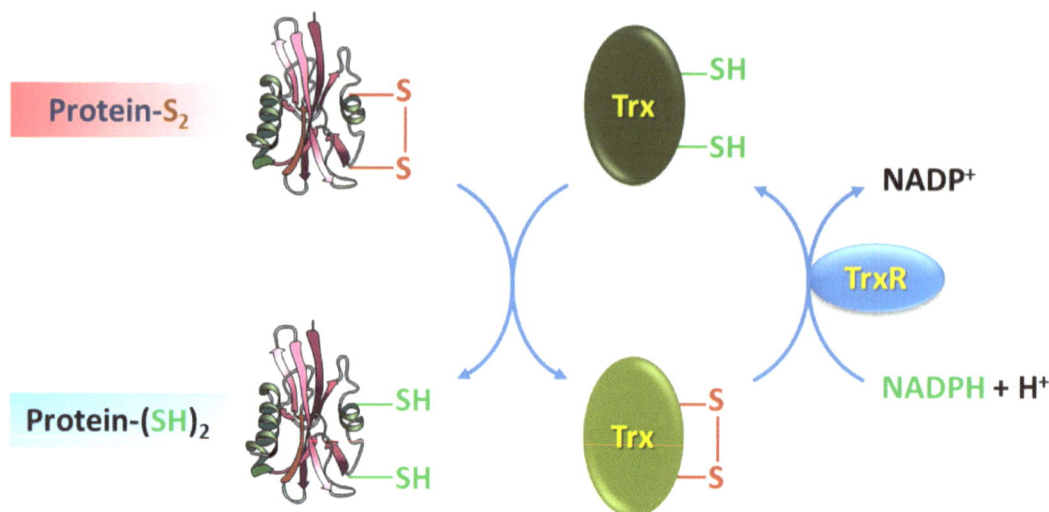

FIGURE B.9. Reduction of protein disulfide bridge by thioredoxin (Trx). As illustrated, during the reduction reaction, the sulfhydryl groups on Trx are oxidized to form a disulfide bridge. The oxidized Trx is then reduced back to Trx by thioredoxin reductase (TrxR) using NADPH as the electron donor.

5.1. Thioredoxin

5.1.1. General Characteristics

Thioredoxin (Trx) is a general term for a family of small redox proteins (~12 kDa) that undergo NADPH-dependent reduction by thioredoxin reductase and in turn reduce the disulfide bridge in target proteins. There are at least three Trxs in mammals: Trx1, Trx2, and sperm Trx (Sp-Trx, also designated as p32^{TrxL}). Trxs 1 and 2 are the most extensively studied Trx isoforms in biology and medicine. They are ubiquitously distributed in mammalian tissues. Trx1 is predominantly located in the cytosol, and can be excreted into the extracellular space or translocate into the nuclei, whereas Trx2 is present in the mitochondria. In humans, Trx1 and Trx2 are localized on chromosomes 9q13 and 22q13.1, respectively.

5.1.2. Biochemistry

Trxs are redox proteins that undergo NADPH-dependent reduction by thioredoxin reductase and in turn reduce oxidized cysteine groups on proteins. Trxs have a conserved Cys-Gly-Pro-Cys redox catalytic site that is responsible for reducing the protein disulfide bridge. As a result, the two cysteine residues of the Trxs are oxidized to form disulfide (i.e., the oxidized form of Trxs). The oxidized Trxs are then reduced back to Trxs via thioredoxin reductase using NADPH as the electron donor (**Figure B.9**).

5.1.3. Biological Functions

The primary function of Trxs is to serve as an antioxidant defense against oxidative stress. Trxs are also involved in the regulation of cell signaling, causing both beneficial and detrimental effects.

5.1.3.1. ANTIOXIDANT FUNCTIONS

Trxs possess antioxidant activities via various potential mechanisms. These include that: (1) Trxs directly scavenge ROS; (2) Trxs act as cofactors for peroxiredoxins which are important enzymes for the detoxification of H_2O_2 and organic hydroperoxides; (3) Trxs act as cofactors for methionine sulfoxide reductases, enzymes involved in repairing oxidative protein damage and protecting against oxidative injury; and (4) Trxs may also serve as electron donors for GPx3 (plasma glutathione peroxidase), an enzyme involved in the detoxification of ROS in extracellular environment [66]. However, due to the low concentrations of Trxs in plasma, this reaction may not contribute much to the antioxidant activities of Trxs. As a mitochondrial protein, Trx2 plays an important role in protecting against mitochondrial oxidative stress and associated tissue injury [102, 103].

TABLE B.3. Basic characteristics of mammalian peroxiredoxin (Prx) isozymes

Isozyme	Subgroup	Cellular Location	Chromosomal Localization
Prx1	Typical 2-Cys	Cytosol	1p34.1
Prx2	Typical 2-Cys	Cytosol	19p13.2
Prx3	Typical 2-Cys	Mitochondria	10q25-q26
Prx4	Typical 2-Cys	Endoplasmic reticulum, extracellular space	Xp22.11
Prx5	Atypical 2-Cys	Cytosol, mitochondria, nuclei, peroxisomes	11q13
Prx6	1-Cys	Cytosol	1q25.1

5.1.3.2. CELL SIGNALING

In addition to serving as a cofactor for various mammalian enzymes, including ribonucleotide reductase, peroxiredoxins, and GPx3, Trxs, especially Trx1 can reduce and activate a number of transcription factors (e.g., NF-κB, AP-1, SP-1) that regulate various cellular processes. Trxs also bind to and modify the activities of various other cellular proteins, including those involved in apoptosis. Recently, both Trx1 and Trx2 have been shown to regulate protein denitrosylation [104]. Protein denitrosylation, the removal of nitroso (–NO) groups primarily from cysteine residues in proteins, is an important aspect of nitric oxide-based signaling that regulates protein activity and protein-protein interactions [105]. Notably, Trxs may also act as a master regulator of the tricarboxylic acid cycle in plant mitochondria [106].

Trx-mediated redox modulation also contributes to tumorigenesis. As stated above, GSH and thioredoxin antioxidant pathways synergize to drive cancer initiation and progression [51]. Glioma cells recruit and exploit microglia (the resident immune cells of the brain) for their proliferation and invasion ability. A recent study shows that inhibition of the denitrosylation of S-nitrosylated procaspase-3 mediated by Trx2 is a part of the microglial pro-tumoral activation pathway initiated by glioma cancer cells [107].

5.2. Peroxiredoxin

5.2.1. General Characteristics

Peroxiredoxin (Prx) is a general term that refers to a family of small (22–27 kDa) nonseleno peroxidases currently known to possess six mammalian isozymes, namely, Prx1–6. These isozymes are able to reduce H_2O_2, organic hydroperoxides, and possibly peroxy-

nitrite, and thus represent a class of important antioxidants in mammals.

The six Prxs expressed in mammalian cells are classified into three subgroups: (1) typical 2-Cys Prxs including Prx1–4; (2) atypical 2-Cys Prx (Prx5); and (3) 1-Cys Prx (Prx6). Prxs are widely distributed in mammalian tissues, and the subcellular localization varies with the isozymes. Prx1, 2 and 6 are mainly located in the cytosol. Prx3 is restricted to the mitochondrial compartment. Prx4 is present in the endoplasmic reticulum and also secreted into extracellular environment. Prx5 is localized intracellularly to the cytosol, mitochondria, nuclei, and peroxisomes. In humans, Prx1–6 are localized on chromosomes 1p34.1, 19p13.2, 10q25–q26, Xp22.11, 11q13, and 1q25.1, respectively. **Table B.3** summarizes the basic characteristics of the six Prx isozymes in mammals.

5.2.2. Biochemistry

Prxs catalyze the reduction of H_2O_2 and various organic hydroperoxides to form water and alcohols, respectively through the reactive cysteine (Cys) residues of the enzymes (**Figure B.10**). They are able to also reduce peroxynitrite [108, 109].

The typical 2-Cys Prxs (Prx1–4) are homodimers and contain both the N- and C-terminal-conserved Cys residues and require both of them for catalytic function. Atypical 2-Cys Prx (Prx5) is a monomer and contains only the N-terminal Cys but requires one additional nonconserved Cys residue for catalytic activity. 1-Cys Prx (Prx6) is a homodimer and contains only the N-terminal Cys and requires only the N-terminal Cys for catalytic function.

During the reduction of oxidative substrates, the Cys residues of Prxs are oxidized. Thioredoxin provides the electron for reducing the oxidized Prx 1–5,

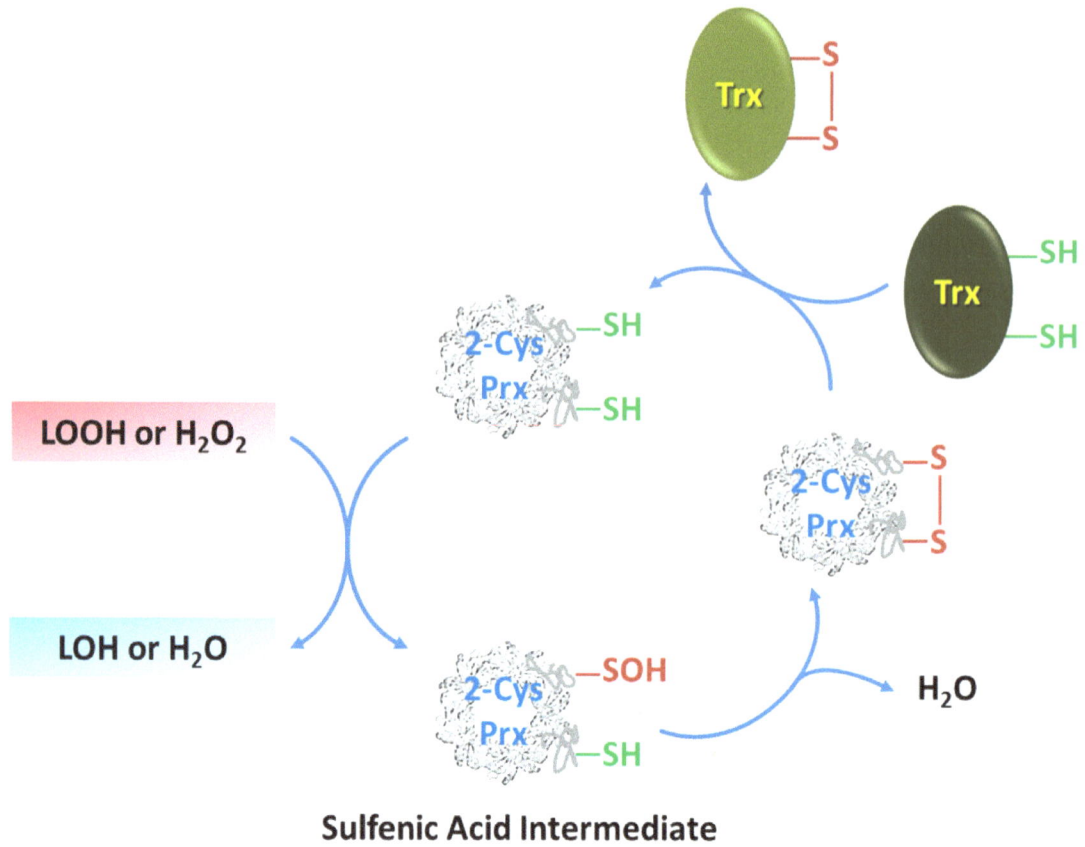

Sulfenic Acid Intermediate

FIGURE B.10. Peroxiredoxin (Prx)-mediated reduction of hydrogen peroxide (H_2O_2) and lipid hydroperoxide (LOOH) using thioredoxin (Trx) as the electron donor. Shown in the illustration is a 2-Cys Prx-catalyzed reduction of H_2O_2 and LOOH to form water and lipid alcohol (LOH), respectively. During the reaction, one sulfhydryl group of the 2-Cys Prx is oxidized to sulfenic acid (SOH) intermediate, followed by the formation of a disulfide bridge (i.e., the oxidized form of Prx). The disulfide bridge is reduced by Trx, and the original Prx is regenerated.

whereas GSH is likely to be employed to reduce the oxidized Prx6 [110].

5.2.3. Biological Functions

5.2.3.1. ANTIOXIDANT FUNCTIONS

Prxs play an important role in the detoxification of H_2O_2 and various organic peroxides as well as per-oxynitrite. This antioxidant function is the basis for this family of enzymes in protecting against oxidative stress and pathogenesis of various types of diseases and coditions that involve an oxidative stress mechanism, such as cardiovascular disorders, diabetes, neurodegeneration, cancer, and aging [111–119].

5.2.3.2. CELL SIGNALING

In addition to their antioxidant function, Prxs are reported to participate in other cellular processes, such as regulation of the activities of transcription factors (e.g., NF-κB, AP-1, p53), and growth factor signaling [120], as well as ROS signaling [121]. With regard to ROS signaling, Prx1 has been shown to regulate the localized levels of H_2O_2 for redox signaling and mitotic progression [122, 123]. Notably, Prx2 and STAT3 form a redox relay for H_2O_2 signaling. In this regard, H_2O_2 oxidizes Prx2, which then interacts with the transcription factor STAT3, resulting in the flow of the oxidative equivalents from Prx2 to STAT3. The redox relay generates di-

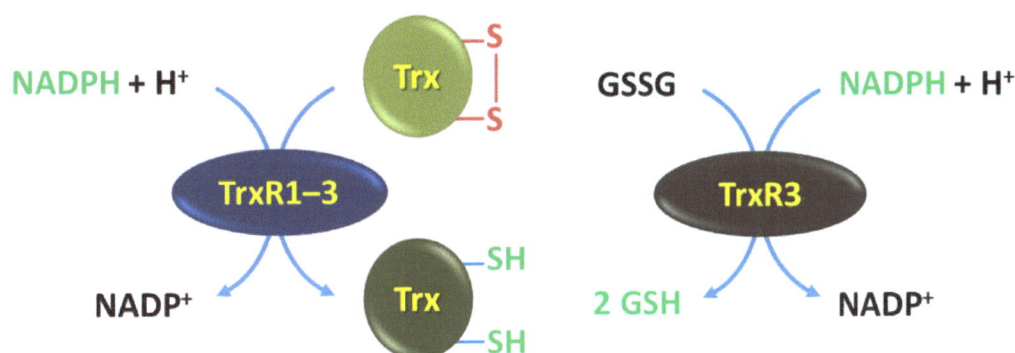

FIGURE B.11. Thioredoxin reductase (TrxR)-mediated reduction of oxidized thioredoxin (Trx) and glutathione disulfide (GSSG). As illustrated, all three isozymes of mammalian TrxR are able to catalyze the reduction of oxidized Trx using NADPH as an electron donor. In addition to catalyzing the reduction of oxidized Trx, TrxR3, known alternatively as thioredoxin glutathione reductase (TGR), also catalyzes the reduction of GSSG to the reduced form of glutathione (GSH) using NADPH as an electron donor.

sulfide-linked STAT3 oligomers with attenuated transcriptional activity [124]. STAT3, a member of the signal transducer and activator of transcription (STAT) protein family, mediates the expression of a variety of genes in response to cell stimuli, and plays a key role in many cellular processes, such as cell growth and apoptosis.

5.3. Thioredoxin Reductase

5.3.1. General Characteristics

Thioredoxin reductase (TrxR) refers to a class of enzymes that catalyze the reduction of oxidized thioredoxins. TrxRs belong to a pyridine nucleotide disulfide oxidoreductase family. There are three major isozymes of TrxR in mammals: TrxR1, TrxR2, and TrxR3, which is commonly known as thioredoxin glutathione reductase (TGR). Similar to thioredoxin-1 and -2, TrxR1 is present in the cytosol and nuclei, and TrxR2 is localized in the mitochondria. Both TrxR1 and TrxR2 are widely distributed in mammalian tissues. TrxR3 possesses both thioredoxin reductase and glutathione reductase activities, and as such is also known as TGR. TrxR3 is abundant in the testis. It is also expressed in other tissues, including the lung, kidney, heart, and brain. In mammals, the genes for TrxR1, TrxR2, and TrxR3 are denoted as Txnrd1, Txnrd2, and Txnrd3, respectively. In humans, Txnrd1, Txnrd2, and Txnrd3 are localized on

chromosomes 12q23–q24.1, 22q11.21, and 3q21.3, respectively.

5.3.2. Biochemistry

Mammalian TrxRs exist as homodimers. Each subunit is ~54–58 kDa in size and contains one FAD binding domain, one NADPH binding domain, and one interface domain required for dimerization. TrxRs are selenoproteins that catalyze the reduction of oxidized thioredoxins using NADPH as an electron donor. TrxR3 also catalyzes the reduction of GSSG to GSH, and thus possesses the glutathione reductase activity [125] (**Figure B.11**). TrxR3 is found to have an additional protein-disulfide isomerase function in sperm cells, and as such may play a role in sperm maturation [126]. In addition to thioredoxins and GSSG, TrxRs may also reduce several other substrates, such as glutaredoxin-2 and protein disulfide isomerase, and play an important role in protein folding [127, 128].

5.3.3. Biological Functions

TrxRs possess antioxidant functions that occur via several potential mechanisms. These include that: (1) TrxRs reduce the oxidized form of thioredoxins to the active form. As discussed earlier, thioredoxins play an important role in antioxidant defenses via serving as a cofactor for various antioxidant enzymes;

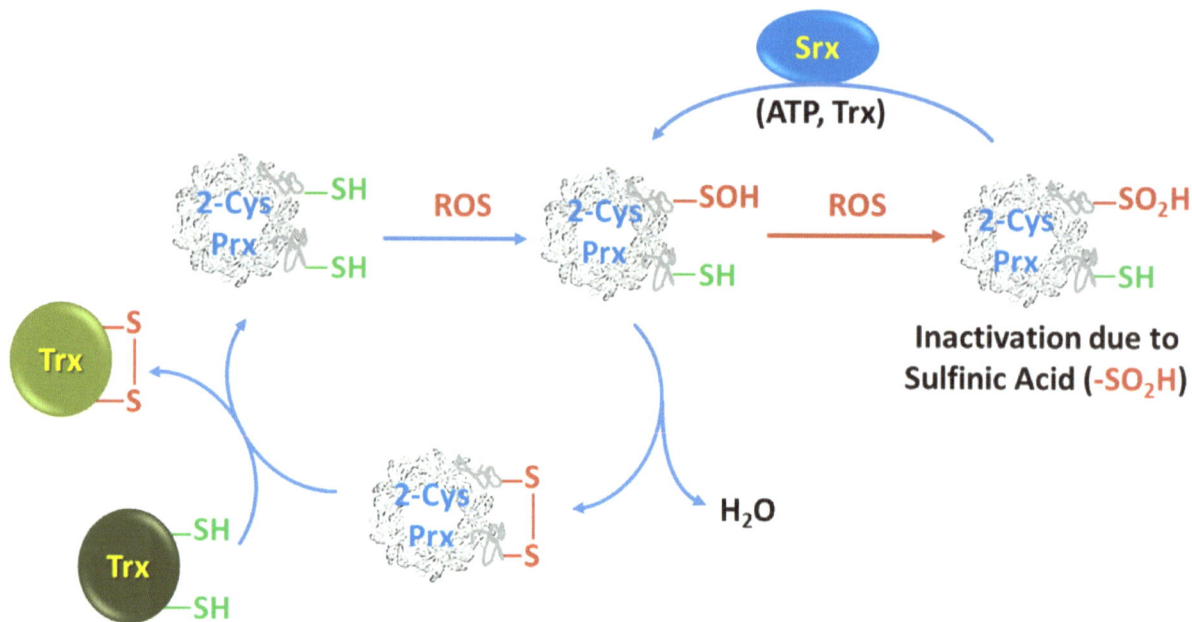

FIGURE B.12. Hyperoxidation of peroxiredoxin (Prx) by reactive oxygen species (ROS) to form sulfinic acid, and sulfiredoxin (Srx)-mediated reduction of the Prx sulfinic acid to sulfenic acid. During normal reduction of ROS (e.g., peroxides), the cysteine residue of Prx is oxidized to sulfenic acid (–SOH), which then leads to the formation of a disulfide bridge, that can be reduced by thioredoxin (Trx). However, under excessive oxidative conditions, the sulfenic acid can be further oxidized to sulfinic acid (–SO$_2$H), leading to inactivation of the enzyme. Srx catalyzes the reduction of sulfinic acid to sulfenic acid. This reaction is dependent on adenosine triphosphate (ATP) and utilizes Trx or reduced form of glutathione (not shown in the diagram) as the electron donor.

(2) TrxRs may also be involved in the regulation of heme oxygenase-1 (HO-1) [129]. HO-1 is a critical antioxidant and anti-inflammatory enzyme in mammalian tissues; and (3) TrxRs may support the antioxidant function of various small molecule antioxidants, including ascorbate, α-tocopherol, and coenzyme Q [130, 131]. Indeed, the mitochondrial TrxR2 acts to protect against mitochondrial oxidative stress and associated myocardial injury [132–134].

5.4. Sulfiredoxin

5.4.1. General Characteristics

Sulfiredoxin (Srx or Srx1) is a recently identified small molecular mass (~13 kDa) antioxidant enzyme that catalyzes the reduction of sulfinic peroxiredoxins (Prxs) in the presence of ATP [135]. Srx is only found in eukaryotic cells. This is thought to be due to the role of Srx in the restoration of hyperoxidized Prxs, whose counterparts in prokaryotes are not sen-

sitive to oxidative inactivation. Srx is ubiquitously expressed in mammalian tissues [136]. It is primarily present in the cytosol and also found to undergo translocation to the mitochondria [137]. In humans, Srx is localized on chromosome 20p13.

5.4.2. Biochemistry

Srx binds to 2-Cys Prxs, forming a complex, as evidenced by their co-immunoprecipitation and structural studies [138]. As stated above, Prxs are antioxidant enzymes that exert cytoprotective effects in many models of oxidative stress. However, under highly oxidizing conditions Prxs can be inactivated through hyperoxidation of their active site cysteine residue to form sulfinic acid (–SO$_2$H). This hyperoxidized form of Prxs cannot be reduced by thioredoxins, and is thus considered as an inactivated state. Srx acts by catalyzing the ATP-dependent formation of a sulfinic acid phosphoric ester on Prxs, which is then reduced by thiol equivalents, such as thioredoxins or glutathione, thereby reactivating the hyperoxidized Prxs [139] (**Figure B.12**). In addition, Srx has been found to catalyze deglutathionylation of proteins, including 2-Cys Prxs [140, 141]. Deglutathionylation is an important mechanism of post-translational modifications of proteins, including signaling molecules, and has been implicated in cell redox homeostasis and growth regulation.

5.4.3. Biological Functions

The major biological function of Srx is to protect against oxidative stress primarily via reactivating Prxs [119, 137]. Recently, Srx is shown to act as a Prx2 denitrosylase, removing –SNO from Prx2 in an ATP-dependent manner [142]. S-Nitrosylation of Prx2, a peroxidase widely expressed in mammalian neurons, inhibits both its enzymatic activity and protective function against oxidative stress injury. Hence, Srx may reactivate Prx enzymes via at least two separate pathways, namely, sulfinic reduction and denitrosylation.

Srx may also play a role in ROS redox signaling. In this context, H_2O_2 released from mitochondria regulates various cell signaling pathways and Prx3 is a major antioxidant enzyme in controlling the levels of mitochondrial H_2O_2. Srx is found to undergo translocation to mitochondria and reactivate mitochondrial Prx3, and this interaction results in an oscillatory H_2O_2 release from the organelle for mediating cell metabolic signaling [143, 144].

6. OTHER ANTIOXIDANT ENZYMES

This section considers several other antioxidant enzymes of biological significance. These include methionine sulfoxide reductase, heme oxygenase, NADPH:quinone oxidoreductase, and paraoxonase.

6.1. Methionine Sulfoxide Reductase

6.1.1. General Characteristics

Mammalian methionine sulfoxide reductase (Msr) refers to two structurally unrelated classes of thiol-dependent enzymes, namely, MsrA and MsrB that catalyze the reduction of methionine S-sulfoxide and methionine R-sulfoxide, respectively. Mammals have a single MsrA gene, and the encoded Msr enzyme can exist in two forms, one in cytosol and the other in mitochondria. In contrast, there are three MsrB isozymes in mammals, namely, MsrB1, MsrB2

and MsrB3. MsrB1 is a selenoprotein and present in the cytosol and nuclei. MsrB2 resides in mitochondria. MsrB3 can be localized in mitochondria or endoplasmic reticulum. Msr isozymes are ubiquitously expressed in mammalian tissues, but their expression levels vary in different tissues. The highest expression levels of MsrA have been reported in the liver, kidney, and brain. MsrB1, like MsrA, is highly expressed in the liver and kidney, whereas highest expression levels of MsrB2 and MsrB3 are found in the heart and skeletal muscle.

Among the four Msr isozymes (MsrA, MsrB1, MsrB2, and MsrB3) only MsrB1 is a selenoprotein, and is shown to have the highest catalytic activity due to the selenocysteine in the active site. MsrB1 is also known as selenoprotein R (Sel R). The other Msr isozymes have cysteine residues in the active sites instead of selenocysteine. Msrs are low molecular weight proteins with molecular masses of approximately 25 kDa for MsrA, and 12 kDa for MsrB1, and 20 kDa for MsrB2 and MsrB3. In humans, the genes for MsrA, MsrB1, MsrB2, and MsrB3 are localized on chromosomes 8p23.1, 16p13.3, 10p12, and 12q14.3, respectively.

6.1.2. Biochemistry

MsrA and MsrB catalyze the reduction of methionine S-sulfoxide and methione R-sulfoxide, respectively, to form the normal methionine using thioredoxin as the electron donor (**Figure B.13**). Mammalian MsrA has three conserved cysteine residues, which participate in the reaction as catalytic and resolving cysteines. A sulfenic acid intermediate at the catalytic cysteine is generated when this cysteine residue attacks the sulfur of methionine S-sulfoxide. Subsequently, the thiol-disulfide exchange involving the two resolving cysteine residues results in the formation of a disulfide bond on the enzyme surface, which is finally reduced by thioredoxin.

Mammalian MsrB1 has one conserved cysteine residue in the N-terminal portion and the catalytic selenocysteine in the C-terminal region. During catalysis, the selenocysteine is converted to selenenic acid intermediate upon interacting with the sulfur of methionine R-sulfoxide, and the selenenic acid intermediate rearranges to form seleneylsulfide with the help of the resolving cysteine residue. The seleneylsulfide is reduced to selenocysteine by thioredoxin. In contrast, mammalian MsrB2 and MsrB3 have only one conserved cysteine residue and seem to have evolved a different catalytic mechanism for the direct reduction of the sulfenic acid intermediate

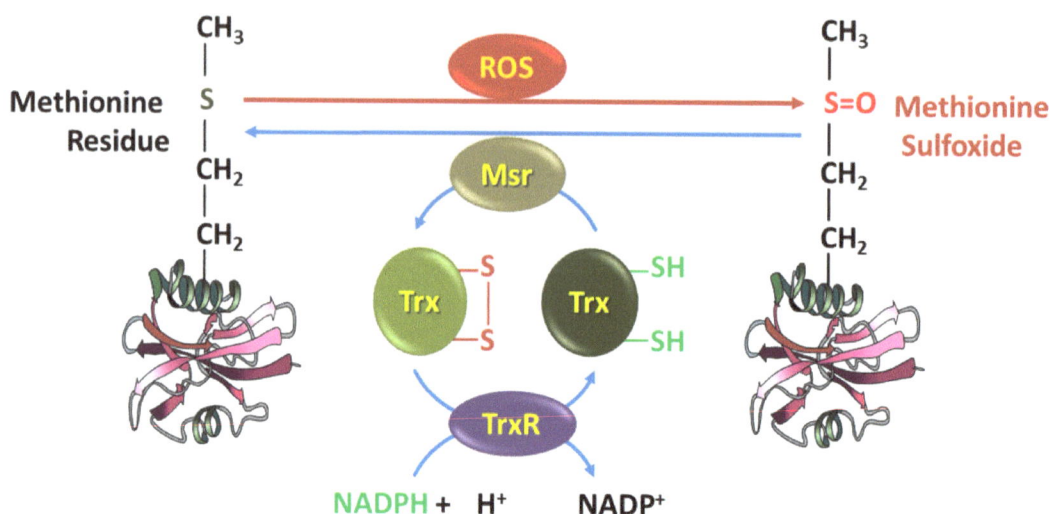

FIGURE B.13. Methionine sulfoxide reductase (Msr)-catalyzed reduction of protein methionine sulfoxide. As illustrated, upon exposure to reactive oxygen species (ROS), the protein methionine residue may be oxidized to methionine sulfoxide, resulting in oxidative protein damage and dysfunction. This can be reversed by Msr-catalyzed reduction using thioredoxin (Trx) as an electron donor. Thioredoxin reductase (TrxR) then regenerates the Trx from its oxidized form using NADPH as a reducing equivalent. It should be noted that Msr-catalyzed reduction is stereospecific (not depicted in the illustration) with MsrA and MsrB catalyzing the reduction of methionine S-sulfoxide and methionine R-sulfoxide, respectively, to form the normal methionine.

by thioredoxin. Although thioredoxin is the most important cellular cofactor for mammalian Msr isozymes, other thiol equivalents may also be utilized as reductants under certain experimental conditions. These include dithiothreitol, thionein, and selenocystamine [145, 146]. Moreover, under certain conditions, MsrA may also function as a stereospecific methionine oxidase, producing S-methionine sulfoxide as its product [147].

6.1.3. Biological Functions

The primary function of Msr enzymes is to repair oxidative protein damage. Oxidative modifications of proteins have been implicated in various degenerative disease conditions and aging. As compared with most other amino acid residues in proteins, methionine is particularly susceptible to oxidation by ROS, giving rise to a diastereomeric mixture of methionine sulfoxides, namely, methionine S-sulfoxide and methionine R-sulfoxide. By reducing methionine sulfoxide to methionine, Msr enzymes protect against oxidative stress [148–150] and associated conditions, including cardiovascular disorders [151, 152], hearing loss [153, 154], and aging [155, 156].

By reducing methionine oxide in target proteins, Msrs may also play a role in regulating other cellular processes, such as actin dynamics [157, 158]. In conjunction with Mical proteins, methionine R-sulfoxide reductase B1 (MsrB1) regulates mammalian actin assembly via stereoselective methionine oxidation and reduction in a reversible, site-specific manner. Two methionine residues in actin are specifically converted to methionine R-sulfoxide by Mical1 and Mical2 and reduced back to methionine by selenoprotein MsrB1, supporting actin disassembly and assembly, respectively [158].

6.2. Heme Oxygenase

6.2.1. General Characteristics

Mammalian heme oxygenase (HO) refers to a family of two major isozymes, namely, HO-1 and HO-2 that catalyze the first and rate-limiting step in the oxidative degradation of heme to eventually produce bilirubin along with the release of carbon monoxide and ferrous iron. HO-1 is also known as the inducible form, and HO-2 as the constitutively expressed form. Expression of HO-1 occurs at low levels in most tis-

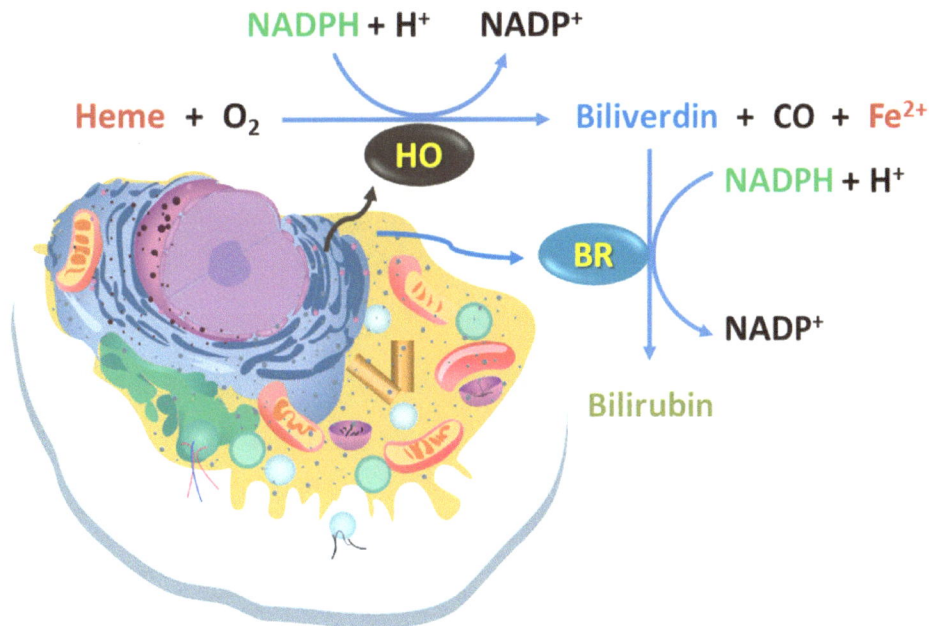

FIGURE B.14. Heme oxygenase (HO)-catalyzed degradation of heme. As illustrated, endoplasmic reticulum-associated HO catalyzes the degradation of heme to form biliverdin along with the release of carbon monoxide (CO) and ferrous iron. Biliverdin is further converted to bilirubin by cytosolic biliverdin reductase (BR). NADPH serves as the electron donor for both HO- and BR-catalyzed reactions.

sues under physiological conditions with the exception of the spleen (the site of red blood cell hemoglobin turnover) and several other unique cell types (e.g., renal inner medullary cells, Kupffer cells in the liver, Purkinje cells in the cerebellum, and $CD4^+/CD25^+$ regulatory T cells). HO-2 is constitutively expressed in mammalian tissues under physiological conditions, with the highest levels found in the brain and testes. The molecular masses for HO-1 and HO-2 are 32 and 36 kDa, respectively. In mammalian cells, HO-1 and HO-2 are mainly associated with endoplasmic reticulum. HO-1 is also reported to localize to distinct subcellular compartments, including the plasma membrane caveolae, mitochondria, and nuclei. A putative third isozyme of HO, namely, HO-3 is reported to be expressed in rat tissues. However, the in vivo significance of HO-3 is unclear. In humans, HO-1 and HO-2 genes are localized on chromosomes 22q13.1 and 16p13.3, respectively.

6.2.2. Biochemistry

Both HO-1 and HO-2 catalyze the first and rate-limiting step in the oxidative degradation of heme to form the open-chain tetrapyrrole biliverdin with concurrent release of iron (Fe^{2+}) and carbon monoxide (CO). This reaction requires molecular oxygen as well as reducing equivalents from NADPH cytochrome P450 reductase. The HO reaction displays regiospecificity for the heme molecule, such that only the α-isomer of biliverdin is produced. The biliverdin formed is subsequently reduced to bilirubin by biliverdin reductase (**Figure B.14**)

6.2.3. Biological Functions

HO isozymes possess antioxidative and anti-inflammatory activities, which result, at least partly, from: (1) the enzymatic degradation of heme, an oxidative species; (2) formation of biliverdin and bilirubin, two antioxidant molecules; and (3) production of carbon monoxide, an anti-inflammatory molecule. Due to the prooxidant activity of iron (e.g., participation in Fenton reaction, leading to the formation of hydroxyl radical), the iron released from HO-catalyzed reaction would seem to lead to detrimental effects. However, induction of HO activity and release of iron are usually associated with concurrent

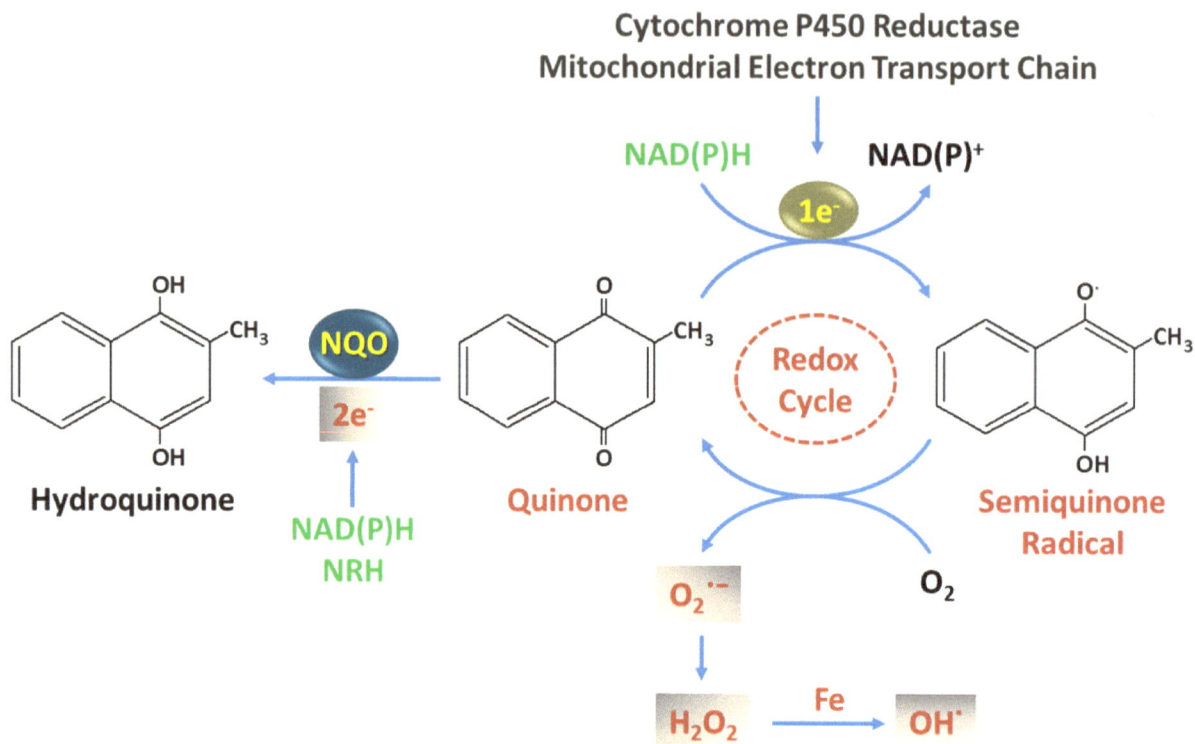

FIGURE B.15. NAD(P)H:quinone oxidoreductase (NQO)-catalyzed two-electron reduction of menadione, a quinone compound. As illustrated, NQO enzymes catalyze two-electron reduction of the quinone to hydroquinone. This prevents the quinone from undergoing one-electron reduction catalyzed by enzymes, such as cytochrome P450 reductase or mitochondrial electron transport chain enzyme complexes. One-electron reduction of the quinone leads to the formation of semiquinone radical. The semiquinone radical readily reduces oxygen to superoxide ($O_2^{\cdot-}$), which may subsequently lead to the formation of other reactive oxygen species, such as hydrogen peroxide (H_2O_2) and hydroxyl radical ($OH^{\cdot}$). NADPH serves as the electron donor for NQO1, wheras NQO2 uses dihydronicotinamide riboside (NRH) as the electron donor.

induction of ferritin, an iron-chelating protein. Induction of ferritin thus minimizes the prooxidant potential of the released iron. The reaction products biliverdin, bilirubin, and carbon monoxide primarily mediate the antioxidative and anti-inflammatory activities of the HO isozymes in protecting against the pathogenesis of various disease conditions, including cardiovascular diseases [159–162], inflammatory disorders [163, 164], and neuronal injury [165–167]. A recent study shows that HO-2 is a cellular myristate-binding protein that negatively regulates both retrovirus replication and host inflammatory responses [168].

While HO isozymes are generally considered as cytoprotective machineries, these enzymes may also cause detrimental effects under certain conditions.

For instance, nuclear targeting of HO-1 is found to promote cancer cell proliferation and progression independent of its enzymatic activity [169]. On the other hand, fasting-mimicking diet promotes T cell-mediated tumor cytotoxicity via downregulation of HO-1 [170].

6.3. NAD(P)H:Quinone Oxidoreductase

6.3.1. General Characteristics

NAD(P)H:quinone oxidoreductase (NQO) refers to a family of flavoproteins that includes two members, NQO1 and NQO2 in mammals. NQO1 and NQO2 stand for NAD(P)H:quinone oxidoreductase 1 and NRH:quinone oxidoreductase 2, respectively. NQO2

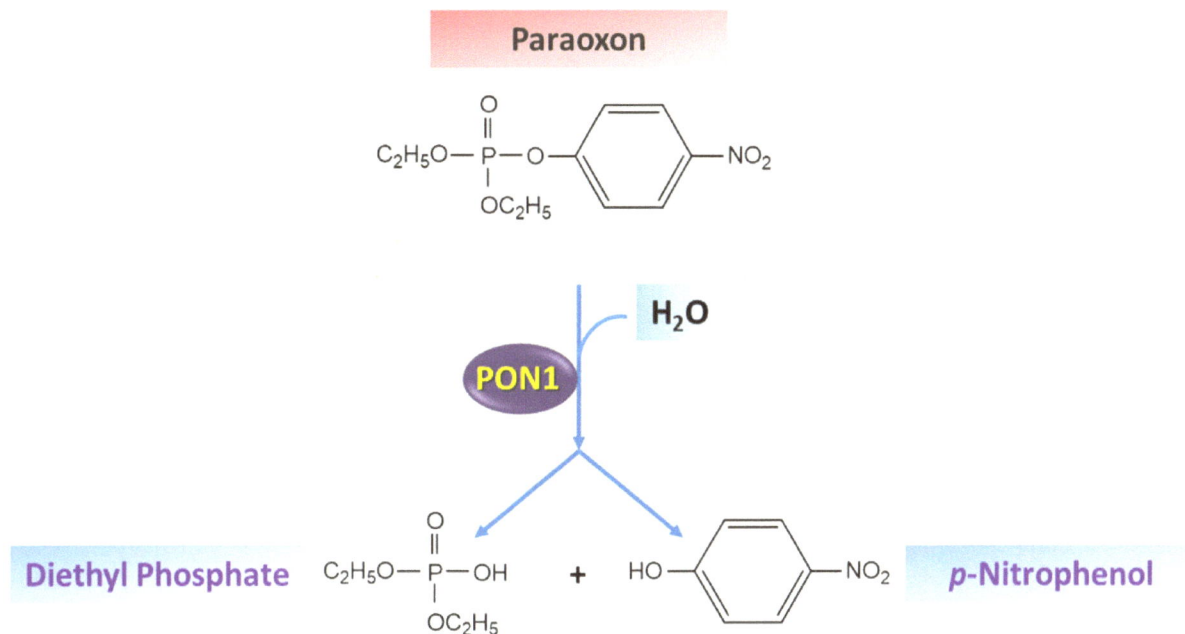

FIGURE B.16. Hydrolysis of paraoxon by paraoxonase 1 (PON1). As illustrated, PON1-catalyzed hydrolysis of paraoxon forms diethyl phosphate and *p*-nitrophenol. This is a classical reaction catalyzed by PON1. In addition, PON1 also catalyzes the degradation of oxidized lipids as well as the hydrolysis of a variety of aromatic and aliphatic lactones.

uses dihydronicotinamide riboside (NRH) rather than NAD(P)H as the electron donor. NQO1 and NQO2 catalyze two-electron reduction of various quinones and derivatives. As described below, these two enzymes also possess other novel biological activities. NQO1 and NQO2 are cytosolic enzymes with a molecular mass of 31 and 25 kDa, respectively. They are widely distributed in mammalian tissues though the highest levels are usually found in the liver. In humans, NQO1 and NQO2 genes are localized on chromosomes 16q22.1 and 6pter–q12, respectively.

6.3.2. Biochemistry

Both NQO1 and NQO2 catalyze two-electron reduction of quinones to hydroquinones, which then undergo conjugation reactions, leading to their excretion from the body. This two-electron reduction reaction prevents the unwanted one-electron reduction of quinones by other enzymes, such as cytochrome P450 reductase. The one-electron reduction results in the formation of reactive semiquinone radicals, and the subsequent formation of ROS via redox cycling (**Figure B.15**). Two-electron reduction of

quinones by NQO enzymes thus prevents the formation of reactive semiquinone radicals and ROS. In addition to quinones, NQO enzymes also catalyze the two-electron reduction of quinoneimines, nitroaromatics, and azo dyes.

6.3.3. Biological Functions

6.3.3.1. PRIMARY BIOLOGICAL FUNCTIONS

The most notable function of NQO enzymes is to metabolize quinone compounds, leading to their detoxification and excretion. In addition, NQO1 may help maintain certain endogenous antioxidants in their reduced and active forms. Both ubiquinone (coenzyme Q) and α-tocopherol-quinone, two important lipid-soluble antioxidants are substrates for NQO1. NQO1 catalyzes the two-electron reduction of ubiquinone and α-tocopherol-quinone to their hydroquinone forms, which then protect against lipid peroxidation of membranes [171, 172].

It is well-known that both NQO1 and NQO2 protect against ROS formation from quinone redox cycling. In addition, NQO1 also directly scavenges superoxide in an NAD(P)H-dependent manner [173]. This effect may be particularly significant in tissues, such as vasculature and myocardium, where NQO1 is highly expressed [174].

Reduction of certain quinones to their hydroquinone form by NQO1 may lead to their bioactivation, producing ROS. This occurs when the hydroquinone form is unstable and autoxidizes to give rise to superoxide. Quinone compounds that are bioactivated by NQO1 include the anticancer agents mitomycin C [175] and beta-lapachone [176].

6.3.3.2. ATYPICAL BIOLOGICAL ACTIVITIES

Several atypical activities of NQO have been identified. These include: (1) stabilization of p53 and other tumor suppressors; (2) as a gatekeeper of the 20s proteasome; and (3) binding to melatonin.

(1) Stabilization of p53 and other tumor suppressors: The p53 tumor suppressor protein suppresses tumorigenesis by mediating either growth arrest or apoptosis in response to stresses, such as DNA damage. NQO1 is shown to play an important role in stabilizing p53 protein via processes including protein-protein interaction that prevents ubiquitin-independent degradation of p53 by 20S proteasome [177, 178]. Stabilization of p53 protein by NQO1 may contribute to the protective role of NQO1 in multistage carcinogenesis. In addition to p53, NQO1 also regulates the ubiquitin-independent 20S proteasomal degradation of p73α and p33, two other tumor suppressors [179, 180].

(2) As a gatekeeper of the 20S proteasome: It has been demonstrated that in murine liver tissue majority of NQO1 is associated with the 20S proteasome, and NQO1 may function as a gatekeeper for protein degradation through the 20S proteasome. More recently, NQO1 is found to protect eukaryotic translation initiation factor (eIF) 4GI from proteasomal degradation, and as such may participate in the regulation of translation [181].

(3) Binding to melatonin: NQO2 has a melatonin-binding site, and as such may mediate some of the biological activities of melatonin, such as the antioxidant effects [182, 183]. However, the exact biological significance of the binding of melatonin to NQO2 remains to be elucidated. Such a binding might also impact the function of NQO2.

6.4. Paraoxonase

6.4.1. General Characteristics

Paraoxonase (PON) refers to a family of enzymes that includes three members in mammals, namely, PON1, PON2, and PON3. PON1 (43 kDa) is synthesized and secreted by the liver, and is primarily associated with high-density lipoprotein (HDL) in the plasma. PON1 catalyzes the breakdown of oxidized lipids, and blocks oxidation of HDL as well as low-density lipoprotein (LDL). PON2 is an intracellular protein that is widely distributed in mammalian tissues. Similar to PON1, PON2 with a molecular mass of 44 kDa also acts as an antioxidant protecting against oxidative stress. PON3 (40 kDa) is primarily expressed in the liver, and associated with HDL in the plasma. Like other members of the paraoxonase gene family, PON3 has significant antioxidant activity in protecting both HDL and LDL from oxidation. In humans, PON1, PON2, and PON3 are localized next to each other on chromosome 7q21.3–22.1.

6.4.2. Biochemistry

6.4.2.1. PON1

PON1 is an excellent example of a multitasking protein, displaying at least three important biochemical functions: (1) hydrolysis of organophosphates (pesticides and nerve agents) leading to their detoxification; (2) protection against lipoprotein oxidation by catalyzing the degradation of oxidized lipids; and (3) catalyzing the hydrolysis of a variety of aromatic and aliphatic lactones as well as the reverse reaction—lactonization of γ- and δ-hydroxycarboxylic acids [184]. PON1 is most noted for its ability to hydrolyze a variety of organophosphate pesticides and nerve agents, including paraoxon, diazoxon, chlorpyrifos-oxon, sarin, and soman [185]. Hydrolysis of these organophosphates by PON1 leads to their detoxification. **Figure B.16** illustrates the chemical reaction of PON1-catalyzed hydrolysis of paraoxon.

6.4.2.2. PON2 AND PON3

PON2 and PON3 lack the ability to hydrolyze organophosphates. However, PON2 and PON3 effectively hydrolyze lactones, and as such also act as lactonases. Similar to PON1, purified PON2 and PON3 are shown to inhibit lipid peroxidation of LDL in vitro. Since PON2 is an intracellular protein and not present in the plasma, it is suggested to act as a protector against cellular oxidative stress. Indeed, intracellular overexpression of PON2 attenuates oxidative stress in vascular cells and protects against cell-mediated oxidation of LDL [186, 187].

6.4.3. Biological Functions

Among the PON isozymes, PON1 has received the most attention with regard to the biological functions. As noted above, the classical function of PON1 is to metabolize organophosphates leading to their detoxification. Due to its close association with HDL, the role of PON1 in cardiovascular homeostasis has been investigated extensively. In humans, polymorphisms of PON1 gene have been shown to be an independent cardiovascular risk factor [188, 189]. PON1 may also determine the efficacy of certain cardiovascular drugs. For example, PON1 is found to be crucial for the bioactivation and also a major determinant of the clinical efficacy of clopidogrel, a widely used platelet inhibitor for the treatment of coronary heart disease [190]. The protective roles of PON1 as well as PON2 and PON3 have also been demonstrated in animal models of cardiovascular diseases, especially atherosclerosis [191–195].

7. SUMMARY AND CAVEATS

This appendix surveys common mammalian antioxidants with regard to their basic biochemical properties and biological functions. As stated throughout the appendix, an antioxidant molecule may also possess other biochemical properties and biological functions independent of its antioxidant activity. This is not surprising as most, if not all, cellular biomolecules are multifunctional. As such, it is important to bear in mind some of the common caveats on antioxidants and antioxidant-based modalities for disease intervention.

7.1. Antioxidants as Multitasking Molecules

Many antioxidants have well-established ability to scavenge FRRS, inhibit their formation, or repair the damage caused by FRRS. However, it is important to note that in addition to their effects on FRRS antioxidants, including both protein and non-protein antioxidants may also exert other biological effects irrelevant to their antioxidant activities. For example, the antioxidant enzyme catalase decomposes H_2O_2 to form water and molecular oxygen, a well-known antioxidant activity of catalase. This antioxidant enzyme also exhibits peroxidase and oxidase activities toward a number of other substrates, including alcohols [28]. Another example is α-tocopherol, which is known to inhibit lipid peroxidation by scavenging lipid peroxyl radical. α-Tocopherol has been shown to also exert non-antioxidant effects, such as inhibition of protein kinases [196].

The grape-derived polyphenol resveratrol is popularly recognized as an antioxidant compound providing protective effects in a wide variety of pathophysiological conditions, including cardiovascular injury, diabetes, and metabolic syndrome [197, 198]. These beneficial effects of resveratrol appear to result largely from its interaction with specific cellular targets, such as SIRT1 and cAMP phosphodiesterases independent of its antioxidant activity [197, 199, 200].

Thus, the response of a biological system to a particular antioxidant molecule may result from: (1) the antioxidative activity of the molecule; (2) the non-antioxidative activity of the molecule; or (3) the combined antioxidative and non-antioxidative activities. In free radical biology and medicine, another important consideration is that many antioxidants, such as GSH and GST are also important factors in the detoxification of electrophilic species, including reactive aldehydes. Reactive aldehydes are produced from lipid peroxidation elicited by FRRS, and they also cause damage to biomolecules.

7.2. Antioxidants as Double-Edged Swords

Like FRRS, antioxidants may also be double-edged swords. On the one hand, antioxidants protect against oxidative stress and associated tissue injury. On the other hand, under certain conditions, antioxidants may cause deleterious effects. For example, increasing some antioxidants (e.g., GSH and thioredoxin) or persistent activation of the antioxidant-regulator Nrf2 may promote cancer cell proliferation and metastasis [201–205]. Cancer cells typically produce higher levels of ROS than normal cells. Such elevated ROS levels, when they are moderate, are used as signaling molecules to promote cancer cell growth. On the other hand, when the levels of ROS go beyond moderate, these reactive species may actually become cytotoxic and thus inhibit cancer cell growth. Indeed, either overexpression of endogenous antioxidants or supplementation of exogenous antioxidants has been found to promote tumorigenesis and cancer metastasis in certain experimental models [201, 206].

The above new findings suggest that too much antioxidant defense might promote cancer development, which is in contrast to the conventional belief that antioxidants are always beneficial to health. This notion, on the one hand, reveals the complexity of ROS biology, and on the other hand, points to the need for taking such a complexity into consideration when devising strategies for the intervention of diseases involving an ROS-dependent mechanism.

7.3. Issues with Genetic Manipulations of Antioxidant Genes

Transgenic overexpression or knockout of specific antioxidant genes is frequently used to study the biological activities of endogenous antioxidant proteins in experimental animals. While these genetic animal models provide the most convincing evidence regarding the biological functions of particular antioxidant enzymes, interpretation of the data should be done with caution. This is because deletion of one antioxidant gene may lead to the compensatory upregulation of others. Likewise, overexpression of one antioxidant gene may also lead to downregulation of others. Thus, the changes in the phenotypes of these genetic animal models likely result from the combined actions of all the antioxidants whose expression is altered due to the genetic manipulation of a single antioxidant gene.

Another notion regarding transgenic overexpression of antioxidant genes is that the levels of the overexpressed antioxidant proteins are usually several or even over ten-fold higher than the basal physiological levels. The physiological significance of such dramatically overexpressed antioxidant proteins thus needs to be evaluated with caution. Regardless of the caveats, genetic manipulation of antioxidant genes in experimental animals continues to serve as an important approach to understanding the biology of endogenous antioxidants.

REFERENCES

1. Han BH, Zhou ML, Johnson AW, Singh I, Liao F, Vellimana AK, Nelson JW, Milner E, Cirrito JR, Basak J, Yoo M, Dietrich HH, et al. Contribution of reactive oxygen species to cerebral amyloid angiopathy, vasomotor dysfunction, and microhemorrhage in aged Tg2576 mice. *Proc Natl Acad Sci USA* 2015; 112(8):E881–90.
2. Zhang J, Malik A, Choi HB, Ko RW, Dissing-Olesen L, MacVicar BA. Microglial CR3 activation triggers long-term synaptic depression in the hippocampus via NADPH oxidase. *Neuron* 2014; 82(1):195–207.
3. Brennan AM, Suh SW, Won SJ, Narasimhan P, Kauppinen TM, Lee H, Edling Y, Chan PH, Swanson RA. NADPH oxidase is the primary source of superoxide induced by NMDA receptor activation. *Nat Neurosci* 2009; 12(7):857–63.
4. Desco MC, Asensi M, Marquez R, Martinez-Valls J, Vento M, Pallardo FV, Sastre J, Vina J. Xanthine oxidase is involved in free radical production in type 1 diabetes: protection by allopurinol. *Diabetes* 2002; 51(4):1118–24.
5. Mellin V, Isabelle M, Oudot A, Vergely-Vandriesse C, Monteil C, Di Meglio B, Henry JP, Dautreaux B, Rochette L, Thuillez C, Mulder P. Transient reduction in myocardial free oxygen radical levels is involved in the improved cardiac function and structure after long-term allopurinol treatment initiated in established chronic heart failure. *Eur Heart J* 2005; 26(15):1544–50.
6. Rajendra NS, Ireland S, George J, Belch JJ, Lang CC, Struthers AD. Mechanistic insights into the therapeutic use of high-dose allopurinol in angina pectoris. *J Am Coll Cardiol* 2011; 58(8):820–8.
7. Noubade R, Wong K, Ota N, Rutz S, Eidenschenk C, Valdez PA, Ding J, Peng I, Sebrell A, Caplazi P, DeVoss J, Soriano RH, et al. NRROS negatively regulates reactive oxygen species during host defence and autoimmunity. *Nature* 2014; 509(7499):235–9.
8. Wisnovsky S, Jean SR, Kelley SO. Mitochondrial DNA repair and replication proteins revealed by targeted chemical probes. *Nat Chem Biol* 2016; 12(7):567–73.
9. Thomas JP, Maiorino M, Ursini F, Girotti AW. Protective action of phospholipid hydroperoxide glutathione peroxidase against membrane-damaging lipid peroxidation: in situ reduction of phospholipid and cholesterol hydroperoxides. *J Biol Chem* 1990; 265(1):454–61.
10. Cao X, Li C, Xiao S, Tang Y, Huang J, Zhao S, Li X, Li J, Zhang R, Yu W. Acetylation promotes TyrRS nuclear translocation to prevent oxidative damage. *Proc Natl Acad Sci USA* 2017; 114(4):687–92.
11. Arsenijevic D, Onuma H, Pecqueur C, Raimbault S, Manning BS, Miroux B, Couplan E, Alves-Guerra MC, Goubern M, Surwit R, Bouillaud F, Richard D, et al. Disruption of the uncoupling protein-2 gene in mice reveals a role in immunity and reactive oxygen species

production. *Nat Genet* 2000; 26(4):435–9.

12. Gao X, Dinkova-Kostova AT, Talalay P. Powerful and prolonged protection of human retinal pigment epithelial cells, keratinocytes, and mouse leukemia cells against oxidative damage: the indirect antioxidant effects of sulforaphane. *Proc Natl Acad Sci USA* 2001; 98(26):15221–6.

13. Talalay P, Fahey JW, Healy ZR, Wehage SL, Benedict AL, Min C, Dinkova-Kostova AT. Sulforaphane mobilizes cellular defenses that protect skin against damage by UV radiation. *Proc Natl Acad Sci USA* 2007; 104(44):17500–5.

14. Pekovic-Vaughan V, Gibbs J, Yoshitane H, Yang N, Pathiranage D, Guo B, Sagami A, Taguchi K, Bechtold D, Loudon A, Yamamoto M, Chan J, et al. The circadian clock regulates rhythmic activation of the NRF2/glutathione-mediated antioxidant defense pathway to modulate pulmonary fibrosis. *Genes Dev* 2014; 28(6):548–60.

15. Kerns ML, Hakim JM, Lu RG, Guo Y, Berroth A, Kaspar RL, Coulombe PA. Oxidative stress and dysfunctional NRF2 underlie pachyonychia congenita phenotypes. *J Clin Invest* 2016; 126(6):2356–66.

16. Nguyen T, Nioi P, Pickett CB. The Nrf2-antioxidant response element signaling pathway and its activation by oxidative stress. *J Biol Chem* 2009; 284(20):13291–5.

17. Chorley BN, Campbell MR, Wang X, Karaca M, Sambandan D, Bangura F, Xue P, Pi J, Kleeberger SR, Bell DA. Identification of novel NRF2-regulated genes by ChIP-Seq: influence on retinoid X receptor alpha. *Nucleic Acids Res* 2012; 40(15):7416–29.

18. Malhotra D, Portales-Casamar E, Singh A, Srivastava S, Arenillas D, Happel C, Shyr C, Wakabayashi N, Kensler TW, Wasserman WW, Biswal S. Global mapping of binding sites for Nrf2 identifies novel targets in cell survival response through ChIP-Seq profiling and network analysis. *Nucleic Acids Res* 2010; 38(17):5718–34.

19. Li Y, Huang TT, Carlson EJ, Melov S, Ursell PC, Olson JL, Noble LJ, Yoshimura MP, Berger C, Chan PH, Wallace DC, Epstein CJ. Dilated cardiomyopathy and neonatal lethality in mutant mice lacking manganese superoxide dismutase. *Nat Genet* 1995; 11(4):376–81.

20. Garratt M, Pichaud N, Glaros EN, Kee AJ, Brooks RC. Superoxide dismutase deficiency impairs olfactory sexual signaling and alters

bioenergetic function in mice. *Proc Natl Acad Sci USA* 2014; 111(22):8119–24.

21. Rosen DR, Siddique T, Patterson D, Figlewicz DA, Sapp P, Hentati A, Donaldson D, Goto J, O'Regan JP, Deng HX, et al. Mutations in Cu/Zn superoxide dismutase gene are associated with familial amyotrophic lateral sclerosis. *Nature* 1993; 362(6415):59–62.

22. Yim MB, Kang JH, Yim HS, Kwak HS, Chock PB, Stadtman ER. A gain-of-function of an amyotrophic lateral sclerosis-associated Cu,Zn-superoxide dismutase mutant: an enhancement of free radical formation due to a decrease in Km for hydrogen peroxide. *Proc Natl Acad Sci USA* 1996; 93(12):5709–14.

23. Bidhendi EE, Bergh J, Zetterstrom P, Andersen PM, Marklund SL, Brannstrom T. Two superoxide dismutase prion strains transmit amyotrophic lateral sclerosis-like disease. *J Clin Invest* 2016; 126(6):2249–53.

24. Hemachandra LP, Shin DH, Dier U, Iuliano JN, Engelberth SA, Uusitalo LM, Murphy SK, Hempel N. Mitochondrial superoxide dismutase has a protumorigenic role in ovarian clear cell carcinoma. *Cancer Res* 2015; 75(22):4973–84.

25. Hart PC, Mao M, de Abreu AL, Ansenberger-Fricano K, Ekoue DN, Ganini D, Kajdacsy-Balla A, Diamond AM, Minshall RD, Consolaro ME, Santos JH, Bonini MG. MnSOD upregulation sustains the Warburg effect via mitochondrial ROS and AMPK-dependent signalling in cancer. *Nat Commun* 2015; 6:6053.

26. Tsang CK, Liu Y, Thomas J, Zhang Y, Zheng XF. Superoxide dismutase 1 acts as a nuclear transcription factor to regulate oxidative stress resistance. *Nat Commun* 2014; 5:3446.

27. Rindler PM, Plafker SM, Szweda LI, Kinter M. High dietary fat selectively increases catalase expression within cardiac mitochondria. *J Biol Chem* 2013; 288(3):1979–90.

28. Vetrano AM, Heck DE, Mariano TM, Mishin V, Laskin DL, Laskin JD. Characterization of the oxidase activity in mammalian catalase. *J Biol Chem* 2005; 280(42):35372–81.

29. Schriner SE, Linford NJ, Martin GM, Treuting P, Ogburn CE, Emond M, Coskun PE, Ladiges W, Wolf N, Van Remmen H, Wallace DC, Rabinovitch PS. Extension of murine life span by overexpression of catalase targeted to mitochondria. *Science* 2005; 308(5730):1909–11.

30. Dai DF, Santana LF, Vermulst M, Tomazela DM, Emond MJ, MacCoss MJ, Gollahon K, Martin GM, Loeb LA, Ladiges WC, Rabinovitch

PS. Overexpression of catalase targeted to mitochondria attenuates murine cardiac aging. *Circulation* 2009; 119(21):2789–97.

31. Lee HY, Choi CS, Birkenfeld AL, Alves TC, Jornayvaz FR, Jurczak MJ, Zhang D, Woo DK, Shadel GS, Ladiges W, Rabinovitch PS, Santos JH, et al. Targeted expression of catalase to mitochondria prevents age-associated reductions in mitochondrial function and insulin resistance. *Cell Metab* 2010; 12(6):668–74.

32. Goth L, Eaton JW. Hereditary catalase deficiencies and increased risk of diabetes. *Lancet* 2000; 356(9244):1820–1.

33. Corrall RJ, Rodman HM, Margolis J, Landau BR. Stereospecificity of the oxidation of ethanol by catalase. *J Biol Chem* 1974; 249(10):3181–2.

34. Handler JA, Thurman RG. Redox interactions between catalase and alcohol dehydrogenase pathways of ethanol metabolism in the perfused rat liver. *J Biol Chem* 1990; 265(3):1510–5.

35. Clancy RM, Levartovsky D, Leszczynska-Piziak J, Yegudin J, Abramson SB. Nitric oxide reacts with intracellular glutathione and activates the hexose monophosphate shunt in human neutrophils: evidence for S-nitrosoglutathione as a bioactive intermediary. *Proc Natl Acad Sci USA* 1994; 91(9):3680–4.

36. Liu L, Yan Y, Zeng M, Zhang J, Hanes MA, Ahearn G, McMahon TJ, Dickfeld T, Marshall HE, Que LG, Stamler JS. Essential roles of S-nitrosothiols in vascular homeostasis and endotoxic shock. *Cell* 2004; 116(4):617–28.

37. Anders MW. Chemical toxicology of reactive intermediates formed by the glutathione-dependent bioactivation of halogen-containing compounds. *Chem Res Toxicol* 2008; 21(1):145–59.

38. Meister A. Glutathione-ascorbic acid antioxidant system in animals. *J Biol Chem* 1994; 269(13):9397–400.

39. Ishikawa T, Casini AF, Nishikimi M. Molecular cloning and functional expression of rat liver glutathione-dependent dehydroascorbate reductase. *J Biol Chem* 1998; 273(44):28708–12.

40. Alegre-Cebollada J, Kosuri P, Giganti D, Eckels E, Rivas-Pardo JA, Hamdani N, Warren CM, Solaro RJ, Linke WA, Fernandez JM. S-Glutathionylation of cryptic cysteines enhances titin elasticity by blocking protein folding. *Cell* 2014; 156(6):1235–46.

41. Banci L, Ciofi-Baffoni S, Gajda K, Muzzioli R, Peruzzini R, Winkelmann J. N-Terminal domains mediate [2Fe-2S] cluster transfer from glutaredoxin-3 to anamorsin. *Nat Chem Biol* 2015; 11(10):772–8.

42. Giacco F, Du X, D'Agati VD, Milne R, Sui G, Geoffrion M, Brownlee M. Knockdown of glyoxalase 1 mimics diabetic nephropathy in nondiabetic mice. *Diabetes* 2014; 63(1):291–9.

43. Xue M, Weickert MO, Qureshi S, Kandala NB, Anwar A, Waldron M, Shafie A, Messenger D, Fowler M, Jenkins G, Rabbani N, Thornalley PJ. Improved glycemic control and vascular function in overweight and obese subjects by glyoxalase 1 inducer formulation. *Diabetes* 2016; 65(8):2282–94.

44. Yang G, Cancino GI, Zahr SK, Guskjolen A, Voronova A, Gallagher D, Frankland PW, Kaplan DR, Miller FD. A Glo1-methylglyoxal pathway that is perturbed in maternal diabetes regulates embryonic and adult neural stem cell pools in murine offspring. *Cell Rep* 2016; 17(4):1022–36.

45. Hovatta I, Tennant RS, Helton R, Marr RA, Singer O, Redwine JM, Ellison JA, Schadt EE, Verma IM, Lockhart DJ, Barlow C. Glyoxalase 1 and glutathione reductase 1 regulate anxiety in mice. *Nature* 2005; 438(7068):662–6.

46. Distler MG, Plant LD, Sokoloff G, Hawk AJ, Aneas I, Wuenschell GE, Termini J, Meredith SC, Nobrega MA, Palmer AA. Glyoxalase 1 increases anxiety by reducing GABAA receptor agonist methylglyoxal. *J Clin Invest* 2012; 122(6):2306–15.

47. Reniere ML, Whiteley AT, Hamilton KL, John SM, Lauer P, Brennan RG, Portnoy DA. Glutathione activates virulence gene expression of an intracellular pathogen. *Nature* 2015; 517(7533):170–3.

48. Hall M, Grundstrom C, Begum A, Lindberg MJ, Sauer UH, Almqvist F, Johansson J, Sauer-Eriksson AE. Structural basis for glutathione-mediated activation of the virulence regulatory protein PrfA in Listeria. *Proc Natl Acad Sci USA* 2016; 113(51):14733–8.

49. Tew KD. Glutathione-associated enzymes in anticancer drug resistance. *Cancer Res* 1994; 54(16):4313–20.

50. Tew KD. Glutathione-associated enzymes in anticancer drug resistance. *Cancer Res* 2016; 76(1):7–9.

51. Harris IS, Treloar AE, Inoue S, Sasaki M, Gorrini C, Lee KC, Yung KY, Brenner D, Knobbe-Thomsen CB, Cox MA, Elia A, Berger T, et al. Glutathione and thioredoxin antioxidant pathways synergize to drive cancer initiation and

progression. *Cancer Cell* 2015; 27(2):211–22.

52. Lien EC, Lyssiotis CA, Juvekar A, Hu H, Asara JM, Cantley LC, Toker A. Glutathione biosynthesis is a metabolic vulnerability in PI₃K/Akt-driven breast cancer. *Nat Cell Biol* 2016; 18(5):572–8.

53. Nguyen VD, Saaranen MJ, Karala AR, Lappi AK, Wang L, Raykhel IB, Alanen HI, Salo KE, Wang CC, Ruddock LW. Two endoplasmic reticulum PDI peroxidases increase the efficiency of the use of peroxide during disulfide bond formation. *J Mol Biol* 2011; 406(3):503–15.

54. Utomo A, Jiang X, Furuta S, Yun J, Levin DS, Wang YC, Desai KV, Green JE, Chen PL, Lee WH. Identification of a novel putative non-selenocysteine containing phospholipid hydroperoxide glutathione peroxidase (NPGPx) essential for alleviating oxidative stress generated from polyunsaturated fatty acids in breast cancer cells. *J Biol Chem* 2004; 279(42):43522–9.

55. Chang YC, Yu YH, Shew JY, Lee WJ, Hwang JJ, Chen YH, Chen YR, Wei PC, Chuang LM, Lee WH. Deficiency of NPGPx, an oxidative stress sensor, leads to obesity in mice and human. *EMBO Mol Med* 2013; 5(8):1165–79.

56. Wei PC, Hsieh YH, Su MI, Jiang X, Hsu PH, Lo WT, Weng JY, Jeng YM, Wang JM, Chen PL, Chang YC, Lee KF, et al. Loss of the oxidative stress sensor NPGPx compromises GRP78 chaperone activity and induces systemic disease. *Mol Cell* 2012; 48(5):747–59.

57. Ursini F, Heim S, Kiess M, Maiorino M, Roveri A, Wissing J, Flohe L. Dual function of the selenoprotein PHGPx during sperm maturation. *Science* 1999; 285(5432):1393–6.

58. Yang WS, SriRamaratnam R, Welsch ME, Shimada K, Skouta R, Viswanathan VS, Cheah JH, Clemons PA, Shamji AF, Clish CB, Brown LM, Girotti AW, et al. Regulation of ferroptotic cancer cell death by GPX4. *Cell* 2014; 156(1–2):317–31.

59. Dixon SJ, Lemberg KM, Lamprecht MR, Skouta R, Zaitsev EM, Gleason CE, Patel DN, Bauer AJ, Cantley AM, Yang WS, Morrison B, 3rd, Stockwell BR. Ferroptosis: an iron-dependent form of nonapoptotic cell death. *Cell* 2012; 149(5):1060–72.

60. Yang WS, Kim KJ, Gaschler MM, Patel M, Shchepinov MS, Stockwell BR. Peroxidation of polyunsaturated fatty acids by lipoxygenases drives ferroptosis. *Proc Natl Acad Sci USA* 2016; 113(34):E4966–75.

61. Kagan VE, Mao G, Qu F, Angeli JP, Doll S, Croix CS, Dar HH, Liu B, Tyurin VA, Ritov VB, Kapralov AA, Amoscato AA, et al. Oxidized arachidonic and adrenic PEs navigate cells to ferroptosis. *Nat Chem Biol* 2017; 13(1):81–90.

62. Friedmann Angeli JP, Schneider M, Proneth B, Tyurina YY, Tyurin VA, Hammond VJ, Herbach N, Aichler M, Walch A, Eggenhofer E, Basavarajappa D, Radmark O, et al. Inactivation of the ferroptosis regulator Gpx4 triggers acute renal failure in mice. *Nat Cell Biol* 2014; 16(12):1180–91.

63. Chen L, Hambright WS, Na R, Ran Q. Ablation of the ferroptosis inhibitor glutathione peroxidase 4 in neurons results in rapid motor neuron degeneration and paralysis. *J Biol Chem* 2015; 290(47):28097–106.

64. Chabory E, Damon C, Lenoir A, Kauselmann G, Kern H, Zevnik B, Garrel C, Saez F, Cadet R, Henry-Berger J, Schoor M, Gottwald U, et al. Epididymis seleno-independent glutathione peroxidase 5 maintains sperm DNA integrity in mice. *J Clin Invest* 2009; 119(7):2074–85.

65. Shema R, Kulicke R, Cowley GS, Stein R, Root DE, Heiman M. Synthetic lethal screening in the mammalian central nervous system identifies Gpx6 as a modulator of Huntington's disease. *Proc Natl Acad Sci USA* 2015; 112(1):268–72.

66. Bjornstedt M, Xue J, Huang W, Akesson B, Holmgren A. The thioredoxin and glutaredoxin systems are efficient electron donors to human plasma glutathione peroxidase. *J Biol Chem* 1994; 269(47):29382–4.

67. Sies H, Sharov VS, Klotz LO, Briviba K. Glutathione peroxidase protects against peroxynitrite-mediated oxidations: a new function for selenoproteins as peroxynitrite reductase. *J Biol Chem* 1997; 272(44):27812–7.

68. Imai H, Hakkaku N, Iwamoto R, Suzuki J, Suzuki T, Tajima Y, Konishi K, Minami S, Ichinose S, Ishizaka K, Shioda S, Arata S, et al. Depletion of selenoprotein GPx4 in spermatocytes causes male infertility in mice. *J Biol Chem* 2009; 284(47):32522–32.

69. Ingold I, Aichler M, Yefremova E, Roveri A, Buday K, Doll S, Tasdemir A, Hoffard N, Wurst W, Walch A, Ursini F, Friedmann Angeli JP, et al. Expression of a catalytically inactive mutant form of glutathione peroxidase 4 (Gpx4) confers a dominant-negative effect in male fertility. *J Biol Chem* 2015; 290(23):14668–78.

70. Karplus PA, Schulz GE. Refined structure of glutathione reductase at 1.54 A resolution. *J Mol*

Biol 1987; 195(3):701–29.

71. Meister A. Glutathione metabolism and its selective modification. *J Biol Chem* 1988; 263(33):17205–8.

72. Morgan B, Ezerina D, Amoako TN, Riemer J, Seedorf M, Dick TP. Multiple glutathione disulfide removal pathways mediate cytosolic redox homeostasis. *Nat Chem Biol* 2013; 9(2):119–25.

73. Yang Y, Cheng JZ, Singhal SS, Saini M, Pandya U, Awasthi S, Awasthi YC. Role of glutathione S-transferases in protection against lipid peroxidation: overexpression of hGSTA2-2 in K562 cells protects against hydrogen peroxide-induced apoptosis and inhibits JNK and caspase 3 activation. *J Biol Chem* 2001; 276(22):19220–30.

74. Hiratsuka A, Yamane H, Yamazaki S, Ozawa N, Watabe T. Subunit Ya-specific glutathione peroxidase activity toward cholesterol 7-hydroperoxides of glutathione S-transferases in cytosols from rat liver and skin. *J Biol Chem* 1997; 272(8):4763–9.

75. Singh SP, Janecki AJ, Srivastava SK, Awasthi S, Awasthi YC, Xia SJ, Zimniak P. Membrane association of glutathione S-transferase mGSTA4-4, an enzyme that metabolizes lipid peroxidation products. *J Biol Chem* 2002; 277(6):4232–9.

76. Curtis JM, Grimsrud PA, Wright WS, Xu X, Foncea RE, Graham DW, Brestoff JR, Wiczer BM, Ilkayeva O, Cianflone K, Muoio DE, Arriaga EA, et al. Downregulation of adipose glutathione S-transferase A4 leads to increased protein carbonylation, oxidative stress, and mitochondrial dysfunction. *Diabetes* 2010; 59(5):1132–42.

77. Conklin DJ, Guo Y, Jagatheesan G, Kilfoil PJ, Haberzettl P, Hill BG, Baba SP, Guo L, Wetzelberger K, Obal D, Rokosh DG, Prough RA, et al. Genetic deficiency of glutathione S-transferase P increases myocardial sensitivity to ischemia-reperfusion injury. *Circ Res* 2015; 117(5):437–49.

78. Schroer KT, Gibson AM, Sivaprasad U, Bass SA, Ericksen MB, Wills-Karp M, Lecras T, Fitzpatrick AM, Brown LA, Stringer KF, Hershey GK. Downregulation of glutathione S-transferase pi in asthma contributes to enhanced oxidative stress. *J Allergy Clin Immunol* 2011; 128(3):539–48.

79. Whitworth AJ, Theodore DA, Greene JC, Benes H, Wes PD, Pallanck LJ. Increased glutathione S-transferase activity rescues dopaminergic neuron loss in a Drosophila model of Parkinson's disease. *Proc Natl Acad Sci USA* 2005; 102(22):8024–9.

80. Kim K, Kim SH, Kim J, Kim H, Yim J. Glutathione S-transferase omega 1 activity is sufficient to suppress neurodegeneration in a Drosophila model of Parkinson disease. *J Biol Chem* 2012; 287(9):6628–41.

81. Henderson CJ, Smith AG, Ure J, Brown K, Bacon EJ, Wolf CR. Increased skin tumorigenesis in mice lacking pi class glutathione S-transferases. *Proc Natl Acad Sci USA* 1998; 95(9):5275–80.

82. Ritchie KJ, Henderson CJ, Wang XJ, Vassieva O, Carrie D, Farmer PB, Gaskell M, Park K, Wolf CR. Glutathione transferase pi plays a critical role in the development of lung carcinogenesis following exposure to tobacco-related carcinogens and urethane. *Cancer Res* 2007; 67(19):9248–57.

83. Ritchie KJ, Walsh S, Sansom OJ, Henderson CJ, Wolf CR. Markedly enhanced colon tumorigenesis in Apc(Min) mice lacking glutathione S-transferase Pi. *Proc Natl Acad Sci USA* 2009; 106(49):20859–64.

84. Townsend DM, Manevich Y, He L, Hutchens S, Pazoles CJ, Tew KD. Novel role for glutathione S-transferase pi: regulator of protein S-glutathionylation following oxidative and nitrosative stress. *J Biol Chem* 2009; 284(1):436–45.

85. Adler V, Yin Z, Fuchs SY, Benezra M, Rosario L, Tew KD, Pincus MR, Sardana M, Henderson CJ, Wolf CR, Davis RJ, Ronai Z. Regulation of JNK signaling by GSTp. *EMBO J* 1999; 18(5):1321–34.

86. Wang T, Arifoglu P, Ronai Z, Tew KD. Glutathione S-transferase P1-1 (GSTP1-1) inhibits c-Jun N-terminal kinase (JNK1) signaling through interaction with the C terminus. *J Biol Chem* 2001; 276(24):20999–1003.

87. Okamura T, Antoun G, Keir ST, Friedman H, Bigner DD, Ali-Osman F. Phosphorylation of glutathione S-transferase P1 (GSTP1) by epidermal growth factor receptor (EGFR) promotes formation of the GSTP1-c-Jun N-terminal kinase (JNK) complex and suppresses JNK downstream signaling and apoptosis in brain tumor cells. *J Biol Chem* 2015; 290(52):30866–78.

88. Beer SM, Taylor ER, Brown SE, Dahm CC,

Costa NJ, Runswick MJ, Murphy MP. Glutaredoxin 2 catalyzes the reversible oxidation and glutathionylation of mitochondrial membrane thiol proteins: implications for mitochondrial redox regulation and antioxidant defense. *J Biol Chem* 2004; 279(46):47939–51.

89. Wells WW, Xu DP, Yang YF, Rocque PA. Mammalian thioltransferase (glutaredoxin) and protein disulfide isomerase have dehydroascorbate reductase activity. *J Biol Chem* 1990; 265(26):15361–4.

90. Song JJ, Rhee JG, Suntharalingam M, Walsh SA, Spitz DR, Lee YJ. Role of glutaredoxin in metabolic oxidative stress: glutaredoxin as a sensor of oxidative stress mediated by H_2O_2. *J Biol Chem* 2002; 277(48):46566–75.

91. Daily D, Vlamis-Gardikas A, Offen D, Mittelman L, Melamed E, Holmgren A, Barzilai A. Glutaredoxin protects cerebellar granule neurons from dopamine-induced apoptosis by dual activation of the ras-phosphoinositide 3-kinase and jun N-terminal kinase pathways. *J Biol Chem* 2001; 276(24):21618–26.

92. Murata H, Ihara Y, Nakamura H, Yodoi J, Sumikawa K, Kondo T. Glutaredoxin exerts an antiapoptotic effect by regulating the redox state of Akt. *J Biol Chem* 2003; 278(50):50226–33.

93. Prinarakis E, Chantzoura E, Thanos D, Spyrou G. S-Glutathionylation of IRF3 regulates IRF3-CBP interaction and activation of the IFN beta pathway. *EMBO J* 2008; 27(6):865–75.

94. Shelton MD, Kern TS, Mieyal JJ. Glutaredoxin regulates nuclear factor kappa-B and intercellular adhesion molecule in Muller cells: model of diabetic retinopathy. *J Biol Chem* 2007; 282(17):12467–74.

95. Brautigam L, Schutte LD, Godoy JR, Prozorovski T, Gellert M, Hauptmann G, Holmgren A, Lillig CH, Berndt C. Vertebrate-specific glutaredoxin is essential for brain development. *Proc Natl Acad Sci USA* 2011; 108(51):20532–7.

96. Brautigam L, Jensen LD, Poschmann G, Nystrom S, Bannenberg S, Dreij K, Lepka K, Prozorovski T, Montano SJ, Aktas O, Uhlen P, Stuhler K, et al. Glutaredoxin regulates vascular development by reversible glutathionylation of sirtuin 1. *Proc Natl Acad Sci USA* 2013; 110(50):20057–62.

97. Holmgren A. Hydrogen donor system for *Escherichia coli* ribonucleoside-diphosphate reductase dependent upon glutathione. *Proc Natl Acad Sci USA* 1976; 73(7):2275–9.

98. Zahedi Avval F, Holmgren A. Molecular mechanisms of thioredoxin and glutaredoxin as hydrogen donors for mammalian S phase ribonucleotide reductase. *J Biol Chem* 2009; 284(13):8233–40.

99. Banci L, Brancaccio D, Ciofi-Baffoni S, Del Conte R, Gadepalli R, Mikolajczyk M, Neri S, Piccioli M, Winkelmann J. [2Fe-2S] cluster transfer in iron-sulfur protein biogenesis. *Proc Natl Acad Sci USA* 2014; 111(17):6203–8.

100. Ye H, Jeong SY, Ghosh MC, Kovtunovych G, Silvestri L, Ortillo D, Uchida N, Tisdale J, Camaschella C, Rouault TA. Glutaredoxin 5 deficiency causes sideroblastic anemia by specifically impairing heme biosynthesis and depleting cytosolic iron in human erythroblasts. *J Clin Invest* 2010; 120(5):1749–61.

101. Wingert RA, Galloway JL, Barut B, Foott H, Fraenkel P, Axe JL, Weber GJ, Dooley K, Davidson AJ, Schmid B, Paw BH, Shaw GC, et al. Deficiency of glutaredoxin 5 reveals Fe-S clusters are required for vertebrate haem synthesis. *Nature* 2005; 436(7053):1035–39.

102. Huang Q, Zhou HJ, Zhang H, Huang Y, Hinojosa-Kirschenbaum F, Fan P, Yao L, Belardinelli L, Tellides G, Giordano FJ, Budas GR, Min W. Thioredoxin-2 inhibits mitochondrial reactive oxygen species generation and apoptosis stress kinase-1 activity to maintain cardiac function. *Circulation* 2015; 131(12):1082–97.

103. Holzerova E, Danhauser K, Haack TB, Kremer LS, Melcher M, Ingold I, Kobayashi S, Terrile C, Wolf P, Schaper J, Mayatepek E, Baertling F, et al. Human thioredoxin 2 deficiency impairs mitochondrial redox homeostasis and causes early-onset neurodegeneration. *Brain* 2016; 139(Pt 2):346–54.

104. Benhar M, Forrester MT, Hess DT, Stamler JS. Regulated protein denitrosylation by cytosolic and mitochondrial thioredoxins. *Science* 2008; 320(5879):1050–4.

105. Benhar M, Forrester MT, Stamler JS. Protein denitrosylation: enzymatic mechanisms and cellular functions. *Nat Rev Mol Cell Biol* 2009; 10(10):721–32.

106. Daloso DM, Muller K, Obata T, Florian A, Tohge T, Bottcher A, Riondet C, Bariat L, Carrari F, Nunes-Nesi A, Buchanan BB, Reichheld JP, et al. Thioredoxin, a master regulator of the tricarboxylic acid cycle in plant mitochondria. *Proc Natl Acad Sci USA* 2015; 112(11):E1392–400.

107. Shen X, Burguillos MA, Osman AM, Frijhoff J, Carrillo-Jimenez A, Kanatani S, Augsten M, Saidi D, Rodhe J, Kavanagh E, Rongvaux A, Rraklli V, et al. Glioma-induced inhibition of caspase-3 in microglia promotes a tumor-supportive phenotype. *Nat Immunol* 2016; 17(11):1282–90.

108. Bryk R, Griffin P, Nathan C. Peroxynitrite reductase activity of bacterial peroxiredoxins. *Nature* 2000; 407(6801):211–5.

109. Manta B, Hugo M, Ortiz C, Ferrer-Sueta G, Trujillo M, Denicola A. The peroxidase and peroxynitrite reductase activity of human erythrocyte peroxiredoxin 2. *Arch Biochem Biophys* 2009; 484(2):146–54.

110. Chen JW, Dodia C, Feinstein SI, Jain MK, Fisher AB. 1-Cys peroxiredoxin, a bifunctional enzyme with glutathione peroxidase and phospholipase A2 activities. *J Biol Chem* 2000; 275(37):28421–7.

111. Manevich Y, Sweitzer T, Pak JH, Feinstein SI, Muzykantov V, Fisher AB. 1-Cys peroxiredoxin overexpression protects cells against phospholipid peroxidation-mediated membrane damage. *Proc Natl Acad Sci SA* 2002; 99(18):11599–604.

112. Lee TH, Kim SU, Yu SL, Kim SH, Park DS, Moon HB, Dho SH, Kwon KS, Kwon HJ, Han YH, Jeong S, Kang SW, et al. Peroxiredoxin II is essential for sustaining life span of erythrocytes in mice. *Blood* 2003; 101(12):5033–8.

113. Neumann CA, Krause DS, Carman CV, Das S, Dubey DP, Abraham JL, Bronson RT, Fujiwara Y, Orkin SH, Van Etten RA. Essential role for the peroxiredoxin Prdx1 in erythrocyte antioxidant defence and tumour suppression. *Nature* 2003; 424(6948):561–5.

114. Matsushima S, Ide T, Yamato M, Matsusaka H, Hattori F, Ikeuchi M, Kubota T, Sunagawa K, Hasegawa Y, Kurihara T, Oikawa S, Kinugawa S, et al. Overexpression of mitochondrial peroxiredoxin-3 prevents left ventricular remodeling and failure after myocardial infarction in mice. *Circulation* 2006; 113(14):1779–86.

115. Fang J, Nakamura T, Cho DH, Gu Z, Lipton SA. S-Nitrosylation of peroxiredoxin 2 promotes oxidative stress-induced neuronal cell death in Parkinson's disease. *Proc Natl Acad Sci USA* 2007; 104(47):18742–7.

116. De Haes W, Frooninckx L, Van Assche R, Smolders A, Depuydt G, Billen J, Braeckman BP, Schoofs L, Temmerman L. Metformin promotes lifespan through mitohormesis via the peroxiredoxin PRDX-2. *Proc Natl Acad Sci USA* 2014; 111(24):E2501–9.

117. Pacifici F, Arriga R, Sorice GP, Capuani B, Scioli MG, Pastore D, Donadel G, Bellia A, Caratelli S, Coppola A, Ferrelli F, Federici M, et al. Peroxiredoxin 6, a novel player in the pathogenesis of diabetes. *Diabetes* 2014; 63(10):3210–20.

118. Molin M, Yang J, Hanzen S, Toledano MB, Labarre J, Nystrom T. Life span extension and H_2O_2 resistance elicited by caloric restriction require the peroxiredoxin Tsa1 in *Saccharomyces cerevisiae*. *Mol Cell* 2011; 43(5):823–33.

119. Hanzen S, Vielfort K, Yang J, Roger F, Andersson V, Zamarbide-Fores S, Andersson R, Malm L, Palais G, Biteau B, Liu B, Toledano MB, et al. Lifespan control by redox-dependent recruitment of chaperones to misfolded proteins. *Cell* 2016; 166(1):140–51.

120. Choi MH, Lee IK, Kim GW, Kim BU, Han YH, Yu DY, Park HS, Kim KY, Lee JS, Choi C, Bae YS, Lee BI, et al. Regulation of PDGF signalling and vascular remodelling by peroxiredoxin II. *Nature* 2005; 435(7040):347–53.

121. Netto LE, Antunes F. The Roles of Peroxiredoxin and thioredoxin in hydrogen peroxide sensing and in signal transduction. *Mol Cells* 2016; 39(1):65–71.

122. Woo HA, Yim SH, Shin DH, Kang D, Yu DY, Rhee SG. Inactivation of peroxiredoxin I by phosphorylation allows localized H_2O_2 accumulation for cell signaling. *Cell* 2010; 140(4):517–28.

123. Lim JM, Lee KS, Woo HA, Kang D, Rhee SG. Control of the pericentrosomal H_2O_2 level by peroxiredoxin I is critical for mitotic progression. *J Cell Biol* 2015; 210(1):23–33.

124. Sobotta MC, Liou W, Stocker S, Talwar D, Oehler M, Ruppert T, Scharf AN, Dick TP. Peroxiredoxin-2 and STAT3 form a redox relay for H_2O_2 signaling. *Nat Chem Biol* 2015; 11(1):64–70.

125. Sun QA, Kirnarsky L, Sherman S, Gladyshev VN. Selenoprotein oxidoreductase with specificity for thioredoxin and glutathione systems. *Proc Natl Acad Sci USA* 2001; 98(7):3673–8.

126. Su D, Novoselov SV, Sun QA, Moustafa ME, Zhou Y, Oko R, Hatfield DL, Gladyshev VN. Mammalian selenoprotein thioredoxin-glutathione reductase: roles in disulfide bond

formation and sperm maturation. *J Biol Chem* 2005; 280(28):26491–8.

127. Poet GJ, Oka OB, van Lith M, Cao Z, Robinson PJ, Pringle MA, Arner ES, Bulleid NJ. Cytosolic thioredoxin reductase 1 is required for correct disulfide formation in the ER. *EMBO J* 2017.

128. Lundstrom J, Holmgren A. Protein disulfide-isomerase is a substrate for thioredoxin reductase and has thioredoxin-like activity. *J Biol Chem* 1990; 265(16):9114–20.

129. Trigona WL, Mullarky IK, Cao Y, Sordillo LM. Thioredoxin reductase regulates the induction of haem oxygenase-1 expression in aortic endothelial cells. *Biochem J* 2006; 394(Pt 1):207–16.

130. Xia L, Nordman T, Olsson JM, Damdimopoulos A, Bjorkhem-Bergman L, Nalvarte I, Eriksson LC, Arner ES, Spyrou G, Bjornstedt M. The mammalian cytosolic selenoenzyme thioredoxin reductase reduces ubiquinone: a novel mechanism for defense against oxidative stress. *J Biol Chem* 2003; 278(4):2141–6.

131. May JM, Mendiratta S, Hill KE, Burk RF. Reduction of dehydroascorbate to ascorbate by the selenoenzyme thioredoxin reductase. *J Biol Chem* 1997; 272(36):22607–10.

132. Horstkotte J, Perisic T, Schneider M, Lange P, Schroeder M, Kiermayer C, Hinkel R, Ziegler T, Mandal PK, David R, Schulz S, Schmitt S, et al. Mitochondrial thioredoxin reductase is essential for early postischemic myocardial protection. *Circulation* 2011; 124(25):2892–902.

133. Sibbing D, Pfeufer A, Perisic T, Mannes AM, Fritz-Wolf K, Unwin S, Sinner MF, Gieger C, Gloeckner CJ, Wichmann HE, Kremmer E, Schafer Z, et al. Mutations in the mitochondrial thioredoxin reductase gene TXNRD2 cause dilated cardiomyopathy. *Eur Heart J* 2011; 32(9):1121–33.

134. Stanley BA, Sivakumaran V, Shi S, McDonald I, Lloyd D, Watson WH, Aon MA, Paolocci N. Thioredoxin reductase-2 is essential for keeping low levels of H_2O_2 emission from isolated heart mitochondria. *J Biol Chem* 2011; 286(38):33669–77.

135. Biteau B, Labarre J, Toledano MB. ATP-dependent reduction of cysteine-sulphinic acid by *S. cerevisiae* sulphiredoxin. *Nature* 2003; 425(6961):980–4.

136. Chang TS, Jeong W, Woo HA, Lee SM, Park S, Rhee SG. Characterization of mammalian sulfiredoxin and its reactivation of hyperoxidized peroxiredoxin through reduction of cysteine sulfinic acid in the active site to cysteine. *J Biol Chem* 2004; 279(49):50994–1001.

137. Noh YH, Baek JY, Jeong W, Rhee SG, Chang TS. Sulfiredoxin translocation into mitochondria plays a crucial role in reducing hyperoxidized peroxiredoxin III. *J Biol Chem* 2009; 284(13):8470–7.

138. Jonsson TJ, Johnson LC, Lowther WT. Structure of the sulphiredoxin-peroxiredoxin complex reveals an essential repair embrace. *Nature* 2008; 451(7174):98–101.

139. Jonsson TJ, Murray MS, Johnson LC, Lowther WT. Reduction of cysteine sulfinic acid in peroxiredoxin by sulfiredoxin proceeds directly through a sulfinic phosphoryl ester intermediate. *J Biol Chem* 2008; 283(35):23846–51.

140. Findlay VJ, Townsend DM, Morris TE, Fraser JP, He L, Tew KD. A novel role for human sulfiredoxin in the reversal of glutathionylation. *Cancer Res* 2006; 66(13):6800–6.

141. Park JW, Mieyal JJ, Rhee SG, Chock PB. Deglutathionylation of 2-Cys peroxiredoxin is specifically catalyzed by sulfiredoxin. *J Biol Chem* 2009; 284(35):23364–74.

142. Sunico CR, Sultan A, Nakamura T, Dolatabadi N, Parker J, Shan B, Han X, Yates JR, 3rd, Masliah E, Ambasudhan R, Nakanishi N, Lipton SA. Role of sulfiredoxin as a peroxiredoxin-2 denitrosylase in human iPSC-derived dopaminergic neurons. *Proc Natl Acad Sci USA* 2016; 113(47):E7564–E71.

143. Kil IS, Ryu KW, Lee SK, Kim JY, Chu SY, Kim JH, Park S, Rhee SG. Circadian oscillation of sulfiredoxin in the mitochondria. *Mol Cell* 2015; 59(4):651–63.

144. Kil IS, Lee SK, Ryu KW, Woo HA, Hu MC, Bae SH, Rhee SG. Feedback control of adrenal steroidogenesis via H_2O_2-dependent, reversible inactivation of peroxiredoxin III in mitochondria. *Mol Cell* 2012; 46(5):584–94.

145. Lowther WT, Brot N, Weissbach H, Honek JF, Matthews BW. Thiol-disulfide exchange is involved in the catalytic mechanism of peptide methionine sulfoxide reductase. *Proc Natl Acad Sci USA* 2000; 97(12):6463–8.

146. Sagher D, Brunell D, Hejtmancik JF, Kantorow M, Brot N, Weissbach H. Thionein can serve as a reducing agent for the methionine sulfoxide reductases. *Proc Natl Acad Sci USA* 2006; 103(23):8656–61.

147. Lim JC, You Z, Kim G, Levine RL. Methionine sulfoxide reductase A is a stereospecific

methionine oxidase. *Proc Natl Acad Sci USA* 2011; 108(26):10472–7.

148. Moskovitz J, Flescher E, Berlett BS, Azare J, Poston JM, Stadtman ER. Overexpression of peptide-methionine sulfoxide reductase in *Saccharomyces cerevisiae* and human T cells provides them with high resistance to oxidative stress. *Proc Natl Acad Sci USA* 1998; 95(24):14071–5.

149. Kantorow M, Hawse JR, Cowell TL, Benhamed S, Pizarro GO, Reddy VN, Hejtmancik JF. Methionine sulfoxide reductase A is important for lens cell viability and resistance to oxidative stress. *Proc Natl Acad Sci USA* 2004; 101(26):9654–9.

150. Yermolaieva O, Xu R, Schinstock C, Brot N, Weissbach H, Heinemann SH, Hoshi T. Methionine sulfoxide reductase A protects neuronal cells against brief hypoxia/reoxygenation. *Proc Natl Acad Sci USA* 2004; 101(5):1159–64.

151. Shao B, Cavigiolio G, Brot N, Oda MN, Heinecke JW. Methionine oxidation impairs reverse cholesterol transport by apolipoprotein A-I. *Proc Natl Acad Sci USA* 2008; 105(34):12224–9.

152. Purohit A, Rokita AG, Guan X, Chen B, Koval OM, Voigt N, Neef S, Sowa T, Gao Z, Luczak ED, Stefansdottir H, Behunin AC, et al. Oxidized Ca^{2+}/calmodulin-dependent protein kinase II triggers atrial fibrillation. *Circulation* 2013; 128(16):1748–57.

153. Ahmed ZM, Yousaf R, Lee BC, Khan SN, Lee S, Lee K, Husnain T, Rehman AU, Bonneux S, Ansar M, Ahmad W, Leal SM, et al. Functional null mutations of MSRB3 encoding methionine sulfoxide reductase are associated with human deafness DFNB74. *Am J Hum Genet* 2011; 88(1):19–29.

154. Kwon TJ, Cho HJ, Kim UK, Lee E, Oh SK, Bok J, Bae YC, Yi JK, Lee JW, Ryoo ZY, Lee SH, Lee KY, et al. Methionine sulfoxide reductase B3 deficiency causes hearing loss due to stereocilia degeneration and apoptotic cell death in cochlear hair cells. *Hum Mol Genet* 2014; 23(6):1591–601.

155. Moskovitz J, Bar-Noy S, Williams WM, Requena J, Berlett BS, Stadtman ER. Methionine sulfoxide reductase (MsrA) is a regulator of antioxidant defense and lifespan in mammals. *Proc Natl Acad Sci USA* 2001; 98(23):12920–5.

156. Ruan H, Tang XD, Chen ML, Joiner ML, Sun G, Brot N, Weissbach H, Heinemann SH, Iverson L, Wu CF, Hoshi T. High-quality life extension by the enzyme peptide methionine sulfoxide reductase. *Proc Natl Acad Sci USA* 2002; 99(5):2748–53.

157. Hung RJ, Spaeth CS, Yesilyurt HG, Terman JR. SelR reverses Mical-mediated oxidation of actin to regulate F-actin dynamics. *Nat Cell Biol* 2013; 15(12):1445–54.

158. Lee BC, Peterfi Z, Hoffmann FW, Moore RE, Kaya A, Avanesov A, Tarrago L, Zhou Y, Weerapana E, Fomenko DE, Hoffmann PR, Gladyshev VN. MsrB1 and MICALs regulate actin assembly and macrophage function via reversible stereoselective methionine oxidation. *Mol Cell* 2013; 51(3):397–404.

159. Duckers HJ, Boehm M, True AL, Yet SF, San H, Park JL, Clinton Webb R, Lee ME, Nabel GJ, Nabel EG. Heme oxygenase-1 protects against vascular constriction and proliferation. *Nat Med* 2001; 7(6):693–8.

160. Juan SH, Lee TS, Tseng KW, Liou JY, Shyue SK, Wu KK, Chau LY. Adenovirus-mediated heme oxygenase-1 gene transfer inhibits the development of atherosclerosis in apolipoprotein E-deficient mice. *Circulation* 2001; 104(13):1519–25.

161. Hinkel R, Lange P, Petersen B, Gottlieb E, Ng JK, Finger S, Horstkotte J, Lee S, Thormann M, Knorr M, El-Aouni C, Boeksltegers P, et al. Heme oxygenase-1 gene therapy provides cardioprotection via control of post-ischemic inflammation: an experimental study in a pre-clinical pig model. *J Am Coll Cardiol* 2015; 66(2):154–65.

162. Wenzel P, Rossmann H, Muller C, Kossmann S, Oelze M, Schulz A, Arnold N, Simsek C, Lagrange J, Klemz R, Schonfelder T, Brandt M, et al. Heme oxygenase-1 suppresses a pro-inflammatory phenotype in monocytes and determines endothelial function and arterial hypertension in mice and humans. *Eur Heart J* 2015; 36(48):3437–46.

163. Tzima S, Victoratos P, Kranidioti K, Alexiou M, Kollias G. Myeloid heme oxygenase-1 regulates innate immunity and autoimmunity by modulating IFN-beta production. *J Exp Med* 2009; 206(5):1167–79.

164. Chung SW, Liu X, Macias AA, Baron RM, Perrella MA. Heme oxygenase-1-derived carbon monoxide enhances the host defense response to microbial sepsis in mice. *J Clin Invest* 2008; 118(1):239–47.

165. Pamplona A, Ferreira A, Balla J, Jeney V, Balla G, Epiphanio S, Chora A, Rodrigues CD, Gregoire IP, Cunha-Rodrigues M, Portugal S, Soares MP, et al. Heme oxygenase-1 and carbon monoxide suppress the pathogenesis of experimental cerebral malaria. *Nat Med* 2007; 13(6):703–10.

166. Chora AA, Fontoura P, Cunha A, Pais TF, Cardoso S, Ho PP, Lee LY, Sobel RA, Steinman L, Soares MP. Heme oxygenase-1 and carbon monoxide suppress autoimmune neuroinflammation. *J Clin Invest* 2007; 117(2):438–47.

167. Schallner N, Pandit R, LeBlanc R, 3rd, Thomas AJ, Ogilvy CS, Zuckerbraun BS, Gallo D, Otterbein LE, Hanafy KA. Microglia regulate blood clearance in subarachnoid hemorrhage by heme oxygenase-1. *J Clin Invest* 2015; 125(7):2609–25.

168. Zhu Y, Luo S, Sabo Y, Wang C, Tong L, Goff SP. Heme oxygenase 2 binds myristate to regulate retrovirus assembly and TLR4 signaling. *Cell Host Microbe* 2017.

169. Hsu FF, Yeh CT, Sun YJ, Chiang MT, Lan WM, Li FA, Lee WH, Chau LY. Signal peptide peptidase-mediated nuclear localization of heme oxygenase-1 promotes cancer cell proliferation and invasion independent of its enzymatic activity. *Oncogene* 2015; 34(18):2360–70.

170. Di Biase S, Lee C, Brandhorst S, Manes B, Buono R, Cheng CW, Cacciottolo M, Martin-Montalvo A, de Cabo R, Wei M, Morgan TE, Longo VD. Fasting-mimicking diet reduces HO-1 to promote t cell-mediated tumor cytotoxicity. *Cancer Cell* 2016; 30(1):136–46.

171. Beyer RE, Segura-Aguilar J, Di Bernardo S, Cavazzoni M, Fato R, Fiorentini D, Galli MC, Setti M, Landi L, Lenaz G. The role of DT-diaphorase in the maintenance of the reduced antioxidant form of coenzyme Q in membrane systems. *Proc Natl Acad Sci USA* 1996; 93(6):2528–32.

172. Siegel D, Bolton EM, Burr JA, Liebler DC, Ross D. The reduction of alpha-tocopherolquinone by human NAD(P)H:quinone oxidoreductase: the role of alpha-tocopherolhydroquinone as a cellular antioxidant. *Mol Pharmacol* 1997; 52(2):300–5.

173. Siegel D, Gustafson DL, Dehn DL, Han JY, Boonchoong P, Berliner LJ, Ross D. NAD(P)H:quinone oxidoreductase 1: role as a superoxide scavenger. *Mol Pharmacol* 2004; 65(5):1238–47.

174. Zhu H, Jia Z, Mahaney JE, Ross D, Misra HP, Trush MA, Li Y. The highly expressed and inducible endogenous NAD(P)H:quinone oxidoreductase 1 in cardiovascular cells acts as a potential superoxide scavenger. *Cardiovasc Toxicol* 2007; 7(3):202–11.

175. Adikesavan AK, Barrios R, Jaiswal AK. In vivo role of NAD(P)H:quinone oxidoreductase 1 in metabolic activation of mitomycin C and bone marrow cytotoxicity. *Cancer Res* 2007; 67(17):7966–71.

176. Pink JJ, Planchon SM, Tagliarino C, Varnes ME, Siegel D, Boothman DA. NAD(P)H:quinone oxidoreductase activity is the principal determinant of beta-lapachone cytotoxicity. *J Biol Chem* 2000; 275(8):5416–24.

177. Asher G, Lotem J, Cohen B, Sachs L, Shaul Y. Regulation of p53 stability and p53-dependent apoptosis by NADH quinone oxidoreductase 1. *Proc Natl Acad Sci USA* 2001; 98(3):1188–93.

178. Anwar A, Dehn D, Siegel D, Kepa JK, Tang LJ, Pietenpol JA, Ross D. Interaction of human NAD(P)H:quinone oxidoreductase 1 (NQO1) with the tumor suppressor protein p53 in cells and cell-free systems. *J Biol Chem* 2003; 278(12):10368–73.

179. Asher G, Tsvetkov P, Kahana C, Shaul Y. A mechanism of ubiquitin-independent proteasomal degradation of the tumor suppressors p53 and p73. *Genes Dev* 2005; 19(3):316–21.

180. Garate M, Wong RP, Campos EI, Wang Y, Li G. NAD(P)H quinone oxidoreductase 1 inhibits the proteasomal degradation of the tumour suppressor p33(ING1b). *EMBO Rep* 2008; 9(6):576–81.

181. Alard A, Fabre B, Anesia R, Marboeuf C, Pierre P, Susini C, Bousquet C, Pyronnet S. NAD(P)H quinone-oxydoreductase 1 protects eukaryotic translation initiation factor 4GI from degradation by the proteasome. *Mol Cell Biol* 2010; 30(4):1097–105.

182. Nosjean O, Ferro M, Coge F, Beauverger P, Henlin JM, Lefoulon F, Fauchere JL, Delagrange P, Canet E, Boutin JA. Identification of the melatonin-binding site MT3 as the quinone reductase 2. *J Biol Chem* 2000; 275(40):31311–7.

183. Mailliet F, Ferry G, Vella F, Thiam K, Delagrange P, Boutin JA. Organs from mice deleted for NRH:quinone oxidoreductase 2 are deprived of the melatonin binding site MT3. *FEBS Lett* 2004; 578(1–2):116–20.

184. Draganov DI, Teiber JF, Speelman A, Osawa Y, Sunahara R, La Du BN. Human paraoxonases (PON1, PON2, and PON3) are lactonases with overlapping and distinct substrate specificities. *J Lipid Res* 2005; 46(6):1239–47.

185. Chambers JE. PON1 multitasks to protect health. *Proc Natl Acad Sci USA* 2008; 105(35):12639–40.

186. Horke S, Witte I, Wilgenbus P, Kruger M, Strand D, Forstermann U. Paraoxonase-2 reduces oxidative stress in vascular cells and decreases endoplasmic reticulum stress-induced caspase activation. *Circulation* 2007; 115(15):2055–64.

187. Ng CJ, Wadleigh DJ, Gangopadhyay A, Hama S, Grijalva VR, Navab M, Fogelman AM, Reddy ST. Paraoxonase-2 is a ubiquitously expressed protein with antioxidant properties and is capable of preventing cell-mediated oxidative modification of low density lipoprotein. *J Biol Chem* 2001; 276(48):44444–9.

188. Ruiz J, Blanche H, James RW, Garin MC, Vaisse C, Charpentier G, Cohen N, Morabia A, Passa P, Froguel P. Gln-Arg192 polymorphism of paraoxonase and coronary heart disease in type 2 diabetes. *Lancet* 1995; 346(8979):869–72.

189. Regieli JJ, Jukema JW, Doevendans PA, Zwinderman AH, Kastelein JJ, Grobbee DE, van der Graaf Y. Paraoxonase variants relate to 10-year risk in coronary artery disease: impact of a high-density lipoprotein-bound antioxidant in secondary prevention. *J Am Coll Cardiol* 2009; 54(14):1238–45.

190. Bouman HJ, Schomig E, van Werkum JW, Velder J, Hackeng CM, Hirschhauser C, Waldmann C, Schmalz HG, ten Berg JM, Taubert D. Paraoxonase-1 is a major determinant of clopidogrel efficacy. *Nat Med* 2011; 17(1):110–6.

191. Shih DM, Gu L, Xia YR, Navab M, Li WF, Hama S, Castellani LW, Furlong CE, Costa LG, Fogelman AM, Lusis AJ. Mice lacking serum paraoxonase are susceptible to organophosphate toxicity and atherosclerosis. *Nature* 1998; 394(6690):284–7.

192. Tward A, Xia YR, Wang XP, Shi YS, Park C, Castellani LW, Lusis AJ, Shih DM. Decreased atherosclerotic lesion formation in human serum paraoxonase transgenic mice. *Circulation* 2002; 106(4):484–90.

193. Ng CJ, Bourquard N, Grijalva V, Hama S, Shih DM, Navab M, Fogelman AM, Lusis AJ, Young S, Reddy ST. Paraoxonase-2 deficiency aggravates atherosclerosis in mice despite lower apolipoprotein-B-containing lipoproteins: anti-atherogenic role for paraoxonase-2. *J Biol Chem* 2006; 281(40):29491–500.

194. Shih DM, Xia YR, Wang XP, Wang SS, Bourquard N, Fogelman AM, Lusis AJ, Reddy ST. Decreased obesity and atherosclerosis in human paraoxonase 3 transgenic mice. *Circ Res* 2007; 100(8):1200–7.

195. She ZG, Zheng W, Wei YS, Chen HZ, Wang AB, Li HL, Liu G, Zhang R, Liu JJ, Stallcup WB, Zhou Z, Liu DP, et al. Human paraoxonase gene cluster transgenic overexpression represses atherogenesis and promotes atherosclerotic plaque stability in ApoE-null mice. *Circ Res* 2009; 104(10):1160–8.

196. Tasinato A, Boscoboinik D, Bartoli GM, Maroni P, Azzi A. d-alpha-Tocopherol inhibition of vascular smooth muscle cell proliferation occurs at physiological concentrations, correlates with protein kinase C inhibition, and is independent of its antioxidant properties. *Proc Natl Acad Sci USA* 1995; 92(26):12190–4.

197. Park SJ, Ahmad F, Philp A, Baar K, Williams T, Luo H, Ke H, Rehmann H, Taussig R, Brown AL, Kim MK, Beaven MA, et al. Resveratrol ameliorates aging-related metabolic phenotypes by inhibiting cAMP phosphodiesterases. *Cell* 2012; 148(3):421–33.

198. Jimenez-Gomez Y, Mattison JA, Pearson KJ, Martin-Montalvo A, Palacios HH, Sossong AM, Ward TM, Younts CM, Lewis K, Allard JS, Longo DL, Belman JP, et al. Resveratrol improves adipose insulin signaling and reduces the inflammatory response in adipose tissue of rhesus monkeys on high-fat, high-sugar diet. *Cell Metab* 2013; 18(4):533–45.

199. Milne JC, Lambert PD, Schenk S, Carney DP, Smith JJ, Gagne DJ, Jin L, Boss O, Perni RB, Vu CB, Bemis JE, Xie R, et al. Small molecule activators of SIRT1 as therapeutics for the treatment of type 2 diabetes. *Nature* 2007; 450(7170):712–6.

200. Lagouge M, Argmann C, Gerhart-Hines Z, Meziane H, Lerin C, Daussin F, Messadeq N, Milne J, Lambert P, Elliott P, Geny B, Laakso M, et al. Resveratrol improves mitochondrial function and protects against metabolic disease by activating SIRT1 and PGC-1alpha. *Cell* 2006; 127(6):1109–22.

201. DeNicola GM, Karreth FA, Humpton TJ, Gopinathan A, Wei C, Frese K, Mangal D, Yu KH, Yeo CJ, Calhoun ES, Scrimieri F, Winter

JM, et al. Oncogene-induced Nrf2 transcription promotes ROS detoxification and tumorigenesis. *Nature* 2011; 475(7354):106–9.

202. Mitsuishi Y, Taguchi K, Kawatani Y, Shibata T, Nukiwa T, Aburatani H, Yamamoto M, Motohashi H. Nrf2 redirects glucose and glutamine into anabolic pathways in metabolic reprogramming. *Cancer Cell* 2012; 22(1):66–79.

203. Zavattari P, Perra A, Menegon S, Kowalik MA, Petrelli A, Angioni MM, Follenzi A, Quagliata L, Ledda-Columbano GM, Terracciano L, Giordano S, Columbano A. Nrf2, but not beta-catenin, mutation represents an early event in rat hepatocarcinogenesis. *Hepatology* 2015; 62(3):851–62.

204. Chio, II, Jafarnejad SM, Ponz-Sarvise M, Park Y, Rivera K, Palm W, Wilson J, Sangar V, Hao Y, Ohlund D, Wright K, Filippini D, et al. NRF2 promotes tumor maintenance by modulating mRNA translation in pancreatic cancer. *Cell* 2016; 166(4):963–76.

205. Wang H, Liu X, Long M, Huang Y, Zhang L, Zhang R, Zheng Y, Liao X, Wang Y, Liao Q, Li W, Tang Z, et al. NRF2 activation by antioxidant antidiabetic agents accelerates tumor metastasis. *Sci Transl Med* 2016; 8(334):334ra51.

206. Piskounova E, Agathocleous M, Murphy MM, Hu Z, Huddlestun SE, Zhao Z, Leitch AM, Johnson TM, DeBerardinis RJ, Morrison SJ. Oxidative stress inhibits distant metastasis by human melanoma cells. *Nature* 2015; 527(7577):186–91.

Glossary of Essentials of Free Radical Biology and Medicine

CITATION | *Hopkins RZ and Li YR. Essentials of Free Radical Biology and Medicine. Cell Med Press, Raleigh, NC, USA. 2017. http://dx.doi.org/10.20455/efrbm.2017.glossary*

A

Alkoxyl radical (RO· or LO·): A reactive oxygen species that is typically formed during lipid peroxidation and acts as a potent oxidizing species.

Antioxidant enzyme mimetics: Synthetic small molecular mass compounds that catalytically metabolize reactive oxygen species, including superoxide, hydrogen peroxide, and peroxynitrite. The most commonly used antioxidant enzyme mimetics are metalloporphyrin compounds. For example, MnTBAP and MnTMPyP act as superoxide dismutase and catalase mimetics, and FeTMPyP, FeTMPS, and FeTPPS act as peroxynitrite decomposition catalysts.

Antioxidant response element (ARE): see Nuclear factor E2-related factor 2 (Nrf2)

Antioxidant: Any substance that, when present at a level of biological, physiological, or pharmacological relevance, can prevent, reduce, or repair the oxidant (e.g., reactive oxygen species)-induced damage of a target biomolecule.

Antioxidative/anti-inflammatory defenses: Due to the fact that reactive oxygen species and inflammation are intimately intertwined, many antioxidant enzymes or proteins, as well as non-protein antioxidants also possess anti-inflammatory activities. Hence, the compound term "antioxidative/anti-inflammatory defenses" is sometimes used to describe these antioxidative molecules. The most notable example of an antioxidative/anti-inflammatory enzyme is heme oxygenase-1 (see Section 6.2 of Appendix B).

Antioxidative/phase 2 proteins: see Phase 2 enzymes (phase 2 proteins)

Antoine-Laurent Lavoisier (1743–1794): A French chemist, who along with Carl Wilhelm Scheele (1742–1786) and Joseph Priestley (1733–1804), discovered oxygen in the 1770s.

Aquaporins (AQP): Commonly known as water channels, which represent a family of integral membrane proteins that serve as channels in the transfer of water, and in some cases, small polar solutes (e.g., glycerol, amino acids, sugars) across the membrane. Currently, there are at least 13 aquaporins in mammals, namely, AQP1–13. Some aquaporins, such as AQP3, AQP8, and AQP9, also transport hydrogen peroxide across cell membrane.

B

Biological ozone: see Ozone (O_3)

Biological system: The term is frequently used, but often ill-defined in the field of free radical biology and medicine. In this book, the term biological system is tentatively defined as a system consisting of biological entities or processes, such as organisms, organs, tissues, cells, or biomolecules, or combinations of them. A biomolecule is a molecule produced by living cells, e.g., a protein, carbohydrate, lipid, or nucleic acid.

Biomarker: A characteristic that is objectively measured and evaluated as an indicator of normal biological processes, pathogenic processes, or pharmacological responses to a therapeutic intervention. Oxidative stress biomarker may be defined as a molecular change in a biological molecule (e.g., a lipid, protein, or DNA molecule) that has arisen from attack by reactive oxygen species and related reactive species, and such a molecular change can be objectively measured and evaluated as an indicator of disease pathogenesis and development. According to this definition, a valid oxidative stress biomarker should be predictive of disease pathogenesis and disease progression.

Biomolecule: see Biological system

C

Caenorhabditis elegans: A widely used model organism to study animal development and others. This soil nematode offers great potential for genetic analysis, partly because of its rapid (3-day) life cycle, small size (1.5 mm-long adult), and ease of laboratory cultivation. This organism is also commonly used to study the impact of reactive oxygen species on longevity.

Cancer photodynamic therapy: Using photosensitizers and visible light in combination with molecular oxygen to produce reactive oxygen species to kill the cancer cells. Photodynamic therapy (PDT) is also used in the management of other disease conditions, including acne, certain dermatitis, and infections.

Carbon monoxide (CO): An environmental pollutant as well as an endogenously produced gaseous signaling molecule in biological systems. Heme oxygenase is currently the only mammalian enzyme found to produce carbon monoxide.

Carl Wilhelm Scheele (1742−1786): A Swedish chemist, who along with Joseph Priestley (1733−1804) and Antoine-Laurent Lavoisier (1743−1794), discovered oxygen in the 1770s.

Carotenoids: Carotenoids are a family of compounds of over six hundred fat-soluble plant pigments that provide much of the color we see in nature. The major carotenoids in human diets include β-carotene, α-carotene, lycopene, lutein, zeaxanthin,

β-cryptoxanthin, and astaxanthin. Many, if not all, carotenoids are potent scavengers of singlet oxygen in biological systems.

Causal relationship: see Risk factor

Cell senescence: The phenomenon by which normal diploid cells lose the ability to divide, normally after certain numbers of cell divisions in vitro. Free radicals and related reactive species can cause cell senescence.

Cell signal transduction: see Cell signaling

Cell signaling: The ability of cells to detect changes in their environment to generate an appropriate physiological response upon information processing. Cell signaling and cell signal transduction are frequently used interchangeably in the literature. Signaling molecules are the protein and non-protein molecules involved in cell signaling. Second messengers are small signaling molecules (e.g., cyclic adenosine monophosphate [cAMP], Ca^{2+}, and diacylglycerol) that are generated upon receptor activation by the extracellular stimulus (also known as extracellular signaling molecule or first messenger) and diffuse away from their source, spreading the signal to other parts of the cell. Certain reactive oxygen species, such as nitric oxide and hydrogen peroxide, act as second messengers.

Cell transformation: The change that a normal cell undergoes as it becomes malignant. Free radicals and related reactive species can cause cell transformation.

Cystathionine β-synthase (CBS): see Hydrogen sulfide (H_2S)

Cystathionine γ-lyase (CSE): see Hydrogen sulfide (H_2S)

D

Death rate or mortality rate: The relative frequency with which death occurs within some specified interval of time in a population. Mortality rate is typically expressed as number of deaths per 100,000 individuals per year.

Disease incidence: The number of new cases of a disease that develop in a population per unit of time. The unit of time for incidence is not necessarily one year although we often discuss incidence in terms of one year.

Disease prevalence: An estimate of how many people have a disease at a given point or period in time. Prevalence is sometimes expressed as a percentage of population.

Dismutation: A reaction between two identical molecules in which one is reduced and the other oxidized.

Dose-response relationship: The change in effect on, or response of, an organism caused by differing levels of exposure (or doses) to a factor (usually a chemical, a drug, or a pathogen) after a certain exposure time.

E

Electrophile (electrophilic species): An electron-deficient species that undergoes covalent reactions by accepting an electron pair from an electron-rich biomolecule, such as a protein or DNA molecule. The electron-rich biomolecule is known as a nucleophile. α,β-Unsaturated aldehydes are good examples of electrophiles produced in biological systems as a result of lipid peroxidation.

Electrophile response element (EpRE): see Nuclear factor E2-related factor 2 (Nrf2)

eNOS uncoupling: see Uncoupling of endothelial nitric oxide synthase (eNOS)

Epidemiology: The study of the distribution and determinants of health-related states or events in specified populations and the application of this study to control health problems. The objectives of epidemiology include: (1) identification of the etiology or cause of a disease and the relevant risk factors; (2) determination of the extent of disease found in the community; (3) study of the natural history and prognosis of disease; (4) evaluation of both existing and newly developed preventive and therapeutic measures and modes of health care delivery; and (5) providing the foundation for developing public policy relating to environmental problems, genetic issues, and other considerations regarding disease prevention and health promotion.

EPR spectrometer: see Paramagnetism

EPR: see Paramagnetism

ESR: see Paramagnetism

F

Fenton reaction: see Haber–Weiss reaction

Fenton-type reaction: see Haber–Weiss reaction

Ferritin: A 24-subunit intracellular protein whose principal role within mammalian cells is the storage of iron in a nontoxic, but bioavailable, form.

First messenger: see Cell signaling

Flavonoids: see Phenolic compounds

Free radical biology and medicine: The study of free radicals and related reactive species and antioxidants in biological systems and their roles in human health and disease.

Free radical paradigm: A recently coined term to define the scope of free radical biology and medicine and offer a framework for understanding the basic biology of free radicals and related reactive species and antioxidants, as well as their roles in human health and disease.

Free radical: Any chemical species capable of independent existence that contains one or more unpaired electrons. An unpaired electron refers to the one that occupies an atomic or molecular orbital by itself. Hydrogen atom ($H^\bullet$) is the simplest free radical as it contains only one electron (which is certainly unpaired). A superscript dot ($^\bullet$) is frequently used to indicate the unpaired electron and denote that the species is a free radical.

G

Genome: see Redox proteome

Genomics: see Redox proteome

Glucose 6-phosphate dehydrogenase (G6PD): see Pentose phosphate pathway

γ-Glutamylcysteine ligase (γGCL): Also known as γ-glutamylcysteine synthetase (γGCS), the key enzyme involved in the biosynthesis of reduced glutathione (GSH). It catalyzes the formation of γ-glutamylcysteine from the reaction of glutamate and cysteine. Glutathine synthetase (GSS) catalyzes the formation of GSH from the reaction of γ-glutamylcysteine and glycine.

γ-Glutamylcysteine synthetase (γGCS): see γ-Glutamylcysteine ligase (γGCL)

Glutathione synthetase (GSS): see γ-Glutamylcysteine ligase (γGCL)

Glutaredoxin (Grx): A term that refers to a family of reduced glutathione (GSH)-dependent enzymes that catalyze the reduction of glutathionylated proteins. This reduction reaction is known as deglutathionylation. Protein glutathionylation (also known as protein S-glutathionylation) refers to the covalent attachment of glutathione to a protein cysteine residue via a disulfide bridge. There are currently 4 mammalian Grxs, namely, Grx1, Grx2, Grx3, and Grx5. Grx4 is only present in lower eukaryotes.

Glutathione disulfide (GSSG): see Glutathione

Glutathione peroxidase (GPx): A term that refers to a family of multiple isozymes that catalyze the reduction of H_2O_2 or organic hydroperoxides to water or corresponding alcohols using reduced glutathione (GSH) as an electron donor. Currently there are eight mammalian GPx isozymes, namely, GPx1, 2, 3, 4, 5, 6, 7, and 8. GPx may also decompose peroxynitrite to form nitrite and water.

Glutathione reductase (GR): A homodimeric flavoprotein that catalyzes the formation of reducled glutathione (GSH) from glutathione disulfide (GSSG) at the expense of the reduced form of nicotinamide adenine dinucleotide phosphate (NADPH).

Glutathione S-transferase (GST): A term that refers to a superfamily of enzymes that catalyze the conjugation of reduced glutathione (GSH) to a wide variety of xenobiotics and play important roles in protecting mammalian cells and tissues from electrophilic and oxidative stress. Some GST isozymes also regulate cellular processes via non-GSH conjugation-dependent mechanisms. Mammalian GST isozymes are classified into three main families: (1) cytosolic GSTs; (2) mitochondrial GSTs; and (3) microsomal GSTs.

Glutathione system: A major cellular antioxidant defense system that includes the reduced form of glutathione (GSH), glutathione peroxidase, glutathione reductase, glutathione S-transferase, and glutaredoxin.

Glutathione: A term, if not specifies, typically refers to both the reduced form (GSH) and the oxidized form (GSSG) of glutathione. GSSG is also called glutathione disulfide. GSSG is reduced to GSH by glutathione reductase (GR or GSR).

Great Oxidation Event (GOE): The increase of oxygen in the atmosphere 2.4–2.1 billion years ago. GOE is believed to lead to the emergence of earliest animals on Earth.

H

Haber–Weiss reaction: The reaction between superoxide and hydrogen peroxide to give rise to hydroxyl radical, hydroxide ion, and molecular oxygen. This reaction proceeds slowly and can be dramatically accelerated by iron ions, which is known as iron-catalyzed Haber–Weiss reaction. The iron-catalyzed Haber–Weiss reaction can be written in two sequential sub-reactions: (1) $O_2^{\cdot-} + Fe^{3+} \rightarrow O_2 + Fe^{2+}$, and (2) $Fe^{2+} + H_2O_2 \rightarrow Fe^{3+} + OH^{\cdot} + OH^-$. The second reaction is commonly referred to as the Fenton reaction, which is also frequently called the Fenton chemistry. Other transition metal ions such as Cu^{1+} also react with hydrogen peroxide to form hydroxyl radical, and such reactions are called Fenton-type reactions.

Heme oxygenase (HO): A term that refers to a family of two major isozymes, namely, HO-1 and HO-2 that catalyze the first and rate-limiting step in the oxidative degradation of heme to eventually produce bilirubin along with the release of carbon monoxide and ferrous iron. HO enzymes, especially HO-1 possess potent antioxidative and anti-inflammatory activities.

HO-1: see Heme oxygenase (HO)

Homolysis: Also known as homolytic fission or homolytic cleavage referring to the cleavage of a bond so that each of the molecular fragments between which the bond is broken retains one of the bonding electrons. Thus, the products of homolysis are free radicals.

Hydrogen gas (H_2): A gas that is mainly produced in the gut via bacteria-mediated fermentation of dietary components. It is recognized as a potent antioxidant protecting against diverse disease processes.

Hydrogen peroxide (H_2O_2): One of the most extensively investigated reactive oxygen species produced in biological systems. It is also recognized as a signaling molecule. Hydrogen peroxide occurs ubiquitously in both animal and plant cells, as well as microorganisms. It is also found in Earth's atmosphere as well as interstellar space.

Hydrogen sulfide (H_2S): An environmental pollutant as well as an endogenously produced gaseous signaling molecule in biological systems. H_2S is produced endogenously via enzymatic activity of cystathionine β-synthase (CBS) or cystathionine γ-lyase (CSE), nonenzymatic pathways (such as reduction of thiol-containing molecules), and is also released from intracellular sulfur stores (sulfane sulfur).

Hydroxyl radical (HO˙): Probably the most powerful oxidizing reactive oxygen species in biology and medicine with a standard reduction potential of +2300 mV.

Hypochlorous acid (HOCl): An active ingredient of household bleach. It is also produced in biological systems, especially by phagocytic cells during respiratory burst to kill invading pathogens.

I

Iron-catalyzed Haber–Weiss reaction: see Haber–Weiss reaction

Iron-sulfur cluster [Fe-S]: Iron-sulfur [Fe-S] clusters, including [2Fe-2S], [4Fe-4S], and [3Fe-4S], are ubiquitous and evolutionarily ancient prosthetic groups that are required to sustain fundamental life processes. [Fe-S] clusters participate in electron transfer, substrate binding/activation, iron/sulfur storage, regulation of gene expression, and enzyme activity. [Fe-S] cluster-containing proteins are called iron-sulfur proteins (e.g., aconitase, succinate dehydrogenase), which are typically susceptible to redox modulation by reactive oxygen species.

Iron-sulfur protein: see Iron-sulfur cluster [Fe-S]

J

James Lorrain Smith (1862−1931): A Scottish pathologist who pioneered the oxygen toxicity research in the late 19th century and discovered the fatal pulmonary damage resulting from exposure to hyperoxia. As such, pulmonary oxygen toxicity is also known as the "Lorrain Smith effect".

Joseph Priestley (1733−1804): An English radical Unitarian minister and chemist, who along with Carl Wilhelm Scheele (1742−1786) and Antoine-Laurent Lavoisier (1743−1794), discovered oxygen in the 1770s. Priestley also discovered nitric oxide (NO) in 1772.

L

Lipid peroxidation: Oxidation of lipids, especially polyunsaturated fatty acids (PUFAs). Free radical-triggered lipid peroxidation proceeds through the following three steps: initiation, propagation, and termination. Lipid peroxidation gives rise to secondary reactive species, including alkoxyl and peroxyl radicals, singlet oxygen, and electrophilic aldehydes, among others.

Lorrain Smith effect: see James Lorrain Smith (1862–1931).

M

Metabolome: see Redox proteome

Metabolomics: see Redox proteome

Metallothionein (MT): A term that refers to a superfamily of small molecular mass proteins (6–7 kDa) with high cysteine content and the capacity to bind various heavy metals, including zinc, copper, cadmium, and mercury.

Methionine sulfoxide reductase (Msr): A term that refers to two structurally unrelated classes of thiol-dependent enzymes, namely, MsrA and MsrB that catalyze the reduction of methionine S-sulfoxide and methionine R-sulfoxide, respectively. Msr enzymes are crucial for repairing oxidative protein damage.

Mitochondrial electron transport chain: Also known as mitochondrial electron transport enzyme complexes, including complex I (NADH:ubiquinone oxidoreductase), complex II (succinate:ubiquinone oxidoreductase), complex III (ubiquinone:cytochrome c oxidoreductase), and complex IV (cytochrome c oxidase). Mitochondrial complex V (ATP synthase) is not part of the electron transport chain.

Mortality: The total number of deaths attributable to a given disease in a population during a specific interval of time, usually a year.

N

NAD(P)H:quinone oxidoreductase (NQO): A term that refers to a family of flavoproteins that include two members, NQO1 and NQO2 in mammals. NQO1 and NQO2 stand for NAD(P)H:quinone oxidoreductase 1 and NRH:quinone oxidoreductase 2, respectively. NQO2 uses dihydronicotinamide riboside (NRH) rather than NAD(P)H as the electron donor. Both NQO1 and NQO2 catalyze two-electron reduction of various quinones and derivatives.

NADPH oxidase: see NOX

NF-κB: see Nuclear factor kappaB

Nitration: see Nitrative stress

Nitrative stress: A condition under which the levels of reactive nitrogen species (RNS) overwhelm the capacity of RNS-detoxification mechanisms in a biological system. Nitrative stress is associated with nitration of biomolecules, leading to cell and tissue injury. Nitration refers to the addition of a nitro ($-NO_2$) group to a compound. Nitration can be caused by peroxynitrite and nitrogen dioxide.

Nitric oxide (NO or NO˙): Also called nitric monoxide, a gaseous signaling molecule playing important physiological roles. Overproduction of nitric oxide also contributes to disease process.

Nitrosation: see Nitrosative stress

Nitrosative stress: A condition induced by nitric oxide (NO˙) or related species, leading to the formation of nitrosation of critical protein cysteine thiols (this is commonly known as S-nitrosylation) or nitrosylation of metallocofactors of proteins. Nitrosation refers to the addition of a nitroso ($-NO$)

group to a thiol group of a protein via covalent binding. This is also known as S-nitrosation. On the other hand, nitrosylation refers to the non-covalent binding of a nitrosyl (NO bound to a metal) group to the redox active metal ion center of a protein. However, the above nomenclature is not strictly adopted in the field of free radical biology and medicine. In this context, S-nitrosation and S-nitrosylation are frequently used interchangeably.

Nitrosylation: see Nitrosative stress

NOX/DUOX family: see NOX

NOX: Denoting NADPH oxidase. The NOX enzyme family currently has 5 members, namely, NOX1, NOX2, NOX3, NOX4, and NOX5. The NOX1–5 along with the dual oxidases (DUOX 1 and DUOX 2) are now members of an enzyme family, known as the NOX/DUOX family.

NQO1: see NAD(P)H:quinone oxidoreductase (NQO)

NQO2: see NAD(P)H:quinone oxidoreductase (NQO)

Nrf2: see Nuclear factor E2-related factor 2

Nuclear factor E2-related factor 2 (Nrf2): Nrf2 is a member of the vertebrate Cap'n'Collar (CNC) transcription factor subfamily of basic leucine zipper (bZip) transcription factors. Other members of the CNC subfamily of transcription factors include Nrf1, Nrf3, and p45 NF-E2. Nrf2 plays a central role in regulating both the constitutive and inducible expression of a wide variety of antioxidative/ cytoprotective genes in mammals. Nrf2 normally resides in the cytosolic compartment via association with a cytosolic actin-binding protein, Keap1 (Kelch-like ECH-associated protein 1), which is also known as INrf2 (inhibitor of Nrf2). Keap1 plays a central role in controlling Nrf2 activity. Keap1 exists as dimers inside the cells and functions as a substrate linker protein for the interaction of Cul3/Rbx1-based E3-ubiquitin ligase complex with Nrf2, leading to continuous ubiquitination of Nrf2 and its proteasomal degradation. Hence, the continuous degradation of Nrf2 under basal conditions keeps the Nrf2 level low and thereby maintains low basal levels of Nrf2-regulated genes. When the cells encounter stresses, such as exposure to oxidants or chemical inducers, Nrf2 dissociates from Keap1, becomes stabilized, and then translocates into the nuclei. Inside the nuclei, Nrf2 interacts with other protein factors, including small Maf (sMaf), and binds to the antioxidant response element (ARE), also known as electrophile response element (EpRE), a unique cis-acting regulatory sequence (core sequence:5′-TGACNNNGC-3′) found in the 5′-regulatory region of a number of antioxidative/cytoprotective genes, leading to their increased transcription.

Nuclear factor kappaB (NF-κB): NF-κB (full name: nuclear factor κ-light-chain-enhancer of activated B cells) is a family of transcription factors that regulate diverse cellular processes, including cytokine production and inflammatory responses, cell survival and proliferation, and cell differentiation, among others. NF-κB has been recognized as a member of Rel family of transcription factors. In mammals, there are five different members to compose the NF-κB family: p65 (RelA), RelB, c-Rel, p50/p105 (NF-κB1), and p52/p100 (NF-κB2). The most widely studied form of NF-κB is a heterodimer of the p50 and p65 subunits and is a potent activator of gene transcription. In the literature of free radical biology and medicine, the term NF-κB, if not specified, typically refers to the p50/p65 heterodimer. NF-κB is activated by a wide variety of agents including free radicals and related reactive species.

Nucleophile: see Electrophile

O

Odds ratio: see Odds

Odds: The ratio of the probability of occurrence of an event to that of non-occurrence, or the ratio of the probability that something is so, to the probability that it is not so. Odds ratio (also known as relative risk) is defined as the ratio of the odds of an event in one group to the odds of an event in another group.

One-electron reduction potential: see Reduction potential

Oxidant stress: see Oxidative stress

Oxidative stress biomarker: see Biomarker

Oxidative stress: Condition where the levels of reactive oxygen species (ROS) significantly overwhelm the capacity of antioxidant defenses, leading to potential damage in a biological system. Oxidative stress condition can be caused by either increased ROS formation or decreased activity of antioxidants or both in a biological system. Oxidative stress is recognized as an important contributor to diverse disease processes. The term oxidant stress is interchangeable with oxidative stress, but less commonly used in the literature.

Oxygen free radical: see Reactive oxygen species

Oxygen radical: see Reactive oxygen species

Ozone (O₃): A gas in the stratosphere (commonly known as stratospheric ozone) that protects animals on Earth from solar irradiation. It is also an air pollutant near Earth's surface (commonly known as tropospheric O_3). Ozone has been suggested to be produced in biological systems via an antibody- or amino acid-catalyzed water oxidation pathway. Biologically produced ozone may be part of the innate immunity.

P

Paramagnetism: The magnetic state of a chemical species with one or more unpaired electrons. The unpaired electrons are attracted by a magnetic field due to the electrons' magnetic dipole moments. Hence, free radicals are paramagnetic and can be detected by electron paramagnetic resonance (EPR) spectrometry, also known as electron spin resonance (ESR) spectrometry. The Bruker (www.bruker.com) EMX spectrometer is perhaps the most widely used EPR instrument in the field of free radical research. EPR technique is considered the most specific way for detecting free radicals in biological systems. Due to relatively low sensitivity of EPR detection and the fact that biologically relevant free radicals are typically in low concentrations and very short-lived, it is difficult, if not impossible, to directly detect these free radicals by EPR spectrometry. This dilemma can be circumvented by EPR detection of more stable secondary radical adducts formed by adding exogenous spin traps—molecules that react with primary free radical species to give rise to longer-lasting free radical adducts with characteristic EPR signatures that can accumulate to levels permitting detection. This technique is commonly known as spin-trapping or EPR spin-trapping detection of free radicals.

Paraoxonase (PON): A term that refers to a family of enzymes that includes three members in mammals, namely, PON1, PON2, and PON3. PON enzymes possess antioxidant activities and protect against oxidative stress, especially in cardiovascular system.

Paul Bert (1833−1886): A French physiologist, who pioneered the oxygen toxicity research in the late 19th century. The central nervous system (CNS) effect of hyperoxia is thus also known as the "Paul Bert effect".

Paul Bert effect: see Paul Bert (1833−1886)

Pentose phosphate pathway: A metabolic process that breaks down glucose 6-phosphate to pentose with the production of NADPH. The two enzymes involved in the production of NADPH are glucose 6-phosphate dehydrogenase (G6PD) and 6-phosphogluconate dehydrogenase (6PGD), with the former as the key enzyme of the pathway.

Peroxiredoxin (Prx): A term that refers to family of small (22–27 kDa) nonseleno peroxidases currently known to possess six mammalian isozymes, namely, Prx1–6. Prx isozymes catalyze the decomposition of H_2O_2, organic hydroperoxides, and possibly peroxynitrite.

Peroxyl radical (ROO˙ or LOO˙): A reactive oxygen species that is typically formed during lipid peroxidation and acts as a potent oxidizing species.

Peroxynitrite (ONOO⁻): Also known as peroxynitrite anion that is typically formed from the bi-radical reaction between superoxide and nitrogen oxide in biological systems. Peroxynitrite is a typical example of reactive nitrogen species. It is also classified as a reactive oxygen species.

Phagocytic respiratory burst: see Respiratory burst

Phase 2 enzymes (phase 2 proteins): This ill-defined term is used loosely in the field of free radical biology and medicine to refer to enzymes that are involved in phase 2 biotransformation reactions, with glutathione S-transferase and UDP-glucuronosyltransferase as prototypical examples. Phase 1 and phase 2 reactions are related to biotransformation (also known as metabolism) of xenobiotics. Phase 1 biotransformation reactions include oxidation, reduction, and hydrolysis, whereas phase 2 biotransformation involves primarily conjugation reactions, such as conjugation with endogenous cellular ligands (e.g., glutathione and glucuronic acid). In addition to the classical conjugation enzymes, other enzymes and proteins have also been considered as phase 2 enzymes/proteins in the literature. These include (in alphabetical order) aflatoxin B1 dehydrogenase, dihydrodiol dehydrogenase, epoxide hydrolase, ferritin, γ-glutamylcysteine ligase, heme oxygenase-1, leukotriene B4 dehydrogenase, and NAD(P)H:quinone oxidoreductase 1. Some of the above phase 2 proteins, such as γ-glutamylcysteine ligase, heme oxygenase-1, and ferritin, are typically classified as antioxidants. As such, the compound term, "antioxidative/phase 2 proteins" is seen in the literature to refer to the above protein molecules.

Phenolic compounds: Phenolic compounds, also called phenols or phenolics, are a class of chemicals consisting of one or more hydroxyl group (–OH) bonded directly to one or more six-membered aromatic rings. Monophenols contain one such aromatic hydroxyl group, whereas compounds containing two such hydroxyl groups are called biphenols. Polyphenols are those that contain more than two such hydroxyl groups. Dietary phenolic compounds are usually classified into five classes: (1) flavonoids (e.g., genistein); (2) stilbenes (e.g., resveratrol); (3) phenolic acids (e.g., caffeic acid); (4) lignans (e.g., secoisolariciresinol); and (5) others (e.g., curcumin). Among dietary phenolic compounds, flavonoids are the most commonly studied compounds. Flavonoids are further classified into the following six subclasses: (1) flavonols (e.g., quercetin); (2) flavones (e.g., luteolin); (3) isoflavones (e.g., genistein); (4) flavanones (e.g., taxifolin); (5) anthocyanidins (e.g., delphinidin); and (6) flavanols (e.g., epigallocatechin-3-gallate).

6-Phosphogluconate dehydrogenase (6PGD): see Pentose phosphate pathway

Photodynamic therapy (PDT): see Cancer photodynamic therapy

Photosensitivity reaction: In a photosensitivity reaction, an endogenous photosensitizer molecule (PS) (e.g., a porphyrin, flavin, or quinone molecule) is converted to an excited state (PS*) upon illumination by light. The excitation energy is then transferred to molecular oxygen (O_2), converting it to singlet oxygen, while the photosensitizer molecule returns to the ground state.

Polyphenols: see Phenolic compounds

Protein carbonyl group: A carbon atom double-bonded to an oxygen atom (C=O) in a protein molecule, which can be formed as a consequence of oxidation of the amino acid residues of a protein by reactive oxygen species (ROS). In free radical biology and medicine, protein carbonylation typically refers to the formation of reactive aldehydes or reactive ketones following ROS attack of the protein. Such carbonyl groups can react with 2,4-dinitrophenylhydrazine to form hydrazones, enabling their detection in a biological system as a biomarker for oxidative protein damage.

Protein carbonylation: see Protein carbonyl group

Protein deglutathionylation: see Glutaredoxin (Grx)

Protein S-glutathionylation: Also known as protein glutathionylation; see Glutaredoxin (Grx)

Protein tyrosine nitration: The addition of a nitro ($-NO_2$) group adjacent to the hydroxyl group on the aromatic ring of the tyrosine residue. Protein tyrosin nitration (3-nitrotyrosine) is commonly used as a biomarker for the formation of reactive nitrogen species.

Proteome: see Redox proteome

Proteomics: see Redox proteome

R

Reactive chlorine species (RCS): Chlorine-containing reactive species, with hypochlorous acid (HOCl) as a prototype. A more generalized term, namely, reactive halogen species, is also sometimes encountered in the literature, and this term refers to halogen (e.g., Cl and Br)-containing reactive species that include HOCl and hypobromous acid (HOBr). Both HOCl and HOBr are produced by granulocytes during their respiratory burst.

Reactive halogen species: see Reactive chlorine species

Reactive nitrogen species (RNS): Nitrogen-containing reactive species that include nitric oxide (NO˙), peroxynitrite (ONOO⁻), nitrogen dioxide radical (NO_2˙), and other oxides of nitrogen or nitrogen-containing reactive species. As RNS are almost exclusively oxygen-containing species, by definition, they also belong to ROS. The compound term "reactive oxygen and nitrogen species (ROS/RNS)" is often used to refer to a group of ROS and RNS commonly seen in biological systems.

Reactive oxygen and nitrogen species (ROS/RNS): see Reactive nitrogen species

Reactive oxygen intermediates (ROIs): see Reactive oxygen species

Reactive oxygen metabolites (ROMs): see Reactive oxygen species

Reactive oxygen species (ROS): Oxygen-containing reactive species. It is a collective term to include superoxide (O_2˙⁻), hydrogen peroxide (H_2O_2), hydroxyl radical (OH˙), singlet oxygen ($^1O_2$), peroxyl radical (LOO˙), alkoxyl radical (LO˙), lipid hydroperoxide (LOOH), peroxynitrite (ONOO⁻), nitric oxide (NO), nitrogen dioxide (NO_2˙), carbonate radical (CO_3˙⁻), hypochlorous acid (HOCl), and ozone (O_3). Some ROS, such as superoxide, hydroxyl radical, and nitrogen dioxide are free radicals and hence are also called oxygen free radicals or oxygen radicals. Although the term ROS is most commonly used, other equivalent terms are also available, including reactive oxygen intermediates (ROIs), reactive oxygen metabolites (ROMs), and reactive oxygen.

Reactive oxygen: see Reactive oxygen species

Redox biology: The term redox refers to reduction-oxidation. Redox biology is a relatively new field that is concerned with the study of oxidation-reduction processes associated with living things. Redox homeostasis refers to a dynamic process involving redox reactions to ensure normal physiology in a biological system. Reactive oxygen species and antioxidant molecules are the key players in redox homeostasis. Disruption of redox homeostasis contributes to disease pathophysiology.

Redox homeostasis: see Redox biology

Redox metabolome: see Redox proteome

Redox modulation: see Redox signaling

Redox potential: see Reduction potential

Redox proteome: Components of the proteome that undergo reversible redox reactions and those modified by reactive oxygen species or related chemical entities. Proteome is the entire set of proteins expressed by a genome, cell, tissue, or organism under certain conditions. Proteomics may be simply defined as the large-scale study/analysis of proteins produced by the genome of a particular cell, tissue, or organism. Other related terms include metabolome, metabolomics, redox metabolome, genome, and genomics. Metabolome is simply defined as the total number of metabolites present within a cell, tissue, or organism. Metabolomics is the large-scale study/analysis of the entire set of metabolites present within a cell, tissue, or organism. Redox metabolome is a redox-active subset of the metabolome, with $NADPH/NADP^+$, GSH/GSSG (reduced form of glutathione/oxidized form of glutathione), and cysteine/cystine being specifically relevant to the redox proteome. Genome is the complete set of genes or genetic material present in a cell or organism. Genomics is the study of the genome.

Redox regulation: see Redox signaling

Redox signaling: The process wherein reactive oxygen species (ROS) or related chemical entities act as second messengers to cause physiological cellular responses via redox reactions. It is necessary to emphasize the difference between redox signaling and redox modulation. Redox signaling emphasizes a physiological process, where ROS act as second messengers to mediate responses that are required for proper function and survival of the cell. On the other hand, redox modulation (or redox regulation) refers to a process wherein ROS alter the activity or function of the redox-sensitive molecular targets, including signaling proteins and metabolic enzymes, leading to either physiological or pathophysiological responses.

Redox: see Redox biology

Reduced glutathione (GSH): Also called reduced form of glutathione; see Glutathione

Reduction potential: Reduction potential is also less commonly known as redox potential. If it is measured at standard conditions (see next), the reduction potential is called standard reduction potential. Standard reduction potential (E_0) may be defined as the potential in volts or millivolts generated by a reduction half-reaction of a redox reaction compared to the standard hydrogen electrode at the standard conditions (i.e., 25°C, 1 atmosphere, 1 M concentration). Hence, reduction potential indicates the tendency of a chemical species to acquire electrons and thereby be reduced during the redox reaction. The more positive the reduction potential is, the more likely the chemical species will be reduced. If the reaction involves a single electron transfer, it is called one-electron reduction. A related term is standard oxidation reduction. It can be defined as the potential in volts or millivolts generated by an oxidation half-reaction of a redox reaction compared to the standard hydrogen electrode at the standard conditions.

Respiratory burst: This term typically refers to an increase in oxygen consumption and reactive oxygen species production by phagocytic cells (e.g., macrophages, neutrophils) as a result of the activation of their membrane NADPH oxidase during phagocytosis of microorganisms.

Risk factor: An exposure, behavior, or attribute that, if present and active, clearly increases the probability of a particular disease in a group of people who have the risk factor compared with an otherwise similar group of people who do not. Risk factor is one of the three fundamental types of causal relationships. The other two are sufficient cause and necessary cause. The former refers to that if the factor (cause) is present, the effect (disease) will always occur, and latter refers to that the factor (cause) must be present for the effect (disease) to occur.

RNS: see Reactive nitrogen species

ROS/RNS: see Reactive nitrogen species

ROS: see Reactive oxygen species

S

Second messenger: see Cell signaling

Singlet oxygen ($^1O_2$): An electronically excited form of molecular oxygen. There are two types of singlet oxygen, namely, $(^1\Delta_g)^1O_2$ and $(^1\Sigma_g^+)^1O_2$. The $^1\Sigma_g^+$ form is a free radical of higher energy that undergoes rapid decay rather than chemical reactions. This form of singlet oxygen is thus regarded to be too short-lived to be of any significance in biological systems.

Singlet oxygen is the major active species responsible for the efficacy of photodynamic therapy.

Signaling molecule: see Cell signaling

SOD1: see Superoxide dismutase

SOD2: see Superoxide dismutase

SOD3: see Superoxide dismutase

Spin-trapping (EPR spin-trapping): see Paramagnetism

Standard reduction potential: see Reduction potential

Statistics: The study of the collection, organization, analysis, and interpretation of data.

Stratospheric ozone: see Ozone (O_3)

Sulfiredoxin (Srx): A recently identified small molecular mass (~13 kDa) antioxidant enzyme that catalyzes the reduction of sulfinic peroxiredoxins in the presence of adenosine triphosphate (ATP) and using thioredoxin or reduced glutathione (GSH) as an electron donor.

Superoxide ($O_2^{\cdot-}$): Also known as superoxide anion or superoxide anion radical. It is produced from one electron reduction of molecular oxygen ($O_2 + e^- \rightarrow O_2^{\cdot-}$) in biological systems. Superoxide is also present in oceans, deserts, and the universe (e.g., Mars).

Superoxide dismutase: The term superoxide dismutase (SOD) refers to a family of enzymes that catalyze the dismutation of superoxide to hydrogen peroxide and molecular oxygen. There are three isozymes of SOD in mammalian systems: SOD1 (or CuZnSOD), SOD2 (or MnSOD), and SOD3 (or ECSOD).

T

Thioredoxin (Trx): A term that refers to a family of small redox proteins (~12 kDa) that undergo NADPH-dependent reduction by thioredoxin reductase and in turn reduce the disulfide bridge in target proteins. Currently, there are three mammalian Trx isozymes: Trx1, Trx2, and sperm Trx.

Thioredoxin glutathione reductase (TGR): see Thioredoxin reductase (TrxR)

Thioredoxin reductase (TrxR): A term that refers to a class of enzymes that catalyze the reduction of oxidized thioredoxin. There are three major isozymes of TrxR in mammals: TrxR1, TrxR2, and TrxR3. TrxR3 is commonly known as thioredoxin glutathione reductase (TGR).

Thioredoxin system: Another important antioxidant system that includes thioredoxin, peroxiredoxin, thioredoxin reductase, and sulfiredoxin.

α-Tocopherol: see Vitamin E

Tropospheric ozone: see Ozone (O_3)

U

Uncoupling of endothelial nitric oxide synthase (eNOS): eNOS uncoupling refers to a state, in which eNOS switches from producing nitric oxide (NO) to generating superoxide. Oxidative modification of eNOS and its co-factors by free radicals and related species may cause eNOS uncoupling. The consequence of eNOS uncoupling is two-fold: (1) decreased NO bioavailability, and (2) increased formation of superoxide and peroxynitrite.

Uncoupling proteins (UCP): Members of the anion carrier protein family located in the inner mitochondrial membrane. Currently there are five uncoupling proteins in mammalian cells, namely, UCP1, UCP2, UCP3, UCP4, and UCP5. These proteins act as proton channels or transporters and dissipate the proton gradient across the mitochondrial inner membrane. Uncoupling proteins, especially UCP2, may regulate mitochondrial reactive oxygen species production.

V

Vascular peroxidases (VPO): Recently identified novel heme-containing peroxidases expressed in cardiovascular tissues. VPO1 is highly expressed in both the heart and the vascular wall, whereas VPO2 is highly expressed only in the heart.

Vitamin C: Also known as ascorbic acid or ascorbate which is a water-soluble molecule synthesized endogenously in animals except humans, monkeys, guinea pigs, and several other animal species. Humans lost this capability as a result of a series inactivating mutations of the gene encoding gulonolactone oxidase, a key enzyme in vitamin C biosynthesis. Ascorbic acid ($AscH_2$) has two ionizable hydroxyl groups. At a physiological pH, ascorbic acid exists predominantly as a monoanion, i.e., ascorbate monoanion ($AscH^-$). $AscH^-$ acts as a reducing agent and is converted to ascorbate radical ($Asc^{\cdot-}$, also known as semidehydroascorbate) after donation of one electron. After losing another electron, $Asc^{\cdot-}$ is converted to dehydroascorbate (DHA). DHA can be reduced by either one electron to $Asc^{\cdot-}$ or by two electrons to $AscH^-$.

Vitamin E: Vitamin E is a nutritional term, and natural dietary vitamin E comprises of eight different forms: α-, β-, γ-, and δ-tocopherols and α-, β-, γ-, and δ-tocotrienols. Tocotrienols have unsaturated side-chain, whereas tocopherols contain a phytyl tail with three chiral centers that naturally occur in the RRR configuration. Among the eight forms of dietary vitamin E, α-tocopherol is the predominant form in human tissues due to efficient retention by the liver and distribution to peripheral tissues.

X

Xanthine dehydrogenase (XDH): see Xanthine oxidoreductase

Xanthine oxidase (XO): see Xanthine oxidoreductase

Xanthine oxidoreductase: Xanthine oxidoreductase (XOR) has two interconvertible forms, xanthine dehydrogenase (XDH) and xanthine oxidase (XO). Both forms catalyze the conversion of hypoxanthine to xanthine and xanthine to uric acid. Both forms also catalyze one- and two-electron reduction of molecular oxygen to form superoxide and hydrogen peroxide, respectively, with xanthine oxidase being more active in generating the above reactive oxygen species. The reversible conversion of xanthine dehydrogenase to xanthine oxidase occurs under certain conditions including hypoxia and oxidation of the cysteine thiol groups of the enzyme.

Index of Essentials of Free Radical Biology and Medicine

CITATION | *Hopkins RZ and Li YR. Essentials of Free Radical Biology and Medicine. Cell Med Press, Raleigh, NC, USA. 2017. http://dx.doi.org/10.20455/efrbm.2017.index*

Note: Page numbers followed by f and t indicate figures and tables, respectively.

A

Acyl-CoA oxidases, 94
Alkoxyl radicals, 166, 167, *see also* Reactive oxygen species
D-Amino acid oxidase, 94
Antioxidants
  classification of, 185t, 186, 187
  common types of, 183–210
  definition of, 16, 17, 184, 223,
  gene therapy of, 33, 210
  in disease intervention, 29, 29f, 39, 32–34
  modes of action of, 184–186, 184f
Antioxidative/anti-inflammatory defenses, 16, 17, *see also* Antioxidants
Apoptosis, 65, *see also* Cell death
Ascorbate, 45, 45f, 110, 190, 191f
Ascorbate radical, *see* Ascorbate
D-Aspartate oxidase, 94
Autophagy, 65, *see also* Cell death

C

cAMP, *see* Cyclic adenosine monophosphate
Carbon dioxide, 117, 118f, 167, 168
Carbon monoxide, 168, 169, 169f
Carbonate radical, 117, 118, 118f, 167
Catalase, 188, 189
Causal relationship, 30–32, 31f
CBS, *see* Cystathionine β-synthase

Cell death
  apoptosis, 65
  autophagy, 65
  ferroptosis, 192
  necrosis, 65
  oncosis, 65
Cell senescence, 66
Cell transformation, 66
Chemiluminescence, 159
5-Chloro-2′-deoxycytidine, 146,
8-Chloro-2′-deoxyguanosine, 146, 146f
Circadian rhythm, 98, 203
5-Cl-dC, *see* 5-Chloro-2′-deoxycytidine (5-Cl-dC)
8-Cl-dG, *see* 8-Chloro-2′-deoxyguanosine
CO, *see* Carbon monoxide
CO₂, *see* Carbon dioxide
Copper, see Transition metals
CSE, *see* Cystathionine γ-lyase
CuZnSOD, see Superoxide dismutase
Cyclic adenosine monophosphate, 22
CYP, *see* Cytochrome P450 system
Cystathionine β-synthase, 116, 117f, 170, 170f
Cystathionine γ-lyase, 170, 170f
Cytochrome c oxidase, 130, 131f, 169, 169f, 170, 170f
Cytochrome P450 system, 52, 78, 79f, 94, 169

D

DEPMPO, *see* 5-(Diethoxyphosphoryl)-5-methyl-1-pyrroline *N*-oxide
5-(Diethoxyphosphoryl)-5-methyl-1-pyrroline *N*-oxide, 42f, 43
Dimol emission, 159

www.ingramcontent.com/pod-product-compliance
Lightning Source LLC
Chambersburg PA
CBHW050825220326
41598CB00006B/313